Rare Neurodegenerative Disorders - New Insights

Edited by Liam Chen

Published in London, United Kingdom

Rare Neurodegenerative Disorders - New Insights
http://dx.doi.org/10.5772/intechopen.112607
Edited by Liam Chen

Contributors
Alessio Mylonas, Ali Abdullah Al-yahawi, Ali Gamal Al-kaf, Christiana C. Christodoulou, Christina A. Kousparou, Eleni Zamba Papanicolaou, Guadalupe Vidal-Martinez, Hadi Sasani, Haiyan Lou, İlknur Altuntaş, Mehtap Odabaşı, Oytun Erbas, Pemra Nesil, Ruth G. Perez

First published in London, United Kingdom, 2024 by IntechOpen
IntechOpen is the global imprint of INTECHOPEN LIMITED, registered in England and Wales, registration number: 11086078, 167-169 Great Portland Street, London, W1W 5PF, United Kingdom

British Library Cataloguing-in-Publication Data
A catalogue record for this book is available from the British Library

Additional hard and PDF copies can be obtained from orders@intechopen.com

Rare Neurodegenerative Disorders - New Insights
Edited by Liam Chen
p. cm.
Print ISBN 978-0-85014-805-3
Online ISBN 978-0-85014-804-6
eBook (PDF) ISBN 978-0-85014-806-0

For EU product safety concerns:
IN TECH d.o.o., Prolaz Marije Krucifikse Kozulić 3, 51000 Rijeka, Croatia,
info@intechopen.com or visit our website at intechopen.com.

Meet the editor

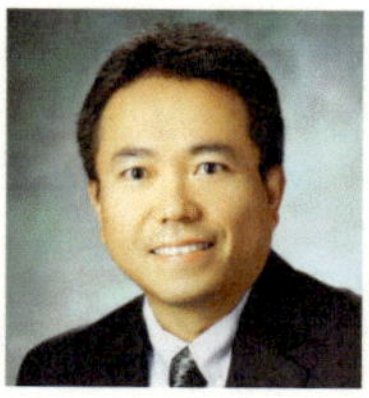

Dr. Liam Chen is a Professor of Pathology and Neurosurgery at the University of Minnesota Medical School, USA, and the director of the Minnesota David Tomassoni Biorepository Center. He is also the director of the Neuropathology Division at the University of Minnesota Medical Center, USA. Dr. Chen received residency and fellowship training at Mass General Brigham Hospital and Harvard Medical School, USA. Dr. Chen has more than 100 scholarly works to his credit, including research articles, reviews, and book chapters. He is an associate editor for several neuropathology journals and a member of many journal editorial boards and national grant review bodies.

Contents

Preface

Rare neurodegenerative disorders represent some of the most challenging and complex conditions in modern medicine. These diseases, while individually rare, collectively affect a significant number of individuals worldwide, leading to debilitating symptoms, loss of cognitive and motor functions, and ultimately, a decline in quality of life. The rarity and heterogeneity of these disorders often make them difficult to diagnose and treat, and they frequently lack effective therapeutic options. This book, *Rare Neurodegenerative Disorders – New Insights*, is a state-of-the-art exploration of the current scientific understanding, research approaches, and therapeutic strategies for addressing these elusive diseases. Each chapter delves into a critical aspect of neurodegenerative disease research, from cutting-edge scientific methodologies to promising treatment avenues. This book offers a broad yet detailed perspective on the ongoing efforts to understand and treat rare neurodegenerative disorders. It is a valuable resource for researchers, clinicians, and students alike, providing both foundational knowledge and insights into the latest advancements in this critical area of medical research. As the field continues to evolve, we hope that this compilation will inspire further exploration and innovation, ultimately leading to more effective therapies and improved quality of life for those affected by these devastating diseases.

Liam Chen
Department of Laboratory Medicine and Pathology,
University of Minnesota Medical School,
Minneapolis, United States

Chapter 1

Omics and Network-Based Approaches in Understanding HD Pathogenesis

Christiana C. Christodoulou and Eleni Zamba Papanicolaou

Abstract

Huntington's Disease (HD) is a rare, progressive neurodegenerative disease caused by CAG repeat expansion in the Huntingtin gene. HD is an incurable disease; therefore, there is a growing need for effective therapeutic treatments and candidate biomarkers for prognosis and diagnosis of HD. Technological advancements over the past couple of years, have led to high-throughput experiments and omics data. The use of System Bioinformatics (SB) approaches, allows for the integration of information across different -omics, this can clarify synergistic relationships across biological molecules, resulting in complex biological networks. SB and network-based approaches, are able to shed light on the potential interactions of genes, proteins, metabolites and pathways participating in HD pathogenesis and how dysregulation of these biological entities, can affect age on onset, disease severity and progression. Moreover, –omics data analysis and network-based approaches can provide better understanding how these biological molecules interact with each other and provides potential drug targets and biomarkers that can be used to treat HD or delay symptom onset; therefore, opening the door towards precision medicine. The aim of the following chapter, is to discuss the most popular -omics related to HD research, and the growing popularity of single cell analysis, repositories and software available for bulk and single cell analysis. In addition, network-based approaches regarding HD will also be mentioned.

Keywords: Huntington's disease, omics, bioinformatics, systems bioinformatics, single cell analysis, network-based approaches

1. Introduction

Huntington's Disease (HD) was first described in 1842 by Charles Oscar Waters and by 1872 a description of the disease was given by George Huntington, who assessed the medical history of several generations of a family exhibiting similar symptoms [1]. In 1983, a linkage on chromosome 4 was performed and by 1993 the Huntingtin (HTT) gene was discovered [1], leading to an increase in the interest of HD. Moreover, the identification of the gene resulted in the development of new animal models, research and therapeutic treatments and drugs to treat HD [1, 2]. HD is the most common monogenic neurological diseases in the developed world [3]. It is a rare, progressive neurodegenerative disease (ND) with autosomal dominant inheritance [1–3] affecting the medium spiny neurons (MSN) of the basal ganglia. HD is characterized by motor, cognitive and behavioral impairment caused by CAG trinucleotide repeat expansion at the N-terminus of the HTT gene responsible for encoding the HTT protein [4].

HD as other NDs, including Alzheimer's disease (AD), Parkinson's disease (PD) and Amyotrophic lateral Sclerosis (ALS) remain incurable [5]. Due to the overwhelming nature of these diseases, high economic and social costs and lack of effective therapeutic treatments [5]. Therefore, there is an increased need for novel biomarkers, pathways, drug targets and new novel pharmacotherapies that will enable the predication, prevention, understanding of disease pathways and most importantly effective treatments for NDs such as HD [5].

In the recent decade, bioinformatics approaches have become of increasing interest especially in NDs as they enable the identification of candidate biomarkers, pathways and mechanisms implicated in disease and potential drugs and their targets [5]. Bioinformatics is a multidisciplinary field utilizing methods from statistics, data-analysis, computer science, mathematics and biology to solve complex biological questions [5]. Bioinformatics is essential for analyzing and interpreting data from high-throughput technologies (DNA- and RNA-sequencing, proteomics, metabolomics, lipidomics etc.) [5, 6]. Due to the large amount of data produced, bioinformatics-based data management, and analysis tools are needed for the extraction, analysis, interpretation, visualization and storage of the data [5]. A relatively new approach is System Bioinformatics (SB), an intersection between systems biology and bioinformatics, which focuses on the integration of information across different -omics levels [6]. The goal of SB is to elucidate synergistic relationships between numerous factors in contrast to representing them as single biological entities, resulting in complex molecular networks of interactions [5]. This allows to better understand how different biological entities interact with one another, thus providing a clear understanding of disease pathogenesis, pathways, genes, proteins, metabolite, lipids and several additional types of biological information interacting together to lead to disease development [5]. Therefore, it is not a surprise that bioinformatics methods are used increasingly in ND research [5, 6].

Cells are complex, heterogenous and show a radical variation at the individual level and recent technological advancements, have enabled cell profiling at the individual level known as single cell analysis (SCA); the analysis of this data using bioinformatics pipelines is a practical solution for researchers; shedding light in understanding diseases, pathogenic mechanisms and the identification of potential biomarkers of diseases. The following chapter will discuss the most popular -omics approaches, SC technologies, data repositories and network-based analysis in HD research.

2. Omics

The past 15 years have seen the affluent use and integration of -omics approaches that include genomics and epigenomics for DNA, transcriptomics for RNA, proteomics for proteins and post-translational modification, metabolomics for metabolites, lipidomics for lipids and several additional -omics approaches (pharmacogenomics, radiomics etc.) [7, 8]. Technological advancement has allowed for the comprehensive measurement and analysis and the global assessment of biological molecules [7, 8] of genes, proteins, metabolites, lipids and several additional omics types within biological fluids, tissues or cells [8, 9], to assist in the understanding and investigation of human health and diseases [7]. These high-throughput technologies can be applied to the biological system and disease of interest to obtain a snapshot of the underlying biology at a resolution which was not previously possible [8], leading to unprecedented ways to better understanding NDs in terms of their pathogenesis, pathways, mechanisms and the interaction between different biological entities. Omics can contribute to biomarker, drug discovery and drug repurposing resulting in novel therapeutic treatments for NDs. Omics data is analyzed using bioinformatics pipelines and tools to obtain a list of genes, proteins, metabolites or lipids from the disease of interest [10], biological interpretation using different bioinformatics approaches **Table 1** (pathway enrichment analysis, protein–protein interaction networks (PPIs), protein-metabolite networks etc.) is vital to gain insight into the mechanisms, pathways and molecules affected in disease. The most common omics and the research conducted in regards to HD will be discussed below (**Figure 1**).

Name	Type	Omics content	Ref	Website (If Available)
Galaxy	Open access	Genomics Transcriptomics Proteomics Metabolomics Metagenomics	[11]	https://usegalaxy.org/
Limma	R-package	Transcriptomics Proteomics Metabolomics	[12]	https://www.bioconductor.org/packages/release/BiocViews.html#___Metabolomics
Ingenuity pathway analysis (IPA)	Commercial Software	Transcriptomics Proteomics Metabolomics	—	—
NextFlow	Software	Genomics Transcriptomics Proteomics Metabolomics	—	https://www.nextflow.io/
EdgeR	R package	Genomics Transcriptomics	[13–15]	—
MaxQuant & Perseus	Open access	Proteomics	[16]	https://www.maxquant.org/
OpenMS	C++ library	Proteomics Metabolomics	[17]	https://openms.de/
MsCoreUtils	R package	Proteomics Metabolomics	[18]	https://www.bioconductor.org/packages/release/bioc/html/MsCoreUtils.html
MetaboAnaylst	Open access & R package	Metabolomics Lipidomics Multi-omics	[19–21]	https://www.metaboanalyst.ca/
MetaCyc	Open access	Metabolomics	[22]	https://metacyc.org/
XCMS	Open access & R package	Metabolomics	[23–25]	https://xcmsonline.scripps.edu/landing_page.php?pgcontent=mainPage
Mzmine	R package	Metabolomics	[26]	http://mzmine.github.io/

Table 1.
Online tools, software and R-packages for omics data analysis.

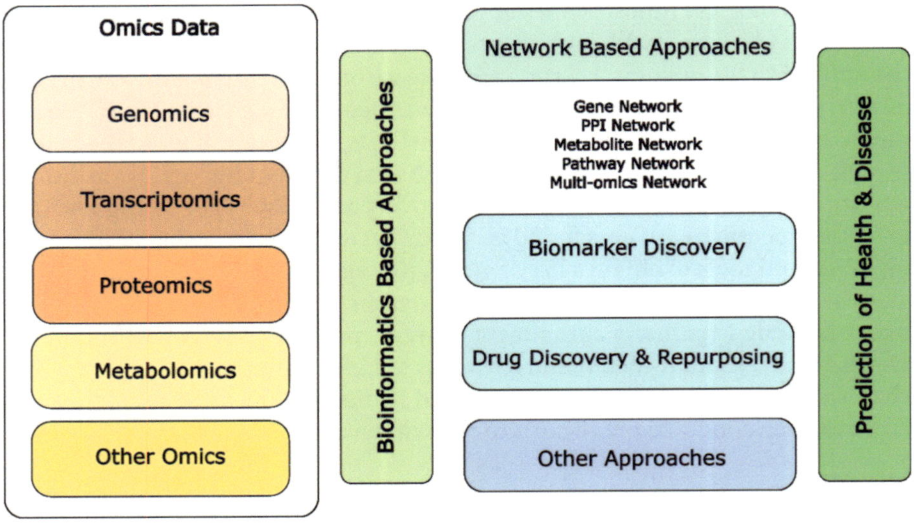

Figure 1.
Omics data types and bioinformatics based approaches.

2.1 Genomics

Since the discovery of the DNA structure by Rosalind Franklin, Frances Crick and James Watson in 1953, there has been a revolution in the field of biological sciences regarding technological advancements such as Sanger sequencing [27–29] and the discovery of the polymerase chain reaction [30] at the beginning of the 21st century. NGS became available, enabling the production of huge amounts of data along with the ability to produce highly efficient, rapid, low-cost approach along with accurate DNA sequencing [31]. Genomics is defined as the interdisciplinary field of biology focusing on genes, their structure, function, evolution, expression, mapping and genome editing [32]. The genome refers to all the genetic material present in any organism, including chromosomal and extrachromosomal DNA, coding and non-coding genes, microRNAs (miRNAs) and single nucleotide polymorphisms (SNPs) [33]. Sequencing of the human genome is important as it can provide insight into: i) gene expression profile of a specific tissue, organ or tumor, ii) human variation and how genomic alterations lead to disease development, iii) identification of genetic modifiers of disease, and iv) determine rate sensitivity to drugs in patients, based on their DNA sequences, this is known as pharmacogenomics [34]. Genomics has the ability to discover and identify genes associated with a disease; making it a vital omics component towards precision medicine. The majority of studies that have taken place regarding HD research have involved either the identification of genetic modifiers that may play a role in the early or delayed onset of HD.

2.1.1 Genomics in HD patients

Marchina et al. [35] investigated the gene expression profiles of fibroblasts of HD patients and healthy controls using microarray technology, and RT-PCR to validate the consistency of the microarray data. Analysis was carried out on nine genes, namely *APC, CDC42EP2, CTNNB1, DNM1L, PLCB4, ROCK1, ROCK2, SSH1*, and *UBE2D3*. These lists of genes, were chosen as some of these genes showed increased differential up-regulation (*PLCB4, APC*) or down-regulation (*SSH1, CDC42EP2*); while other genes were selected due to their possible involvement in HD pathology (*UBE2D3, ROCK1, ROCK2, DNM1L, CTNNB1*) as indicated by previous studies. The *APC, PLCB4, ROCK1*, and *UBE2D3* genes were found to be up-regulated in HD patients in comparison to controls [35]. Some gene ontology (GO) terms identified are, i) transcription, ii) regulation of transcription, DNA-dependent, iii) cell cycle, iv) response to DNA damage stimulus, v) DNA repair, vi) ubiquitin dependent protein catabolic process and vii) DNA recombination. Based on this evidence the gene expression profiles of fibroblasts seem to be altered in HD patients compared to healthy controls [35]. Validation of the differential expressions at the protein level is needed to confirm if fibroblasts can be considered as a suitable model for the identification of HD biomarkers [35].

A study by Wright et al. [36] investigated the gene expression profiles complementing the analysis of genomic modifiers in HD. CAG repeat length is not the only contributing factor to disease onset but genetic modifiers also contribute to disease onset [36]. A genome-wide association study assessing heritable differences in genetically determined expression in diverse tissues, with genome-wide data taken from 4000 HD patients was conducted. In addition, functional validation of prioritized genes was performed in isogenic HD stem cells and post-mortem brain tissue [36]. The genes of *FAN1, GPR161, PMS2 and SUMF2* are associated with age of onset in HD and showed co-localization with gene expression signals in brain tissue [36].

Other genomic studies conducted in HD patients or post-mortem brain tissue include Moss et al. [27], Li et al. [28].

2.1.2 Genomics in HD animal models

One study by Tang et al. [29] performed gene expression profiling on the R6/2 HD transgenic mice model, with varying CAG repeat lengths to reveal genes associated with HD onset and progression [29]. The R6/2 transgenic mice with >300 CAG repeats had prolonged HD progression and a longer lifespan than the parent R6/2 mice with 150 CAG repeats. However, the mechanisms regarding this phenotypic amelioration remains unknown [29].

The expression profiles of the striatum of R6/2 transgenic mice with >300 CAG repeats (R6/2Q300 transgenic mice) and R6/2 transgenic mice with 150 CAG repeats (R6/2Q150 transgenic mice) and littermate wild-type (WT) controls were performed to identify, genes playing an important role, in HD onset and progression. Both R6/2 mouse models demonstrated decreased expression while up-regulated gene expression was seen in R6/2Q300 mice [29]. The up-regulated genes play a role in ubiquitin ligase complex, cell adhesion, protein folding and establishment of protein localization. Increased gene expression for *Lrsam1, Erp29, Nasp, Tap1, Rab9b* and *Pfdn5* was validated using qPCR. Moreover, *Lrsam1* and *Erp29* were significantly up-regulated in R6/2Q300 mice and may have potential neuroprotective effects in primary striatal cultures over-expressing mHTT [29]. Over-expression of *Lrsam1* prevented the loss of NeuN-positive cell bodies in htt171-82Q cultures, associated with a decrease of nuclear HTT aggregates. However, over-expression of *Erp29* demonstrated no significant effect in cells [29]. Therefore, prolonged HD onset and progression seen in R6/2 mice with increased CAG repeat expansions are a result of differential up-regulation in genes involved in protein localization and clearance. These genes may be possible novel therapeutic avenues in decreasing HTT aggregation toxicity and neuronal cell death, with *Lrsam1* being a promising, novel candidate disease modifier [29].

Langfelder et al. [37] integrated genomics and proteomics data to define HTT CAG length networks in HD mice. To gain insight into how mHTT CAG repeat length modifies HD pathogenesis, profiling of mRNA in 600 brain and peripheral tissue samples obtained from HD knock-in mice with increased CAG repeat length was performed [37]. The study found, the repeat length dependent transcriptional signatures were notable in the striatum while the cortex and liver showed less transcriptional signatures [37]. Co-expression networks revealed 13 and 5 striatal and cortical modules, respectively, that were highly correlated with CAG repeat length and age, and are preserved in HD models. The top striatal modules suggest mutant HTT (mHTT) CAG length and age impair the MSN, while a dysregulation of genes and pathways involved in cAMP signaling, cell death, and protocadherin were seen [37]. Proteomics analysis was used to confirm, 790 genes and 5 striatal modules with CAG length-dependent dysregulation was observed at both the RNA and protein level, 22 striatal module genes were validated as modifiers of mHTT toxicities *in vivo* [37].

Other genomics studies in HD animal models or cells include Choudhury et al. [38] and Alcalá-Vida et al. [39].

2.2 Transcriptomics

The transcriptome is the complete set of transcripts within a cell, and their quantity, for a physiological condition or specific developmental stage [40]. Understanding the transcriptome is crucial for interpreting the functional components of the genome and revealing the molecular entities of cells and tissues and also for understanding development and disease pathogenesis [40]. The aim of transcriptomics is to: i) catalog the transcripts, including mRNAs, non-coding RNAs and small RNAs; of all species to determine the transcriptional structure of genes, regarding their start sites, 5′ and 3′ ends, alternative splicing patterns and any additional post-transcriptional modifications; and ii) quantify the fluctuating expression levels of each transcript under different conditions and during development [40]. The development of innovative high-throughput DNA sequencing methods known as RNA Sequencing (RNA-Seq) has allowed the mapping and quantification of transcriptomes. Genomics and transcriptomics are the two most popular omics used for HD research; therefore, it is vital to examine whether peripheral tissues may serve as a possible source of readily accessible biological signatures at not only the DNA and RNA level but also at the protein level and not only. There are numerous studies that have used transcriptomics to perform studies regarding either peripheral tissues, cerebrospinal fluid (CSF) or post-mortem brain tissue samples obtained from HD patients and animal models.

2.2.1 Transcriptomics in HD patients

A study by Neueder et al. [41] investigated the abnormal molecular signatures that characterize inflammation, energy metabolism and vesicle biology in human HD peripheral tissues. Specifically, skeletal muscle, adipose tissue and skin from the quadriceps femoris muscle and blood was collected from 21 pre-HD patients, 20 early motor manifest HD patients and 20 healthy controls. Furthermore, primary fibroblast and myoblast cell lines were established [41]. RNA-Seq and proteomics analysis were used to investigate the involvement of inflammation and energy metabolism in HD pathogenesis.

Initially, RNA-Seq analysis was performed on adipose and muscle tissue from the pre-HD patients (pre-HD), early motor manifest HD patients (early HD) and healthy control groups. In total, 78 and 53 genes were identified to be significantly dysregulated in adipose and skeletal muscle tissue, respectively [41]. Distinctly, only *RPH3A*, *PAX6* and *AC016582.1* were regulated similarly in the pre-HD and early HD groups in comparison to controls. Furthermore, some genes were differentially regulated in both groups [41]. *TBC1D3D*, was differentially regulated in muscle and adipose tissue, the gene was found to be up-regulated in the early HD group in comparison to the pre-HD group [41].

GO enrichment analysis in adipose tissue identified the terms of protein sumoylation (GO: 0016), interleukin-1 mediated signaling pathway (GO:0006470) and cellular response to organic cyclic compound (GO: 0071407) [41]. For the different comparisons, the RE1 silencing TF (REST) target gene was dysregulated only in the pre-HD group, while sumoylation was dysregulated only in the early HD group. Alteration in protein sumoylation is a well-known mechanism and has been implicated in HD pathogenesis [41].

GO analysis in muscle tissue, identified a disruption in homeostatic pathways, including anterograde trans-synaptic signaling (GO: 0098916), regulation of fatty acid oxidation (GO:0046320), regulation of glucose metabolic process (GO:0010906), negative regulation of cell communication (GO:00106458), protein dephosphorylation (GO:0006470), regulation of protein kinase B signaling (GO:0051896) and regulation of MAPK cascade (GO:0043408) particularly in the pre-HD group [41]. *PAX6* is a vital regulator of assorted peripheral and central nervous system processes, it was identified to be highly and gradually up-regulated in both HD groups; therefore, suggesting a compensatory mechanism of muscle regeneration in response to mutant HTT expression [41]. Enrichment analysis of the dysregulated genes in the muscle tissue of the pre-HD group suggest that peroxisome proliferator activated receptor alpha (PPARA) acts as a regulatory protein [41].

In addition, RNA-Seq analysis was also performed on the fibroblast cell lines. Only a few genes were significantly dysregulated between pre-HD and early-HD patient groups compared to healthy controls [41]. Subsequently, GO enrichment analysis resulted in the identification of a few enriched terms, such as phosphorylation (GO:0016310) and regulation of apoptotic processes (GO:0042981) [41]. Interestingly, *TBC1D3D,* was found to be dysregulated not only in adipose and muscle but also in fibroblasts [41]. Furthermore, proteomics analysis was performed on the tissues obtained; however, this will be further discussed in the proteomics section of the chapter.

Miller et al. [42], performed RNA-Seq analysis on myeloid cells of HD patients to identify transcriptional dysregulation associated with proinflammatory pathway activation. Specifically, whole transcriptome analysis of primary monocytes from 30 manifesting HD patients and 31 healthy control subjects, with or without proinflammatory stimulus [42].

HD monocytes exhibit resting proinflammatory transcriptional changes, 12,599 genes were identified to be differentially expressed (DE) and analysis of said data was conducted, to determine the genes significantly altered between HD and control monocytes, whereas the stimulated and unstimulated monocytes were analyzed separately [43]. Analysis of unstimulated monocytes revealed 130 DE genes, of which 101 were up-regulated and 29 down-regulated genes in resting HD monocytes compared to healthy controls. The DE genes were associated with proinflammatory cytokines and chemokines. HD monocytes had significantly increased expression of *IL6, IL12B, IL19, IL23A, CCL8, CCL19, CCL20, CXCL6* and *CSF2* gene transcripts. All transcripts have a > 2-fold increase in mRNA expression [42]. In contrast, the stimulated monocytes showed little indication of differential expression between HD and controls, the genes of *DNAJB13, STAC* and *RASEF* were DE. Furthermore, each of these genes were observed to be DE in unstimulated monocytes [42]. Generally, gene expression differences between HD and controls were lower in the stimulated 116 DE genes in comparison to the unstimulated 130 DE genes in monocytes [43]. Moreover, gene set enrichment analysis (GSEA) was performed for the up- and down regulated gene expression for both the stimulated and unstimulated monocyte datasets [43]. Analysis of unstimulated monocytes revealed a total of 85 enriched gene sets, a majority of pathways relating to innate immunity, inflammatory response, cytokine production and secretion were identified. Furthermore, pathways such as NFkB and JAK/STAT signaling pathways were also identified to be significantly enriched [43]. In comparison to the down-regulated genes, 6 gene sets were identified and included significantly enriched pathways related to vacuole, lysosome and catabolic functions [42]. Interestingly, the simulated dataset did not reveal any enriched gene sets among the up-regulated genes. However, 83 gene sets were significantly enriched among the down-regulated genes, pathways relating to cholesterol homeostasis, cellular components such as cellular membrane, mitochondria and lysosomes [42].

To understand the mechanisms underlying differential gene expression in unstimulated HD monocytes, upstream regulator analysis was performed using the Ingenuity Pathway Analysis (IPA) software. A total of 155 upstream regulators were identified for the unstimulated dataset, of these 125 were predicted to be significantly activated, while 30 were predicted to be significantly inhibited. A large number of molecules associated with intracellular signaling pathways downstream of the TLR4 receptor were represented in the unstimulated group. The following data were consistent with previous studies, showing NFkB dysregulation in HD myeloid cells, the RELA and the NFkB complex were among the top most significant results ranked by z-score activation [43]. Other prominent potential regulators include NFkB1, ERK and p38 MAPKs, in addition to the transcription factor STAT3 [42]. The study suggests that transcriptional changes observed in the RNA-Seq analysis of stimulated and unstimulated HD monocytes is related to the abnormal activation of specific upstream signaling molecules responsible for driving gene expression in unstimulated HD myeloid cells [42]. Furthermore, HD myeloid cells have a proinflammatory phenotype in the absence of stimulation; consistent with the priming effect of mutant huntingtin (mHTT), whereas basal dysfunction results in an exaggerated inflammatory response once a stimulus is encountered [42]. The following data provides an understanding of mHTT pathogenesis, establishing unstimulated myeloid cells as a vital source of HD immune dysfunction, and demonstrating the importance of immunity as a potential HD treatment.

Other transcriptomic studies conducted in HD patients include Seefelder and Kochanek [44], Sinha et al. [45], Mastrokolias et al. [46, 47], Borovecki et al. [48], Lin et al. [40], Cha [49], Moily et al. [43], Mehta et al. [50], Stopa et al. [51] and Runne et al. [52].

2.2.2 Transcriptomics in HD mouse models

Jin et al. [53] investigating the miRNA and mRNA expression profiles of the cerebral cortex of N171-82Q HD mice [53]. There is growing evidence indicating that miRNAs may play a role in HD pathogenesis [53]. During disease progression significant changes of miRNAs in the cerebral cortex were also detected in the striatum of

HD mice [53]. The study revealed that a significant alteration in the miR-200 miRNA family, more specifically, miR-200a and miR-200c in the cerebral cortex and striatum were seen during the early HD stages in N171-82Q mice.

A computational bioinformatics approach was used to integrate miRNA and mRNA profiles. The gene targets were identified using TargetScan, for miR-200a and miR-200C, there are 680 and 462 gene targets respectively. Some of the predicted gene targets for the miRNAs include *KIF3a, NRXN1, PTPRD, TRIM2, ATXN1, KCNA2* and numerous additional targets [53]. The predicted targets play a role in regulating synaptic function, neuronal survival and neurodevelopment. The results of the study suggest that altered miR-200a and miR-200c expression may interrupt protein production involved in neuronal plasticity and survival [53]. Therefore, further investigation of the involvement of dysfunctional miRNA expression in HD is required and this may result in novel approaches for HD therapy.

Hervás-Corpión [54] investigated the early alternations of epigenetic-related transcription in HD mouse models. The gene expression profiles of the cortex, striatum, hippocampus and cerebellum of juvenile R6/1 and N171-82Q mice, were studied, the profiles consisted of tissular and neuronal-specific genes and showed significant correspondence with transcriptional alteration in HD mouse models deficient of epigenetic regulatory genes [54]. A noteworthy case was the conditional knockout of the lysine acetyltransferase CBP in post-mitotic forebrain neurons, the double knockout of the histone methyltransferases Ezh1 and Ezh2, components of the polycomb repressor complex 2 (PRC2), and the conditional mutants of the histone methyltransferases G9a (Ehmt2) and GLP (Ehmt1) [54]. It is likely that the neuronal epigenetic status is compromised prior to HD onset resulting in transcriptional dysregulation [54].

Other transcriptomic studies conducted in HD animal models include Bensale et al. [55], Dickson et al. [56], Reyes-Ortiz [57], Chaves et al. [58] and Huang et al. [59].

2.3 Proteomics

Proteomics is a new omics type that has rapidly developed especially in the fields of therapeutics and biomarkers discovery [60]. Proteomics is defined as the study of interactions, functions, composition and structure of proteins and their cellular activities. The proteome is defined as the complete set of proteins within a cell, tissue, organism or biological fluid. Proteomics allows for a better understanding of the structure and function of an organism than genomics. However, proteomics is much more cumbersome than genomics as the protein expression is altered according to environmental conditions and time. It is approximated that there are almost one million human proteins, many of which contain some form of post-translational modifications [60]. The majority of proteomics studies have been conducted in HD mouse models, there seems to be a lack of human HD proteomics studies. Proteomics can assist in the discovery of new therapies, biomarkers and better understanding of proteins and protein-complexes in disease.

2.3.1 Proteomics in HD patients

The study by Neueder et al. [49] which previously performed transcriptomic analysis as mentioned in Section 2.2.1 also performed proteomics analysis and revealed, 1347, 2671 and 4640 proteins for adipose, muscle and skin tissue respectively [49]. A progressive increase in the number of dysregulated proteins from the pre-HD to early HD stage was observed for all three tissues [49]. In adipose tissue, there was no overlap of commonly dysregulated proteins between the three comparisons. In muscle tissue, syntaxin-binding protein 3 (STXBP3) was up-regulated in both pre- and early-HD samples. Interestingly, the major change was observed in the skin samples, MOB4 was up-regulated in both pre- and early HD samples [49]. A total of 162 and 23 proteins were significantly dysregulated in the early and pre-HD stages respectively.

GO enrichment on adipose dataset (early HD vs. controls) and skin dataset (early HD vs. controls and the comparison of pre-HD vs. early HD), revealed dysregulated lipid metabolism and proteasome function in the adipose tissue dataset. While proteins related to gene expression such RNA processing and translation and amino acid metabolism are mainly affecting in the early HD samples vs. controls [49]. The predicted regulators are all genes involved in gene expression, specifically, lysine acetyltransferase 2A (KAT2A) and the androgen receptor (AR), in a complex with ataxin 7 (ATXN7) which are associated with polyglutamine diseases [49]. The GO terms for pre- and early HD in the skin datasets, included the regulation of cell survival and proliferation. The results obtained from the above study, indicate that alterations in biological signatures at the RNA and protein level point towards the direction of inflammation, energy metabolism and vesicle biology in peripheral tissues in HD. The following biological signatures may act as suitable biomarkers in clinical trials upon further validation.

A proteomics study by Fang et al. [61] integrated five sets of proteomics data profiling the CSF derived from HD affected and unaffected individuals with genomics data profiling, various human and mouse tissue, including the human HD brain [61]. According to the integrated analysis, brain specific proteins were 1.8 times more likely to be observed in CSF compared to plasma. Furthermore, brain specific proteins decrease in HD CSF compared to unaffected CSF [61].

Approximately, 81% of brain specific proteins have quantitative changes that agree with transcriptional changes seen in different HD brain regions, while the proteins identified to increase in HD CSF tend to be liver associated. The protein changes are consistent with microgliosis, astrocytosis and neurodegeneration which are known to occur in HD [61]. The most significantly over and under abundant dysregulated proteins in CSF between HD affected and unaffected individuals, include, chromogranin B (CHGB), isoform I of Sialate O-actelyesterase precursor (SIAE), isoform long of iduronate 2-sulfatase precursor (IDS), Neurexin 3-alpha (NRXN3) Endonuclease domain-containing 1 protein precursor (ENDOD1), major prion protein precursor (PRNP) and several additional proteins have a trend of decreasing with disease progression (controls > HD early > mid-HD). Some of the over abundant proteins identified are, complement component 1, q subunit, c chain precursor (C1QC), hemopexin (HPX), Triosephosphate isomerase (TPI1), Isoform M1 of Pyruvate kinase isozymes M1/M2; Isoform R-type of Pyruvate kinase isozymes R/L (PKM2/PKLR), Lysozyme C precursor (LYZ) and several other proteins, which have shown to have a trend of increasing as the disease progresses (control > HD early > mid HD) [61].

Other proteomics studies conducted in HD patients include, Chen et al. [62], Schönberger et al. [63], Sorolla et al. [64] and Chae et al. [65], McQuade et al. [66] and Dalrymple et al. [67].

2.3.2 Proteomics in mouse models of HD patients

A previous study by Agrawal and Fox [68] performed targeted proteomics analysis to investigate novel proteomic alterations in brain mitochondria to reveal insights into mitochondrial dysfunction in HD mouse models. Mitochondrial dysfunction is one of contributing pathophysiological mechanisms in HD. The following study used R6/2 and YAC128 HD mouse models to represent different HD progression rates to pinpoint HD brain mitochondrial proteomic signatures. Cerebral cortical mitochondrial of HD and WT littermates were compared by 2D SDS–PAGE electrophoresis and MALDI-TOF/TOF mass spectrometry (MS) [68].

Proteomic analyses concluded 17 and 12 DE proteins in 12-week R6/2- and 15-month YAC128 HD mice, respectively compared to controls. The proteins of peroxiredoxin 3, stress–70, DJ–1, isocitrate dehydrogenase [NAD] α subunit and ATP synthase subunit D were DE in both HD mouse models. Pathway analysis was performed using PANTHER [68], the GO molecular function terms obtained for the DE mitochondrial proteins are i) catalytic activity (GO:0003824), binding (GO:0005488) and antioxidant activity (GO:0016209); most GO biological process proteins belonged to metabolic (GO:0008152) and cellular process (GO:0009987) [68]. While for YAC128 mice, the molecular functions of the DE mitochondrial proteins were catalytic activity (GO:0003824) and binding (GO: 0005488); for GO biological processes most of the proteins also belonged to the metabolic (GO:0008152) and cellular process (GO:0009987) and biogenesis (GO:0071840). The results identify a proteomic signature of HD mitochondria in mouse models that includes previously unrecognized proteins [68].

One study by Choudhary et al. [38] performed differential proteomics and genomic profiling of mouse striatal cell model of HD vs. healthy controls. Transcriptional dysregulation is one of the pathogenic mechanisms contributing to HD. Various studies have identified altered gene expression in HD patient brains and animal models. 2D SDS-PAGE/MALDI-MS coupled with 2D-DIGE and real time PCR on an array of genes concentrated on HD pathways to identified altered proteins and gene expression in STHdhQ111/HdhQ111 compared to STHdhQ7/HdhQ7 (wild-type). Seventy-six proteins were annotated in HD cells while 31 proteins were DE by 2D-DIGE. The bioinformatics tool GeneCodis3 [38] was used to perform pathway analysis using KEGG and GO biological terms. The pathways included, unfolded protein binding (GO:0051082), negative regulation of neuron apoptosis (GO:0006916), response to superoxide's (GO:0006950) and several other pathways. The PCR experiments showed altered gene expression of 47 genes. Altogether, 77 genes/proteins were identified in HD cell lines with potential relevance to HD biology [38].

Other proteomic studies conducted in HD animal models and cells include Mees et al. [69], Liu et al. [70], Perluigi et al. [71], Deschepper et al. [72], Culver et al. [73], Cozzolino et al. [74], Vodicka et al. [75], Sap et al. [76], Ratovitski et al. [77] and Zabel et al. [78].

2.4 Metabolomics

Traditionally, a small number of metabolites have been used for the diagnosis of complex metabolic diseases and monogenic complex diseases such as inborn errors of metabolism [79]. Metabolomics is defined as the comprehensive measurement of metabolites within a biological tissue, cell, organ or fluid (CSF, urine, plasma or serum) [79]. The metabolome is the number of metabolites in an organism. Metabolomics is an emerging technology that holds promise for the development and practice of precision medicine. In addition, metabolomics is able to provide detailed characterization of metabolic phenotypes and can enable precision medicine at numerous levels such as characterization of metabolites underlying disease, discovery of new therapeutic targets, biomarker discovery which may be used for prognosis, diagnosis or monitor activity of therapeutics [79]. Similarly with proteomics, the majority of studies in metabolomics and HD are conducted in HD mouse models.

2.4.1 Metabolomics in HD patients

One study by Rosas et al. [80] investigated the plasma metabolome of HD. The study consisted of targeted metabolomics analysis using the plasma obtained from 52 pre-HD, 102 early symptomatic HD and 140 controls [80].

The pathways altered include i) tryptophan, ii) tyrosine, iii) purine, iv) methionine, v) antioxidant pathways and numerous pathways relating to energetic and oxidative stress derived from the gut microbiome. The tryptophan, tyrosine and purine pathways were altered in prodromal and early HD stages. The selective dysregulation of a good few pathways and the increased regulation of other pathways suggest complex alterations in the feedback controls of underlying genes, proteins, enzymes and metabolites. In addition, multivariate statistical modeling demonstrated mutually distinct metabolomics profiles, suggesting that the process determining onset was likely distinct from processes determining progression [80]. Surprisingly, controls, pre-HD and early HD plasma metabolomes were mutually distinct rather than differing, suggesting varying influences during the prodromal and symptomatic disease stages [80].

Numerous metabolites differentiating the control from the pre-HD and early HD metabolomes, are linked to the gut microbiome, suggesting mHTT favors a distinct microbiome. The systemic effects of HD on the gut microbiome may possibly influence energy homeostasis, vitamin and mineral supply, metabolites and neuroimmune functions while impacting HD expression [80]. The gut microbiome derived metabolites were differentiated in the pre-HD metabolome, while the symptomatic HD metabolome was mostly influenced by metabolites likely reflecting mHTT toxicity and neurodegeneration [80]. The study suggests that the pre-HD metabolome is influenced more by the gut microbiome than the HD metabolome, possibly due to the increasing effects of mHTT toxicity and neurodegeneration. The understanding of these complex alterations is a delicate balance between the metabolome and gut microbiome in HD, and they relate to disease onset, severity, progression and phenotypic variability in HD are vital questions for future research and clinical studies in HD [80].

Herman et al. [81] investigated the metabolic alterations in tyrosine and phenylalanine pathways in the CSF of HD patients. The study consisted of 13 pre-HD mHTT carriers and 13 symptomatic HD patients and 42 controls. The comparison of symptomatic HD patient's vs. controls, identified 24 metabolites to be significantly dysregulated, this included the metabolites of Lumichrome, Xanthine, O-succinyl-homoserine, N-acetylproline, Phenylacetate, Isoleucine, L-DOPA, Leucine, Corticosterone, Ophthalmate, Tyrosine, Valine, Salicylate, Phenylalanine and others. Pathway analysis disclosed 5 biochemical pathways affected in symptomatic HD vs. controls namely i) aminoacyl-tRNA biosynthesis; ii) phenylalanine metabolism; iii) valine, leucine and isoleucine biosynthesis; iv) valine, leucine, isoleucine degradation and v) purine metabolism. Phenylalanine metabolism was highly affected in symptomatic HD patients.

Comparing symptomatic HD patient's vs. pre-HD patients, 28 metabolites were revealed to be significantly altered. Some of the metabolites were, L-DOPA, Xanthine, Ophthalmate, Creatinine, Tyrosine, 5-hydroxytryptophan, Adenosine, Phenylalanine, Phenylacetate, Thyroxine, Glutarylcarnitine, O-succinyl-homoserine, Adenine, Isoleucine, Aldosterone/Cortisone and numerous other metabolites. Fourteen of these were able to distinguish symptomatic HD patient's from controls. Univariate analysis illustrated 11 metabolites were dysregulated (L-DOPA, xanthine, ophthalmate, creatinine, tyrosine, 5-hydroxytryptophan, adenosine and phenylalanine) remained significant after correcting for multiple comparison testing. Furthermore, 4-acetamidobutanoate and S-adenosylhomocysteine had been corrected for age dependence. There was a notable longitudinal decrease in O-acetylcarnitine in the symptomatic HD patients. Significantly altered abundances of Ophthalmate, Phenylalanine, 4-quinolinecarboxylic and N,N,N-trimethyl lysine were observed in six pre-HD patients. Pathway analysis, illustrated 8 biological pathways of: i) aminoacyl-tRNA biosynthesis; ii) phenylalanine, tyrosine and tryptophan biosynthesis; iii) valine, leucine and isoleucine biosynthesis; iv) tyrosine metabolism; v) nitrogen metabolism; vi) valine, leucine and isoleucine degradation; vii) phenylalanine metabolism and viii) purine metabolism. Tyrosine and phenylalanine metabolism pathways were significantly altered between symptomatic and pre-HD patients.

To investigate the effects of disease progression, the association between CSF concentration of altered metabolites and measure of disease severity were researched in all mHTT carriers and to a five-year risk onset of developing HD in pre-HD patients. Hierarchical clustering revealed that tyrosine metabolism, including tyrosine, thyroxine, L-DOPA and dopamine, was significantly dysregulated in symptomatic vs. pre-HD patients. These metabolites displayed moderate to strong associations of measures to disease severity and symptoms. Furthermore, Thyroxine and Dopamine were also correlated with the five-year risk of onset in pre-HD patients. Phenylalanine and purine metabolism were also significantly altered, but associated with decreased disease severity. Decreased levels of Lumichrome were frequent in mHTT carriers and concentrations correlated with five-year risk of HD onset in pre-HD carriers. Biochemical profiling illustrates that the CSF metabolome may be used to characterize molecular pathogenesis in HD, and may be vital for future development of HD therapies.

Other metabolomics studies conducted in HD patients include, McGarry et al. [82], Mastrokolias et al. [47], Cheng et al. [83], Graham [84, 85] and Patassini et al. [86].

2.4.2 Metabolomics in HD animal models

Targeted metabolic profiling on plasma of a pre-HD transgenic sheep model in order to identify potential candidate biomarkers was investigated by Skene et al. [87].

One hundred and thirty metabolites were obtained, Alanine, Arginine, Citrulline, Glutamine, Glutamate, Glycine, Histidine, Isoleucine, Phenylalanine, Proline, Tryptophan, Valine, Creatine, Kynurenine, Serotonin and several additional metabolites [87]. Citrulline and Arginine showed significantly increased levels in HD compared to control sheep, both are involved in the urea cycle, although Ornithine was also identified and is part of the urea cycle, no significant difference between HD vs. healthy controls was seen. Citrulline demonstrated the most significant change in transgenic HD sheep. Regarding the 20 amino acids measured, 10 had shown significantly decreased concentration in HD sheep, the branched amino acids (BCAA) of Valine, Leucine and Isoleucine showed the most notable effect, which have been previously identified as potential biomarkers. This was followed by Threonine, Tyrosine, Methionine, Alanine, Asparagine, Phenylalanine and Glutamine. Significant alterations in respect to genotype were distinguished in 89/130 identified metabolites, including Sphingolipids, Biogenic amines, amino acids and Urea. A significant increase in Urea, Arginine, Citrulline, asymmetric and symmetric dimethylarginine and a decrease in Sphingolipids [87].

Quantitative enrichment analysis using MetaboAnalyst [19–21], identified the top five metabolite pathway-associated metabolite sets of: i) aspartate metabolism; ii) arginine and proline metabolism; iii) valine, leucine and isoleucine degradation; iv) fatty acid metabolism and v) urea cycle. The urea cycle and nitric oxide pathways become dysregulated during the early HD stages. Additionally, logistic prediction modeling identified 8 potential biomarkers (Citrulline, Valine, PC aa C40:4, PC aa C36:5, lysoPC a C17:0, SM (OH) C24:1, Threonine, Tetradecenoylcarnitine (C14:1)). In HD sheep, the metabolites of Citrulline, PC aa C36:5 and lysoPC a C17:0 were increased significantly while Valine, PC aa C40:4, SM (OH) C24:1, Threonine and Tetradecenoylcarnitine (C14:1) were significantly decreased compared to control sheep [87]. The degree of sensitivity, using minimally invasive methods, puts forward a novel approach for monitoring disease progression in HD patients.

Andersen et al. [88] investigated the branched amino acids (BCAA) and their metabolism in the cerebral cortex of a R6/2 HD mouse model using metabolomics analysis [88]. Deficiencies in cerebral energy and neurotransmitter are suggested to play a role in neuronal dysfunction in HD. The BCAAs of Valine, Leucine and Isoleucine are vital in cerebral nitrogen homeostasis, neurotransmitter recycling and are utilized as energy substrates in the tricarboxylic acid (TCA) cycle [88]. Decreased levels of BCAAs in HD haven been previously validated in several studies. However, it remains unclear how cerebral BCAA metabolism is regulated in HD.

Isolated cerebral cortical and striatal slices of controls and R6/2 mice were incubated with labeled Leucine and Isoleucine; however, no differences in Leucine or Isoleucine concentration were shown between R6/2 and control striatal or cerebral cortical slices [88]. Suggesting that the cellular uptake of these BCAAs likely remains unaffected in the R6/2 slices compared to controls. Metabolism of Leucine and Isoleucine, entering oxidative metabolism as acetyl CoA, was preserved in R6/2 mice. However, metabolism of Isoleucine, entering the TCA cycle as Succinyl CoA, was increased in the cerebral cortical and striatal slices of R6/2 mice; therefore, suggesting a rise in metabolic influx via the replenishing of Oxaloacetate in the citric acid cycle. Enzyme expression in the BCAA metabolism was assessed, enzymes related to BCAA metabolism displayed an increased expression in the R6/3 brain, particularly enzymes related to Isoleucine metabolism [88]. This indicates that the capacity for cerebral BCAA metabolism, primarily Isoleucine, is heightened in R6/2 brain tissue indicative of alterations in cerebral BCAA homeostasis.

Other metabolomics studies conducted in HD animal models include Chang et al. [89], Chaves et al. [58], Bertrand et al. [90], Verwaest et al. [91], Hashimoto et al. [92], Kumar et al. [93] and Tsang et al. [94].

3. Single cell omics

Organisms and complex tissues are formed by a heterogeneity of cells undergoing cell division, proliferation, differentiation during various physiological states such as development and adulthood [95]. The fate of each cell is intrinsically determined and is influenced both by external factors and by cell–cell interactions [95]. Various processes taking place within individual cells are a result of complex interactions between chromatin, transcripts, proteins, metabolites, lipids and other biological entities [95, 96]. To identify these activity dependent regulatory processes the majority of approaches used include transcriptomics, proteomics, metabolomics or lipidomics methods on tissues, cells and biological fluids [95]. Although the bulk approaches are useful, they have a drawback, as they average the information derived from thousands to millions of cells, leading to masking of cell specific features or features involved in developmental processes [95]. There are some studies of single cell RNA-Seq analysis in HD [97–99].

Over the past few years, the development of methodological approaches for single cell analysis has greatly increased and addressed the drawback of bulk analysis [95]. Single cell analysis (SCA) has recently been included into multi-omics strategies, which brings together concurrent biological information from different molecular modalities and their relationship with individual cells [95]. Furthermore, analyzing cells individually at a higher resolution results in a more accurate representation of cell–cell variations in comparison to bulk analysis measurements [95]. SCA approaches include: i) single cell genomics, ii) single cell epigenomics iii) single cell transcriptomics, iv) single cell proteomics and v) single cell metabolomics. To fully grasp and understand cellular complexity and specificity of cells, tissues or biological fluid microenvironments in physiological or disease conditions, it is important to measure molecular signatures at the single cell resolution [100]. Benefits of SCA include: i) improvements in experimental design and data analysis for single cells for a disease of interest, ii) targeting of specific cell populations therefore elucidating signaling pathways and networks, iii) cell-to cell communication variation for understanding disease onset, progression and therapeutic response, iv) differentiate normal cells and comprised cells at various developmental stages, v) identify cells and their distinctive susceptibilities, vi) clarify neural communication in unprecedented detail, resulting in new strategies to understand and treat NDs [100]. SCA can provide insight for potential biomarkers, therapeutic targets, pathways and mechanisms in disease involvement [100]. **Tables 2** and **3** indicate the databases and tools used for analysis of SCA, while **Table 4** illustrates software and databases for cell-to-cell communication.

Name	Type	Omics content	Ref	Website (If Available)
Gene expression omnibus	Repository	Single cell RNA-Seq	[101]	https://www.ncbi.nlm.nih.gov/geo/
Single cell epression atlas	Repository	Single cell RNA-Seq	[102]	https://www.ebi.ac.uk/gxa/home
Slavov laboratory/ Quantitative biology	Repository/ Database	Single cell Proteomics	[103]	https://slavovlab.net/data_webs.htm
Proteome exchange	Repository/ Database	Single cell Proteomics	[104, 105]	https://www.proteomexchange.org/
Metabolomics workbench	Repository/ Database	Single cell metabolomics	[106]	https://www.metabolomicsworkbench.org/data/index.php

Table 2.
Single cell repositories and databases.

Name	Type	Omics content	Ref	Website (If Available)
Seurat	R package	Single cell RNA-Seq	[107–109]	https://satijalab.org/seurat/
Galaxy	Open access	Single cell RNA-Seq	[11]	https://usegalaxy.org/
scpdata	R package	Single cell Proteomics	—	https://github.com/UCLouvain-CBIO/scpdata

Table 3.
Online tools, software and R-packages for single cell omics analysis.

Name	Type	Omics content	Ref	Website (If Available)
CellChatDB	Open access & R package	Single cell RNA-Seq	[110]	http://www.cellchat.org/
NICHES	R package	Single cell RNA-Seq	[111]	https://github.com/msraredon/NICHES
CITEdb	Open access & R package	Single cell RNA-Seq	[112]	https://citedb.cn/#/index
CellPhoneDB	Open access	Single cell RNA-Seq	[113]	https://www.cellphonedb.org/

Table 4.
Software and databases for cell-to-cell communication.

4. Bioinformatics

In recent years, technological advancements have made great progress in understanding the genetics, transcripts, proteins and metabolites seen in disease, resulting in an explosion of big data, opening endless scientific possibilities [114]. However, this vast amount of data generated has its own challenges related to: i) data storage, ii) software to process such large amounts of data and ii) analysis and biological interpretation of data. In this circumstance, bioinformatics and computational biology have sought to overcome these challenges in big data generation and analysis [114]. Bioinformatics is a multi-interdisciplinary approach combining mathematics, physics, biology and computer science, it is defined as the application of computational methods and tools for the organization, analysis, understanding, visualization and storage of information associated with biological entities [114]. The development of high-throughput technologies such as NGS, RNA-Seq and liquid chromatography-mass spectrometry (LC–MS) and the analysis of data using bioinformatic approaches has opened a host of new possibilities including but not limited to, gene expression studies, methylation patterns, epigenetic markers, proteins, metabolites, lipids and others [114]. In the recent decade, bioinformatics approaches have become of increasing interest especially in NDs for novel biomarkers and drug discovery and pathways [6]. Specifically, a multi-interdisciplinary approach such as SB can enhance the contribution of computational therapeutics and diagnostics for NDs, hence providing a stepping stone towards precision medicine.

In the following section, we look into the tools and databases available for.

-omics in regards to obtaining data and analysis of said data. Moreover, we will discuss network-based approaches used in HD research.

4.1 Omics databases and tools

The databases for obtaining publicly available data of different omics data at the single and bulk -omics level is constantly changing with new data becoming available every day. In addition, the analysis of such data is increasingly important, and various tools, software and R-packages are also developed to assist researchers in the analysis of their data. **Table 5** includes repositories and databases where omics data can be found, not only specific for HD but also for other NDs, as well various diseases. **Table 1** illustrates the tools, software and packages mainly in R, used for analysis of -omics data. The tables contain some of the most popular databases, repositories, software, tools and R-packages used, however there are numerous others resources available which have not been listed.

Name	Type	Omics content	Ref	Website (If Available)
Gene expression omnibus	Repository	Genomics, Epigenomics, Transcriptomics,	[101]	https://www.ncbi.nlm.nih.gov/geo/
Expression atlas	Repository	Genomics	[102, 115]	https://www.ebi.ac.uk/gxa/home
Array express	Repository/ Database	Genomics	[116]	https://www.ebi.ac.uk/biostudies/arrayexpress
European variation archive	Repository/ Database	Genomics	[117]	https://www.ebi.ac.uk/eva/?Home
Ensembl	Database	Genomics	[118]	http://www.ensembl.org/index.html
Database of genomic variants archive	Database	Genomics	—	https://www.ebi.ac.uk/dgva/
European genome-phenome archive	Repository/ Database	Genomics	—	https://ega-archive.org/
Answer ALS	Repository	Genomics Transcriptomics, Proteomics, Metabolomics	[119]	https://dataportahttps://dataportal.answerals.org/home
Huntington's disease in high definition (HDinHD)	Database	Genomics	—	https://www.hdinhd.org/
Enroll HD	Repository/ Database	Genomics Transcriptomics, Proteomics	[120]	https://www.enroll-hd.org/
Parkinson's progression markers initiative	Repository/ Database	Genomics Transcriptomics, Proteomics, Metabolomics	[121]	https://www.ppmi-info.org/
Alzheimer's disease neuroimaging initiative	Repository/ Database	Genetics Radiomics	[122]	https://adni.loni.usc.edu/

Name	Type	Omics content	Ref	Website (If Available)
PRIDE	Database	Proteomics	[123]	https://www.ebi.ac.uk/pride/
Proteome exchange	Repository/ Database	Proteomics	[104, 105]	https://www.proteomexchange.org/
Japan proteome standard	Repository/ Database	Proteomics	[124]	https://jpostdb.org/
Mass spectrometry interactive virtual environment	Repository/ Database	Proteomics	—	https://massive.ucsd.edu/ProteoSAFe/static/massive.jsp
ProteomicsDB	Repository/ Database	Proteomics	[125]	https://www.proteomicsdb.org/
Human peptide atlas	Repository/ Database	Proteomics	[126]	https://peptideatlas.org/
Metabolomics workbench	Repository/ Database	Metabolomics	[106]	https://www.metabolomicsworkbench.org/data/index.php
MetaboLights	Repository/ Database	Metabolomics	[127]	https://www.ebi.ac.uk/metabolights/index
Metabolome exchange	Repository/ Database	Metabolomics	—	http://www.metabolomexchange.org/site/
Human metabolome database	Database	Metabolomics	[128]	https://hmdb.ca/

Table 5.
Omics repositories and databases.

4.2 Network-based approaches

In all living organisms, most cellular components exert their functions via interactions with other components, the entirety of these interactions represents the human interactome [129]. The cells and their response to changes in their environment involve coordinated activity of mRNAs, proteins, metabolites and lipids [130]. The fundamentals of proper cellular function are molecular networks connecting these components to process extra-cellular environmental signals driving dynamic cellular responses [130]. Network-based approaches aim to systematically integrate measurements obtained from high-throughput experiments to gain insight of the cellular functions undergoing changes resulting in disease [130]. Systematic integration of varying biological entities is essential to identify molecular networks controlling normal and disease states, and in time, predict complex phenotypes from molecular markers [130]. Network-based approaches in human disease can lead to multiple biological and clinical applications, over the past decade, there has been an exceptional increase in human-specific molecular interaction data, resulting in a greater understanding of how different biological entities interact with one another, in biological networks and how they play a role in human diseases [129]. Examples of molecular networks are i) PPI networks, ii) metabolic networks, iii) regulatory networks, iv) RNA networks, v) cell–cell interaction networks and vi) multi-omics networks [129].

Few studies have been performed in regards to network and bioinformatic based approaches on HD. Some of these studies will be discussed below.

Chandrasekaran and Bonchev [131], performed network analysis on post-mortem tissue of the cerebellum, frontal cortex and caudate nucleus of HD patients. The microarray dataset, GSE3790, has 44 and 36 HD patients and controls respectively [131]. The dataset consists of both Affymetrix GeneChip Human Genome HG-U133A and B [131]. The seed genes are referred to as the significantly differentially expressed genes (SDEGs) [131]. In the GSE3790 HG-U133A, 617 overlapping seed genes were found between the four sets of SDEGs, while in GSE3790 HG-U133B, 351 seed genes were found [131]. Altogether, 925 seed genes were identified; however, network evaluation was performed only for the SDEGs with a p-value <0.01, with this new cut-off threshold, 531 seed genes were identified and underwent network analysis [131].

Pathway enrichment was performed using Pathway Studio 9.0 software along with the molecular interaction database ResNet 9.0 [131], to construct direct interaction, shortest-path and miRNA regulation networks. Gene prioritizing approaches based on network topological measures, high node connectivity, centrality and guilt by association were applied, based on this approach 19 novel genes were found *CEBPA, CDK1, CX3CL1, EGR1, E2F1, ERBB2, LRP1, HSP90AA1* and *ZNF148*; these genes may be of particular interest to undergo experimental validation [131]. The seed genes underwent GO enrichment analysis using DAVID [131], while the IPA software and Pathway Enrichment Analysis in Pathway studio was used to explore the canonical pathways affected in HD [131]. The pathways identified with DAVID are i) neuron development (GO:0048666), ii) neuron differentiation (GO:0030182), iii) regulation of glucose import (GO:0046324), iv) neuron projection (GO:0043005), v) regulation of lipid catabolic process (GO: 0050994) and various additional GO terms. The KEGG pathways from DAVID are i) HD (hsa: 05016), ii) MAPK signaling (hsa:04010), iii) ErbB signaling (hsa:04012), iv) Alzheimer's Disease (hsa: 05010), v) Amyotrophic Lateral Sclerosis (hsa: 05014) and numerous other pathways [131]. The miRNA regulatory network analysis, found miR-124, mir-135a, miR-141, miR-182 and miR-19a to be the top five scoring miRNA within the network [131]. The SDEGs, miRNA and pathways obtained, in combination with experimental validation can shed light onto possible genes, miRNAs and mechanisms affected in HD, which can lead to targeted therapeutic strategies.

Other network and bioinformatics-based approaches conducted in HD include Sneha et al. [132], Pirhaji et al. [133], Pradhan et al. [134], Xiang et al. [135], Zaho et al. [136], Fu et al. [137], Shirasaki et al. [138], Christodoulou [139–141], and Onisiforou [142].

5. Discussion and conclusion

HD remains one of the most debilitating and incurable ND, as currently there is a lack of effective treatments, although clinical trials have been conducted using different strategies such as gene silencing to decrease mHTT protein production [1–3, 5]. However, these attempts were unsuccessful as in some cases, no difference between the drug and placebo groups or no symptom improvement was observed. Therefore, there is a need for effective drugs to be identified and tested and used as pharmacotherapies for HD. Furthermore, a better understanding of how different biological molecules (genes, proteins, metabolites, lipids etc.) interact with not only each other but also with disease pathways, and possibly drugs is vital to understand how these interactions are affected in HD as it will allow to shed light on why some therapeutic treatments are not effective [5]. Dysregulation, in any specific cell type, biological molecule or pathway can influence the entire biological system leading to disease progression [7].

In the past decade technological advancements has led to high-throughput experiments resulting in -omics data and their analysis. In addition, there is a growing interest in SC-omics, allowing analysis of individual cells at a higher resolution, allowing for the accurate representation of cell–cell variation in tissues [95]. Bioinformatics, specifically network-based approaches, can be applied to investigate and understand in depth the relationship between the different biological molecules and their interaction with the HTT protein, each other and within pathways [5]. The advancement of bioinformatics has led to the progress and identification of novel candidate biomarkers and drugs, affected pathway and mechanisms and genes, proteins and metabolites affected in a disease state compared to controls [5, 6]. In addition, there has been an exponential increase in the number of repositories and database available for both bulk and SC analysis for genomics, transcriptomics, proteomics and metabolomics [95, 100]. In addition, this has resulted in numerous bioinformatics tools, software and R-packages, which have been developed to assist researchers in omics data analysis, in order to have meaningful biological interpretation of the data to make proper conclusions that will possibly lead to the discovery of potential biomarkers and drugs resulting in better prognosis, diagnosis and drug sensitivity of patients [100, 114]. The contribution of SB can provide a stepping stone towards precision medicine and potentially address the absence of HD treatments.

Conflict of interest

The authors declare no conflict of interest.

Additional information

The Cyprus Institute of Neurology and Genetics is a full member of the european reference network for rare neurological diseases (ERN-RND).

Author details

Christiana C. Christodoulou and Eleni Zamba Papanicolaou*
The Cyprus Institute of Neurology and Genetics, Nicosia, Cyprus

*Address all correspondence to: ezamba@cing.ac.cy

References

[1] Roos RA. Huntington's disease: A clinical review. Orphanet Journal of Rare Diseases. 2010;**5**:40. DOI: 10.1186/1750-1172-5-40

[2] Novak MJU, Tabrizi SJ. CliniCal review Huntington's disease. BMJ. 2010:340. DOI: 10.1136/bmj.c3109

[3] Bates GP, Dorsey R, Gusella JF, Hayden MR, Kay C, Leavitt BR, et al. Huntington Disease; 2015

[4] Lanciego JL, Luquin N, Obeso JA. Functional neuroanatomy of the basal ganglia. Cold Springer Harbor Perspective Medicine. 2012;**2**:1-20. DOI: 10.1101/cshperspect.a009621

[5] Paananen J. Bioinformatics in the identification of novel targets and pathways in neurodegenerative diseases. Current Genetics in Medical Report. 2017;**5**:15-21. DOI: 10.1007/s40142-017-0115-8

[6] Oulas A, Minadakis G, Zachariou M, Sokratous K, Bourdakou MM, Spyrou GM. Systems bioinformatics: Increasing precision of Computational Diagnostics and therapeutics through network-based approaches. Briefings in Bioinformatics. 2019;**20**:806-824. DOI: 10.1093/bib/bbx151

[7] Diaz-Ortiz ME, Chen-Plotkin AS. Omics in neurodegenerative disease: Hope or hype? Trends in Genetics. 2020;**36**:152-159

[8] Micheel C, Nass SJ, Omenn GS. Institute of Medicine (U.S.). Committee on the Review of Omics-Based Tests for Predicting Patient Outcomes in Clinical Trials Evolution of Translational Omics : Lessons Learned and the Path Forward; ISBN 9780309224185

[9] Chen C, McGarvey PB, Huang H, Wu CH. Protein bioinformatics infrastructure for the integration and analysis of multiple high-throughput omics data. Advances in Bioinformatics. 2010;**2010**:1-19. DOI: 10.1155/2010/423589

[10] Paszkiewicz KH, Giezen M. Bioinformatics, and infectious disease research. In: Genetics and Evolution of Infectious Diseases. Amsterdam, The Netherlands: Elsevier Inc.; 2011. pp. 523-539

[11] Afgan E, Nekrutenko A, Grüning BA, Blankenberg D, Goecks J, Schatz MC, et al. The galaxy platform for accessible, reproducible and collaborative biomedical analyses: 2022 update. Nucleic Acids Research. 2022;**50**:W345-W351. DOI: 10.1093/nar/gkac247

[12] Ritchie ME, Phipson B, Wu D, Hu Y, Law CW, Shi W, et al. Limma powers differential expression analyses for RNA-sequencing and microarray studies. Nucleic Acids Research. 2015;**43**:e47. DOI: 10.1093/nar/gkv007

[13] Robinson MD, McCarthy DJ, Smyth GK. EdgeR: A Bioconductor package for differential expression analysis of digital gene expression data. Bioinformatics. 2009;**26**:139-140. DOI: 10.1093/bioinformatics/btp616

[14] Chen Y, Lun ATL, Smyth GK. From reads to genes to pathways: Differential expression analysis of RNA-Seq experiments using Rsubread and the EdgeR quasi-likelihood pipeline.

F1000Res. 2016;**5**:1438. DOI: 10.12688/f1000research.8987.1

[15] McCarthy DJ, Chen Y, Smyth GK. Differential expression analysis of multifactor RNA-Seq experiments with respect to biological variation. Nucleic Acids Research. 2012;**40**:4288-4297. DOI: 10.1093/nar/gks042

[16] Tyanova S, Temu T, Cox J. The MaxQuant computational platform for mass spectrometry-based shotgun proteomics. Nature Protocols. 2016;**11**:2301-2319. DOI: 10.1038/nprot.2016.136

[17] Sturm M, Bertsch A, Gröpl C, Hildebrandt A, Hussong R, Lange E, et al. OpenMS - An open-source software framework for mass spectrometry. BMC Bioinformatics. 2008;**9**:1-11. DOI: 10.1186/1471-2105-9-163

[18] Rainer J, Vicini A, Salzer L, Stanstrup J, Badia JM, Neumann S, et al. A modular and expandable ecosystem for metabolomics data annotation in R. Metabolites. 2022;**12**:1-13. DOI: 10.3390/metabo12020173

[19] Xia J, Wishart DS. Metabolomic data processing, analysis, and interpretation using metaboanalyst. Current Protocols in Bioinformatics. 2011;**34**(1);1-48. DOI: 10.1002/0471250953.bi1410s34

[20] Xia J, Sinelnikov IV, Han B, Wishart DS. MetaboAnalyst 3.0-making metabolomics more meaningful. Nucleic Acids Research. 2015;**2015**:1-7. DOI: 10.1093/nar/gkv380

[21] Chong J, Soufan O, Li C, Caraus I, Li S, Bourque G, et al. MetaboAnalyst 4.0: Towards more transparent and integrative metabolomics analysis. Nucleic Acids Research. 2018;**46**:W486-W494. DOI: 10.1093/nar/gky310

[22] Caspi R, Foerster H, Fulcher CA, Kaipa P, Krummenacker M, Latendresse M, et al. The MetaCyc database of metabolic pathways and enzymes and the BioCyc collection of pathway/genome databases. Nucleic Acids Research. 2008;**36**:623-631. DOI: 10.1093/nar/gkm900

[23] Huan T, Forsberg EM, Rinehart D, Johnson CH, Ivanisevic J, Benton HP, et al. Systems biology guided by XCMS online metabolomics. Nature Methods. 2017;**2017**:1-5

[24] Tautenhahn R, Patti GJ, Rinehart D, Siuzdak G. XCMS online: A web-based platform to process untargeted metabolomic data. Analytical Chemistry. 2012;**84**:5035-5039. DOI: 10.1021/ac300698c

[25] Smith CA, Want EJ, O'Maille G, Abagyan R, Siuzdak G. XCMS: Processing mass spectrometry data for metabolite profiling using nonlinear peak alignment, matching, and identification. Analytical Chemistry. 2006;**78**:779-787. DOI: 10.1021/ac051437y

[26] Myers OD, Sumner SJ, Li S, Barnes S, Du X. Detailed investigation and comparison of the XCMS and MZmine 2 chromatogram construction and chromatographic peak detection methods for Preprocessing mass spectrometry metabolomics data. Analytical Chemistry. 2017;**2017**:8689-8695. DOI: 10.1021/acs.analchem.7b01069

[27] Moss DJH, Tabrizi SJ, Mead S, Lo K, Pardiñas AF, Holmans P, et al. Identification of genetic variants associated with Huntington's disease progression: A genome-wide association study. Lancet Neurology. 2017;**16**:701-711. DOI: 10.1016/S1474-4422(17)30161-8

[28] Li S, Tollefsbol TO. DNA Methylation Methods: Global DNA Methylation and Methylomic Analyses. Vol. 187.

Amsterdam, The Netherlands: Elsevier Inc; 2021 ISBN 2059344573

[29] Tang B, Seredenina T, Coppola G, Kuhn A, Geschwind DH, Luthi-Carter R, et al. Gene expression profiling of R6/2 transgenic mice with different CAG repeat lengths reveals genes associated with disease onset and progression in Huntington's disease. Neurobiology of Disease. 2011;**42**:459-467. DOI: 10.1016/j.nbd.2011.02.008

[30] Saiki K, David GH, Susanne S, Stephen SJ, Russell H, Glenn HT, et al. Henry primer-directed enzymatic amplification of DNA with thermostable DNA polymerase. Science. 1979;**1988**(239):487-491

[31] Behjati S, Tarpey PS. What is next generation sequencing? Archives of Disease in Childhood. Education and Practice Edition. 2013;**98**:236-238. DOI: 10.1136/archdischild-2013-304340

[32] Rossi MJ, Kuntala PK, Lai WKM, Yamada N, Badjatia N, Mittal C, et al. A high-resolution protein architecture of the budding yeast genome. Nature. 2021;**592**:309-314. DOI: 10.1038/s41586-021-03314-8

[33] Roth SC. What is genomic medicine? Journal of the Medical Library Association. 2019;**107**:442-448. DOI: 10.5195/jmla.2019.604

[34] Khodadadian A, Darzi S, Haghi-Daredeh S, Eshaghi FS, Babakhanzadeh E, Mirabutalebi SH, et al. Genomics and transcriptomics: The powerful Technologies in Precision Medicine. International Journal of Genetic Medicine. 2020;**13**:627-640

[35] Marchina E, Misasi S, Bozzato A, Ferraboli S, Agosti C, Rozzini L, et al. Gene expression profile in fibroblasts of Huntington's disease patients and controls. Journal of the Neurological Sciences. 2014;**337**:42-46. DOI: 10.1016/j.jns.2013.11.014

[36] Wright GEB, Caron NS, Ng B, Casal L, Casazza W, Xu X, et al. Gene expression profiles complement the analysis of genomic modifiers of the clinical onset of Huntington disease. Human Molecular Genetics. 2020;**29**:2788-2802. DOI: 10.1093/hmg/ddaa184

[37] Langfelder P, Cantle JP, Chatzopoulou D, Wang N, Gao F, Al-Ramahi I, et al. Integrated genomics and proteomics define huntingtin CAG length-dependent networks in mice. Nature Neuroscience. 2016;**19**:623-633. DOI: 10.1038/nn.4256

[38] Choudhury KR, Das S, Bhattacharyya NP. Differential proteomic and genomic profiling of mouse striatal cell model of Huntington's disease and control; probable implications to the disease biology. Journal of Proteomics. 2016;**132**:155-166. DOI: 10.1016/j.jprot.2015.11.007

[39] Alcalá-Vida R, Seguin J, Lotz C, Molitor AM, Irastorza-Azcarate I, Awada A, et al. Age-related and disease locus-specific mechanisms contribute to early remodelling of chromatin structure in Huntington's disease mice. Nature Communications. 2021;**12**:1-16. DOI: 10.1038/s41467-020-20605-2

[40] Lin L, Park JW, Ramachandran S, Zhang Y, Tseng YT, Shen S, et al. Transcriptome sequencing reveals aberrant alternative splicing in Huntington's disease. Human Molecular Genetics. 2016;**25**:3454-3466. DOI: 10.1093/hmg/ddw187

[41] Neueder A, Kojer K, Hering T, Lavery DJ, Chen J, Birth N, et al. Abnormal molecular signatures of inflammation, energy metabolism, and

vesicle biology in human Huntington disease peripheral tissues. Genome Biology. 2022;**23**:1-21. DOI: 10.1186/s13059-022-02752-5

[42] Miller JRC, Lo KK, Andre R, Hensman Moss DJ, Träger U, Stone TC, et al. RNA-Seq of Huntington's disease patient myeloid cells reveals innate transcriptional dysregulation associated with proinflammatory pathway activation. Human Molecular Genetics. 2016;**25**:2893-2904. DOI: 10.1093/hmg/ddw142

[43] Moily NS, Ormsby AR, Stojilovic A, Ramdzan YM, Diesch J, Hannan RD, et al. Transcriptional profiles for distinct aggregation states of mutant huntingtin exon 1 protein unmask New Huntington's disease pathways. Molecular and Cellular Neuroscience. 2017;**83**:103-112. DOI: 10.1016/j.mcn.2017.07.004

[44] Seefelder M, Kochanek S. A Meta-analysis of transcriptomic profiles of Huntington's disease patients. PLoS One. 2021;**16**. DOI: 10.1371/journal.pone.0253037

[45] Sinha M, Mukhopadhyay S, Bhattacharyya NP. Mechanism(s) of alteration of Micro Rna expressions in Huntington's disease and their possible contributions to the observed cellular and molecular dysfunctions in the disease. Neuromolecular Medicine. 2012;**14**:221-243

[46] Mastrokolias A, Ariyurek Y, Goeman JJ, Van Duijn E, Roos RAC, Van Der Mast RC, et al. Huntington's disease biomarker progression profile identified by transcriptome sequencing in peripheral blood. European Journal of Human Genetics. 2015;**23**:1349-1356. DOI: 10.1038/ejhg.2014.281

[47] Mastrokolias A, Pool R, Mina E, Hettne KM, van Duijn E, van der Mast RC, et al. Integration of targeted metabolomics and transcriptomics identifies deregulation of phosphatidylcholine metabolism in Huntington's disease peripheral blood samples. Metabolomics. 2016;**12**. DOI: 10.1007/s11306-016-1084-8

[48] Borovecki F, Lovrecic L, Zhou J, Jeong H, Then F, Rosas HD, et al. Genome-wide expression profiling of human blood reveals biomarkers for Huntington's disease. Proceedings of the National Academy of Sciences of the United States of America. 2005;**102**:11023-11028. DOI: 10.1073/pnas.0504921102

[49] Cha JHJ. Transcriptional signatures in Huntington's disease

[50] Mehta SR, Tom CM, Wang Y, Bresee C, Rushton D, Mathkar PP, et al. Human Huntington's disease IPSC-derived cortical neurons display altered transcriptomics, morphology, and maturation. Cell Reports. 2018;**25**:1081-1096.e6. DOI: 10.1016/j.celrep.2018.09.076

[51] Stopa EG, Tanis KQ, Miller MC, Nikonova EV, Podtelezhnikov AA, Finney EM, et al. Comparative transcriptomics of choroid plexus in Alzheimer's disease, frontotemporal dementia and Huntington's disease: Implications for CSF homeostasis. Fluids Barriers CNS. 2018;**15**. DOI: 10.1186/s12987-018-0102-9

[52] Runne H, Kuhn A, Wild EJ, Pratyaksha W, Kristiansen M, Isaacs JD, et al. Analysis of potential transcriptomic biomarkers for huntington's disease in peripheral blood. Proceedings of the National Academy of Sciences of the United States of America. 4 Sep 2007;**104**(36):1-6. DOI: 10.1073/pnas.0703652104

[53] Jin J, Cheng Y, Zhang Y, Wood W, Peng Q, Hutchison E, et al. Interrogation of brain MiRNA and MRNA expression profiles reveals a molecular

regulatory network that is perturbed by mutant huntingtin. Journal of Neurochemistry. 2012;**123**:477-490. DOI: 10.1111/j.1471-4159.2012.07925.x

[54] Hervás-Corpión I, Guiretti D, Alcaraz-Iborra M, Olivares R, Campos-Caro A, Barco Á, et al. Early alteration of epigenetic-related transcription in Huntington's disease mouse models. Scientific Reports. 2018;**8**. DOI: 10.1038/s41598-018-28185-4

[55] Bensalel J, Xu H, Lu ML, Capobianco E, Wei J. RNA-Seq analysis reveals significant transcriptome changes in huntingtin-null human neuroblastoma cells. BMC Medical Genomics. 2021;**14**. DOI: 10.1186/s12920-021-01022-w

[56] Dickson E, Dwijesha AS, Andersson N, Lundh S, Björkqvist M, Petersén Å, et al. Microarray profiling of hypothalamic gene expression changes in Huntington's disease mouse models. Frontiers in Neuroscience. 2022;**16**. DOI: 10.3389/fnins.2022.1027269

[57] Reyes-Ortiz AM, Abud EM, Burns MS, Wu J, Hernandez SJ, McClure N, et al. Single-nuclei transcriptome analysis of Huntington disease IPSC and mouse astrocytes implicates maturation and functional deficits. iScience. 2023;**26**. DOI: 10.1016/j.isci.2022.105732

[58] Chaves G, Özel RE, Rao NV, Hadiprodjo H, Da Costa Y, Tokuno Z, et al. Metabolic and transcriptomic analysis of Huntington's disease model reveal changes in intracellular glucose levels and related genes. Heliyon. 2017;**3**:e00381. DOI: 10.1016/j.heliyon.2017

[59] Huang L, Fang L, Liu Q, Torshizi AD, Wang K. Integrated analysis on transcriptome and Behaviors defines HTT repeat-dependent network modules in Huntington's disease. Genes Diseases. 2022;**9**:479-493. DOI: 10.1016/j.gendis.2021.05.004

[60] Al-Amrani S, Al-Jabri Z, Al-Zaabi A, Alshekaili J, Al-Khabori M. Proteomics: Concepts and applications in human medicine. World Journal of Biological Chemistry. 2021;**12**:57-69. DOI: 10.4331/wjbc.v12.i5.57

[61] Fang Q, Strand A, Law W, Faca VM, Fitzgibbon MP, Hamel N, et al. Brain-specific proteins decline in the cerebrospinal fluid of humans with Huntington disease. Molecular and Cellular Proteomics. 2009;**8**:451-466. DOI: 10.1074/mcp.M800231-MCP200

[62] Chen S, Lu FF, Seeman P, Liu F. Quantitative proteomic analysis of human substantia Nigra in Alzheimer's disease, Huntington's disease and multiple sclerosis. Neurochemical Research. 2012;**37**:2805-2813. DOI: 10.1007/s11064-012-0874-2

[63] Schönberger SJ, Jezdic D, Faull RLM, Cooper GJS. Proteomic analysis of the human brain in Huntington's disease indicates pathogenesis by molecular processes linked to other neurodegenerative diseases and to Type-2 diabetes. Journal of Huntingtons Diseases. 2013;**2**:89-99. DOI: 10.3233/JHD-120044

[64] Sorolla MA, Reverter-Branchat G, Tamarit J, Ferrer I, Ros J, Cabiscol E. Proteomic and oxidative stress analysis in human brain samples of Huntington disease. Free Radical Biology & Medicine. 2008;**45**:667-678. DOI: 10.1016/j.freeradbiomed.2008.05.014

[65] Chae J et al. Quantitative proteomic analysis of induced pluripotent stem cells derived from a human Huntington's disease patient. Biochemical Journal. 2012;**446**:359-371. DOI: 10.1042/BJ20111495

[66] McQuade LR, Balachandran A, Scott HA, Khaira S, Baker MS, Schmidt U. Proteomics of Huntington's disease-affected human embryonic stem cells reveals an evolving pathology involving mitochondrial dysfunction and metabolic disturbances. Journal of Proteome Research. 2014;**13**:5648-5659. DOI: 10.1021/pr500649m

[67] Dalrymple A, Wild EJ, Joubert R, Sathasivam K, Björkqvist M, Petersén Å, et al. Proteomic profiling of plasma in Huntington's disease reveals neuroinflammatory activation and biomarker candidates. Journal of Proteome Research. 2007;**6**:2833-2840. DOI: 10.1021/pr0700753

[68] Agrawal S, Fox JH. Novel proteomic changes in brain mitochondria provide insights into mitochondrial dysfunction in mouse models of Huntington's disease. Mitochondrion. 2019;**47**:318-329. DOI: 10.1016/j.mito.2019.03.004

[69] Mees I, Li S, Tran H, Ang CS, Williamson NA, Hannan AJ, et al. Phosphoproteomic dysregulation in Huntington's disease mice is rescued by environmental enrichment. Brain Communication. 2022;**4**. DOI: 10.1093/braincomms/fcac305

[70] Liu X, Miller BR, Rebec GV, Clemmer DE. Protein expression in the striatum and cortex regions of the brain for a mouse model of Huntington's disease. Journal of Proteome Research. 2007;**6**:3134-3142. DOI: 10.1021/pr070092s

[71] Perluigi M, Poon HF, Maragos W, Pierce WM, Klein JB, Calabrese V, et al. Proteomic analysis of protein expression and oxidative modification in R6/2 transgenic mice: A model of Huntington disease. Molecular and Cellular Proteomics. 2005;**4**:1849-1861. DOI: 10.1074/mcp.M500090-MCP200

[72] Deschepper M, Hoogendoorn B, Brooks S, Dunnett SB, Jones L. Proteomic changes in the brains of Huntington's disease mouse models reflect pathology and implicate mitochondrial changes. Brain Research Bulletin. 2012;**88**:210-222. DOI: 10.1016/j.brainresbull.2011.01.012

[73] Culver BP, Savas JN, Park SK, Choi JH, Zheng S, Zeitlin SO, et al. Proteomic analysis of Wild-type and mutant huntingtin-associated proteins in mouse brains identifies unique interactions and involvement in protein synthesis. Journal of Biological Chemistry. 2012;**287**:21599-21614. DOI: 10.1074/jbc.M112.359307

[74] Cozzolino F, Landolfi A, Iacobucci I, Monaco V, Caterino M, Celentano S, et al. New label-free methods for protein relative quantification applied to the investigation of an animal model of Huntington disease. PLoS One. 2020;**15**:1-20. DOI: 10.1371/journal.pone.0238037

[75] Vodicka P, Mo S, Tousley A, Green KM, Sapp E, Iuliano M, et al. Mass spectrometry analysis of Wild-type and Knock-in Q140/Q140 Huntington's disease mouse brains reveals changes in glycerophospholipids including alterations in phosphatidic acid and Lyso-phosphatidic acid. Journal of Huntingtons Diseases. 2015;**4**:187-201. DOI: 10.3233/JHD-150149

[76] Sap KA, Guler AT, Bezstarosti K, Bury AE, Juenemann K, Demmers JAA, et al. Global proteome and ubiquitinome changes in the soluble and insoluble fractions of Q175 Huntington mice brains. Molecular and Cellular Proteomics. 2019;**18**:1705-1720. DOI: 10.1074/mcp.RA119.001486

[77] Ratovitski T, Chighladze E, Arbez N, Boronina T, Herbrich S, Cole RN, et al. Huntingtin protein interactions

altered by polyglutamine expansion as determined by quantitative proteomic analysis. Cell Cycle. 2012;**11**:2006-2021. DOI: 10.4161/cc.20423

[78] Zabel C, Klose J. Influence of huntington's disease on the human and mouse proteome. International Review of Neurobiology. 2004;**61**:241-283. DOI: 10.1016/S0074-7742(04)61010-5

[79] Clish CB. Metabolomics: An emerging but powerful tool for precision medicine. Molecular Case Studies. 2015;**1**:a000588. DOI: 10.1101/mcs.a000588

[80] Rosas HD, Doros G, Bhasin S, Thomas B, Gevorkian S, Malarick K, et al. A systems-level "Misunderstanding": The plasma metabolome in Huntington's disease. Annals of Clinical Translational Neurology. 2015;**2**:756-768. DOI: 10.1002/acn3.214

[81] Herman S, Niemelä V, Emami Khoonsari P, Sundblom J, Burman J, Landtblom AM, et al. Alterations in the tyrosine and phenylalanine pathways revealed by biochemical profiling in cerebrospinal fluid of Huntington's disease subjects. Scientific Reports. 2019;**9**:1-13. DOI: 10.1038/s41598-019-40186-5

[82] McGarry A, Gaughan J, Hackmyer C, Lovett J, Khadeer M, Shaikh H, et al. Cross-sectional analysis of plasma and CSF metabolomic markers in Huntington's disease for participants of varying functional disability: A pilot study. Scientific Reports. 2020;**10**:1-13. DOI: 10.1038/s41598-020-77526-9

[83] Cheng ML, Chang KH, Wu YR, Chen CM. Metabolic disturbances in plasma as biomarkers for Huntington's disease. Journal of Nutritional Biochemistry. 2016;**31**:38-44. DOI: 10.1016/j.jnutbio.2015.12.001

[84] Graham SF, Pan X, Yilmaz A, Macias S, Robinson A, Mann D, et al. Targeted biochemical profiling of brain from Huntington's disease patients reveals novel metabolic pathways of interest. Biochimica et Biophysica Acta - Molecular Basis of Disease. 2018;**1864**:2430-2437. DOI: 10.1016/j.bbadis.2018.04.012

[85] Graham SF, Kumar P, Bahado-Singh RO, Robinson A, Mann D, Green BD. Novel metabolite biomarkers of Huntington's disease as detected by high-resolution mass spectrometry. Journal of Proteome Research. 2016;**15**:1592-1601. DOI: 10.1021/acs.jproteome.6b00049

[86] Patassini S, Begley P, Xu J, Church SJ, Reid SJ, Kim EH, et al. Metabolite mapping reveals severe widespread perturbation of multiple metabolic processes in Huntington's disease human brain. Biochimica et Biophysica Acta - Molecular Basis of Disease. 2016;**1862**:1650-1662. DOI: 10.1016/j.bbadis.2016.06.002

[87] Skene DJ, Middleton B, Fraser CK, Pennings JLA, Kuchel TR, Rudiger SR, et al. Metabolic profiling of Presymptomatic Huntington's disease sheep reveals novel biomarkers. Scientific Reports. 2017;**7**:1-16. DOI: 10.1038/srep43030

[88] Andersen JV, Skotte NH, Aldana BI, Nørremølle A, Waagepetersen HS. Enhanced cerebral branched-chain amino acid metabolism in R6/2 mouse model of Huntington's disease. Cellular and Molecular Life Sciences. 2019;**76**:2449-2461. DOI: 10.1007/s00018-019-03051-2

[89] Chang KL, New LS, Mal M, Goh CW, Aw CC, Browne ER, et al. Metabolic profiling of 3-Nitropropionic acid early-stage Huntingtons disease rat model using gas chromatography time-of-flight mass spectrometry. Journal of Proteome Research. 2011;**10**:2079-2087. DOI: 10.1021/pr2000336

[90] Bertrand M, Decoville M, Meudal H, Birman S, Landon C. Metabolomic nuclear magnetic resonance studies at Presymptomatic and symptomatic stages of Huntington's disease on a Drosophila model. Journal of Proteome Research. 2020;**19**:4034-4045. DOI: 10.1021/acs.jproteome.0c00335

[91] Verwaest KA, Vu TN, Laukens K, Clemens LE, Nguyen HP, Van Gasse B, et al. 1H NMR based metabolomics of CSF and blood serum: A metabolic profile for a transgenic rat model of Huntington disease. Biochimica et Biophysica Acta - Molecular Basis of Disease. 2011;**1812**:1371-1379. DOI: 10.1016/j.bbadis.2011.08.001

[92] Hashimoto M, Watanabe K, Miyoshi K, Koyanagi Y, Tadano J, Miyawaki I. Multiplatform metabolomic analysis of the R6/2 mouse model of Huntington's disease. FEBS Open Bio. 2021;**11**:2807-2818. DOI: 10.1002/2211-5463.13285

[93] Kumar KK, Goodwin CR, Uhouse MA, Bornhorst J, Schwerdtle T, Aschner M, et al. Untargeted metabolic profiling identifies interactions between Huntington's disease and neuronal manganese status. Metallomics. 2015;7:363-370. DOI: 10.1039/c4mt00223g

[94] Tsang TM, Woodman B, Mcloughlin GA, Griffin JL, Tabrizi SJ, Bates GP, et al. Metabolic characterization of the R6/2 transgenic mouse model of Huntington's disease by high-resolution MAS 1H NMR spectroscopy. Journal of Proteome Research. 2006;**5**:483-492. DOI: 10.1021/pr050244o

[95] Dimitriu MA, Lazar-Contes I, Roszkowski M, Mansuy IM. Single-cell multiomics techniques: From conception to applications. Front cell. Developmental Biology. 2022;**10**:1-16

[96] Maiuri T, Truant R. Single cell technologies define New therapeutic avenues for Huntington's disease. Neuron. 2020;**107**:768-769

[97] Malaiya S, Cortes-Gutierrez M, Herb BR, Coffey SR, Legg SRW, Cantle JP, et al. Single-nucleus RNA-Seq reveals dysregulation of striatal cell identity due to Huntington's disease mutations. Journal of Neuroscience. 2021;**41**:5334-5352. DOI: 10.1523/JNEUROSCI.2074-20.2021

[98] Al-Dalahmah O, Sosunov AA, Shaik A, Ofori K, Liu Y, Vonsattel JP, et al. Single-nucleus RNA-Seq identifies Huntington disease astrocyte states. Acta Neuropathologica Communications. 2020;**8**:1-21. DOI: 10.1186/s40478-020-0880-6

[99] Lim RG, Al-Dalahmah O, Wu J, Gold MP, Reidling JC, Tang G, et al. Huntington disease oligodendrocyte maturation deficits revealed by single-nucleus RNAseq are rescued by thiamine-biotin supplementation. Nature Communications. 2022;**13**:1-23. DOI: 10.1038/s41467-022-35388-x

[100] Wang D, Bodovitz S. Single cell analysis: The new frontier in "Omics.". Trends in Biotechnology. 2010;**28**:281-290

[101] Clough E, Barrett T. The gene expression omnibus database. In: Methods in Molecular Biology. Vol. 1418. Humana Press Inc.; 2016. pp. 1-18

[102] Papatheodorou I, Moreno P, Manning J, Fuentes AMP, George N, Fexova S, et al. Expression atlas update: From tissues to single cells. Nucleic Acids Research. 2020;**48**:D77-D83. DOI: 10.1093/nar/gkz947

[103] Slavov N. Driving single cell proteomics forward with innovation. Journal of Proteome Research. 2021;**2021**:1-9

[104] Deutsch EW, Csordas A, Sun Z, Jarnuczak A, Perez-Riverol Y, Ternent T, et al. The ProteomeXchange consortium in 2017: Supporting the cultural change in proteomics public data deposition. Nucleic Acids Research. 2017;**45**:D1100-D1106. DOI: 10.1093/nar/gkw936

[105] Deutsch EW, Bandeira N, Sharma V, Perez-Riverol Y, Carver JJ, Kundu DJ, et al. The ProteomeXchange consortium in 2020: Enabling "big data" approaches in proteomics. Nucleic Acids Research. 2020;**48**:D1145-D1152. DOI: 10.1093/nar/gkz984

[106] Sud M, Fahy E, Cotter D, Azam K, Vadivelu I, Burant C, et al. Metabolomics workbench: An international repository for metabolomics data and metadata, metabolite standards, protocols, tutorials and training, and analysis tools. Nucleic Acids Research. 2016;**44**:D463-D470. DOI: 10.1093/nar/gkv1042

[107] Hao Y, Hao S, Andersen-Nissen E, Mauck WM, Zheng S, Butler A, et al. Integrated analysis of multimodal single-cell data. Cell. 2021;**184**:3573-3587.e29. DOI: 10.1016/j.cell.2021.04.048

[108] Stuart T, Butler A, Hoffman P, Hafemeister C, Papalexi E, Mauck WM, et al. Comprehensive integration of single-cell data. Cell. 2019;**177**:1888-1902.e21. DOI: 10.1016/j.cell.2019.05.031

[109] Satija R, Farrell JA, Gennert D, Schier AF, Regev A. Spatial reconstruction of single-cell gene expression data. Nature Biotechnology. 2015;**33**:495-502. DOI: 10.1038/nbt.3192

[110] Jin S, Guerrero-Juarez CF, Zhang L, Chang I, Ramos R, Kuan CH, et al. Inference and analysis of cell-cell communication using CellChat. Nature Communications. 2021;**12**:1-20. DOI: 10.1038/s41467-021-21246-9

[111] Raredon MSB, Yang J, Kothapalli N, Lewis W, Kaminski N, Niklason LE, et al. Comprehensive visualization of cell-cell interactions in single-cell and spatial transcriptomics with NICHES. Bioinformatics. 2023;**39**:1-3. DOI: 10.1093/bioinformatics/btac775

[112] Shan N, Lu Y, Guo H, Li D, Jiang J, Yan L, et al. CITEdb: A manually curated database of cell-cell interactions in human. Bioinformatics. 2022;**38**:5144-5148. DOI: 10.1093/bioinformatics/btac654

[113] Efremova M, Vento-Tormo M, Teichmann SA, Vento-Tormo R. CellPhoneDB: Inferring cell–cell communication from combined expression of multi-subunit ligand–receptor complexes. Nature Protocols. 2020;**15**:1484-1506. DOI: 10.1038/s41596-020-0292-x

[114] Diniz WJS, Canduri F. Bioinformatics: An overview and its applications. Genetics and Molecular Research. 2017;**16**:1-21

[115] Petryszak R, Fonseca AN, et al. Brazma Alvix RNA-Seq gene profiling - A systematic empirical comparison. Binformatics. 2017;**12**:1-10. DOI: 10.1371/journal

[116] Parkinson H, Kapushesky M, Shojatalab M, Abeygunawardena N, Coulson R, Farne A, et al. ArrayExpress – A public database of microarray experiments and gene expression profiles. Nucleic Acids Research. 2007;**35**:747-750. DOI: 10.1093/nar/gkl995

[117] Cezard T, Cunningham F, Hunt SE, Koylass B, Kumar N, Saunders G, et al. The European variation archive: A FAIR resource of genomic variation for all species. Nucleic Acids Research. 2022;**50**:D1216-D1220. DOI: 10.1093/nar/gkab960

[118] Hubbard T, Barker D, Birney E, Cameron G, Chen Y, Clark L, et al. The Ensembl Genome Database Project. 2002;**30**:38-41

[119] Baxi EG, Thompson T, Li J, Kaye JA, Lim RG, Wu J, et al. Answer ALS, a large-scale resource for sporadic and familial ALS combining clinical and multi-omics data from induced pluripotent cell lines. Nature Neuroscience. 2022;**25**:226-237. DOI: 10.1038/s41593-021-01006-0

[120] Sathe S, Ware J, Levey J, Neacy E, Blumenstein R, Noble S, et al. Enroll-HD: An integrated clinical research platform and worldwide observational study for Huntington's disease. Frontiers in Neurology. 2021;**12**:1-10

[121] Marek K, Chowdhury S, Siderowf A, Lasch S, Coffey CS, Caspell-Garcia C, et al. The Parkinson's progression markers initiative (PPMI) – Establishing a PD biomarker cohort. Annals of Clinical Translational Neurology. 2018;**5**:1460-1477. DOI: 10.1002/acn3.644

[122] Petersen RC, Aisen PS, Beckett LA, Donohue MC, Gamst AC, Harvey DJ, et al. Alzheimer's Disease Neuroimaging Initiative (ADNI). Clinical Characterization. 2010;**2010**:201-209

[123] Philip J, Richard C. The PRIDE Proteomics Identifications Database: Data Submission, Query, and Dataset Comparison. In: Thompson JD, Ueffing M, Schaeffer-Reiss C, editors. Methods in Molecular Biology. Vol. 484. Totowa, NJ: Humana Press; 2008

[124] Moriya Y, Kawano S, Okuda S, Watanabe Y, Matsumoto M, Takami T, et al. The Jpost environment: An integrated proteomics data repository and database. Nucleic Acids Research. 2019;**47**:D1218-D1224. DOI: 10.1093/nar/gky899

[125] Samaras P, Schmidt T, Frejno M, Gessulat S, Reinecke M, Jarzab A, et al. ProteomicsDB: A multi-omics and multi-organism resource for life science research. Nucleic Acids Research. 2020;**48**:D1153-D1163. DOI: 10.1093/nar/gkz974

[126] Deutsch EW. The PeptideAtlas project. Methods in Molecular Biology. 2010;**604**:285-296. DOI: 10.1007/978-1-60761-444-9_19

[127] Haug K, Cochrane K, Nainala VC, Williams M, Chang J, Jayaseelan KV, et al. MetaboLights: A resource evolving in response to the needs of its scientific community. Nucleic Acids Research. 2020;**48**:D440-D444. DOI: 10.1093/nar/gkz1019

[128] Wishart DS, Feunang YD, Marcu A, Guo AC, Liang K, Vázquez-Fresno R, et al. HMDB 4.0: The human metabolome database for 2018. Nucleic Acids Research. 2018;**46**:D608-D617. DOI: 10.1093/nar/gkx1089

[129] Barabási AL, Gulbahce N, Loscalzo J. Network medicine: A network-based approach to human disease. Nature Reviews. Genetics. 2011;**12**:56-68

[130] Chasman D, Siahpirani AF, Roy S. Network-based approaches for analysis of complex biological systems. Current Opinion in Biotechnology. 2016;**39**:157-166

[131] Chandrasekaran S, Bonchev D. Network analysis of human post-mortem microarrays reveals novel genes, MicroRNAs, and mechanistic scenarios of potential importance in fighting Huntington's disease. Computational and Structural Biotechnology Journal. 2016;**14**:117-130. DOI: 10.1016/j.csbj.2016.02.001

[132] Sneha NP, Dharshini SAP, Taguchi YH, Gromiha MM. Integrative

Meta-analysis of Huntington's disease transcriptome landscape. Genes (Basel). 2022;**13**:1-20. DOI: 10.3390/genes13122385

[133] Pirhaji L, Milani P, Leidl M, Curran T, Avila-Pacheco J, Clish CB, et al. Revealing disease-associated pathways by network integration of untargeted metabolomics. Nature Methods. 2016;**13**:770-776. DOI: 10.1038/nmeth.3940

[134] Pradhan SS, Thota SM, Rajaratnam S, Bhagavatham SKS, Pulukool SK, Rathnakumar S, et al. Integrated multi-omics analysis of Huntington disease identifies pathways that modulate protein aggregation. DMM Disease Models and Mechanisms. 2022;**15**:1-20. DOI: 10.1242/dmm.049492

[135] Xiang C, Cong S, Liang B, Cong S. Bioinformatic gene analysis for potential therapeutic targets of Huntington's disease in pre-symptomatic and symptomatic stage. Journal of Translational Medicine. 2020;**18**:1-10. DOI: 10.1186/s12967-020-02549-9

[136] Zhao N, Quicksall Z, Asmann YW, Ren Y. Network approaches for omics studies of neurodegenerative diseases. Frontiers in Genetics. 2022;**13**:1-6

[137] Fu MH, Li CL, Lin HL, Tsai SJ, Lai YY, Chang YF, et al. The potential regulatory mechanisms of MIR-196a in Huntington's disease through bioinformatic analyses. PLoS One. 2015;**10**:1-11. DOI: 10.1371/journal.pone.0137637

[138] Shirasaki DI, Greiner ER, Al-Ramahi I, Gray M, Boontheung P, Geschwind DH, et al. Network Organization of the Huntingtin Proteomic Interactome in mammalian brain. Neuron. 2012;**75**:41-57. DOI: 10.1016/j.neuron.2012.05.024

[139] Christodoulou CC, Papanicolaou EZ. Integrated bioinformatics analysis of shared genes, MiRNA, biological pathways and their potential role as therapeutic targets in Huntington's disease stages. International Journal of Molecular Sciences. 2023;**24**:1-29. DOI: 10.3390/ijms24054873

[140] Kakouri AC, Christodoulou CC, Zachariou M, Oulas A, Minadakis G, Demetriou CA, et al. Revealing clusters of connected pathways through multisource data integration in Huntington's disease and spastic Ataxia. IEEE Journal of Biomedical and Health Informatics. 2019;**23**:26-37. DOI: 10.1109/JBHI.2018.2865569

[141] Christodoulou CC, Zachariou M, Tomazou M, Karatzas E, Demetriou CA, Zamba-Papanicolaou E, et al. Investigating the transition of pre-symptomatic to symptomatic Huntington's disease status based on omics data. International Journal of Molecular Sciences. 2020;**21**:1-26. DOI: 10.3390/ijms21197414

[142] Onisiforou A, Spyrou GM. Systems bioinformatics reveals possible relationship between COVID-19 and the development of neurological diseases and neuropsychiatric disorders. Viruses. 2022;**14**:1-28. DOI: 10.3390/v14102270

Chapter 2

Neurological Impact of Type I Interferon Dysregulation

Alessio Mylonas

Abstract

Type I interferons are a class of potent and tightly regulated cytokines important for antiviral and anti-tumoural innate and adaptive immunity. Dysregulated production can have serious neurologic consequences as exemplified in a family of rare diseases called type I interferonopathies. Interferonopathies represent a group of genetically determined conditions characterised by upregulated type I interferon production causing a spectrum of neuroinflammatory and systemic manifestations. This chapter delves into the historical discovery of type I interferons, their role in innate immunity, and the subsequent identification of interferonopathies placing emphasis on the mechanisms of neurologic dysfunction that often dominate the clinical picture. The insights gained from studying these rare diseases offer valuable lessons for neurodegenerative and neuropsychiatric conditions which demonstrate considerable overlap with interferonopathies, underscoring the broader significance of type I interferons in more common neurologic diseases. Relevant therapeutic strategies targeting this pathway are discussed, emphasising the need for brain-penetrant approaches.

Keywords: type I interferon, IFNα, IFNβ, IFNAR, Type I interferonopathies, Aicardi-Goutières syndrome, Alzheimer's disease, Down's syndrome, Systemic lupus erythematosus, Neurolupus, Interferon therapies, Inflammaging, Traumatic brain injury, HIV/AIDS-associated neurocognitive disorders, major depression, anifrolumab, anti-IFNAR1, CXCL10, CXCR3

1. Introduction

Type I interferonopathies, or simply interferonopathies, are a family of rare autoinflammatory diseases typified by overt sustained activation of type I interferon signalling. In their most characteristic appearance, interferonopathies are a form of neuroinflammatory disease with a genetic origin. In recent years, type I interferons have been implicated in an increasing number of neurologic diseases, raising the question of whether a better understanding of interferonopathies can enhance our knowledge of neurodegeneration mechanisms.

In this chapter, interferonopathies and the type I interferon pathway are introduced, and they are contextualised with our current knowledge of the biology and the underlying immunologic mechanisms. This is then examined in relation to the continuously expanding spectrum of neuropsychiatric diseases induced by interferon dysfunction. While interferonopathies are rare monogenic diseases, dysregulation of the type I interferon pathway has important implications for more common polygenic diseases. Our understanding of this pathway, of these rare interferonopathies, and of the more common interferon dysfunction diseases that they have parallels with, has allowed for great advances in the development of interferon as a therapeutic target with potentially great future clinical implications.

1.1 Historical perspective

Type I interferonopathies are a recent concept encompassing a diverse family of diseases. The term was first introduced by Yanick Crow in 2011 who proposed a unifying notion for several Mendelian diseases that share clinical and molecular features and, importantly, which involve type I interferon dysregulation [1]. Yet the history of type I interferonopathies dates all the way back to the early 1980s, when the deleterious effects of interferons were first observed and hypothesised.

The discovery of type I interferons is a fascinating story of scientific serendipity and perseverance. Interferons have been studied since the mid-1950s, when famous Alick Isaacs and Jean Lindenmann reported the discovery of a soluble factor that could interfere with the replication of influenza virus which they named "interferon" [2, 3]. Initially, the two microbiologists were studying the influenza virus and the resulting cytopathic activity in chick cells and remarked that some cells were more resistant to the infection and importantly that this resistance could be transferred. While fraught with resistance and scepticism from the research community, and hampered by technological limitations, this discovery paved the way for unprecedented therapeutic advances. Years later, it was discovered that many different interferons exist, with broadly overlapping induction mechanisms, functions, and biological effects. Importantly, it was discovered that exogenous delivery could be leveraged for therapeutic benefit in patients.

The first human use of interferons occurred in 1973. A non-purified interferon preparation was delivered intranasally to healthy volunteers later exposed to rhinovirus, demonstrating antiviral immunity in humans for the first time [4]. Aside from their antiviral function, anti-tumour activities were described [5] paving the way for the first antitumour use in humans [6] and the first approval of recombinant IFNα therapy for hairy cell leukaemia in 1986. Later, immunoregulatory effects were also unintentionally discovered in multiple sclerosis (MS), an autoimmune disease, reasoned to be triggered by viral infections [7]. Today, type I interferons, the very same subtype that Isaacs and Lindenmann had first discovered, are used in the treatment of many viral infections, cancers, and even multiple sclerosis. They have also become essential for our understanding of the molecular and cellular basis of innate immunity and host-pathogen interactions. In parallel, as their use increased in the clinics, it very quickly became clear that they also induced psychocognitive effects [8–10], and that they may also induce de novo autoimmunity [11].

In 1978, Ion Gresser, a pioneer of research on the antiviral and antitumoral effects of interferons, demonstrated the counterintuitive benefits of IFNα-neutralising immunoglobulins during acute disease caused by infection [12]. This important observation was the first of many that would contrast the beneficial and detrimental of effects of type I interferons [13] and set the tone for the field for years to come. In many respects, this finding also foretold the great medical advances that would later be anti-cytokine therapies, first with anti-TNF in 1992 [14] and today with the first approved anti-interferon signalling therapies [15].

Around the same time, Jean Aicardi and Françoise Goutières reported eight children with severe early onset encephalopathy, characterised by calcification of the basal ganglia, white matter abnormalities, and calcification of the basal ganglia [16], but the underlying pathomechanism remained unclear. Fuelled by great interest in viral immunity, and the effects of interferons, Aicardi and colleagues investigated the cerebrospinal fluid and sera of these patients, and found that they had high levels of IFNα in both, yet could not attribute a viral aetiology to this [17]. It was many years later that Yanick Crow, Thomas Lindahl, and colleagues attributed to the Aicardi-Goutieres syndrome (AGS) to loss-of-function mutations of the *TREX1* gene encoding a DNA exonuclease [18] and of the *RNASEH2A*, *RNASEH2B*, and *RNASEH2C* genes encoding subunits of the RNA endonuclease RNASEH2 [19]. AGS would later be recognised as the archetypical type I interferonopathy, and one of many which are still being discovered (**Figure 1**).

1.2 Definition and classification of interferonopathies

Few cohort studies have so far been published, and many aspects are derived from case reports. Although type I interferonopathies are defined by similar underlying mechanisms, they are a family of diseases with distinct genetic alterations and a classification has been formulated based on clinical and genetic features (**Table 1**). Broadly, these can be sub-classified as monogenic interferonopathies and non-monogenic type I interferon dysfunction diseases, forming classical interferonopathies, brain vasculopathies, and one autoimmune disease.

Interferonopathies are a monogenic family of diseases caused by mutations in genes involved in the recognition, production, or regulation of type I interferons. These mutations lead to nucleic acid or metabolite accumulation, activating cytosolic nucleic acid sensors. These sensors then induce the production and secretion of type I interferons,

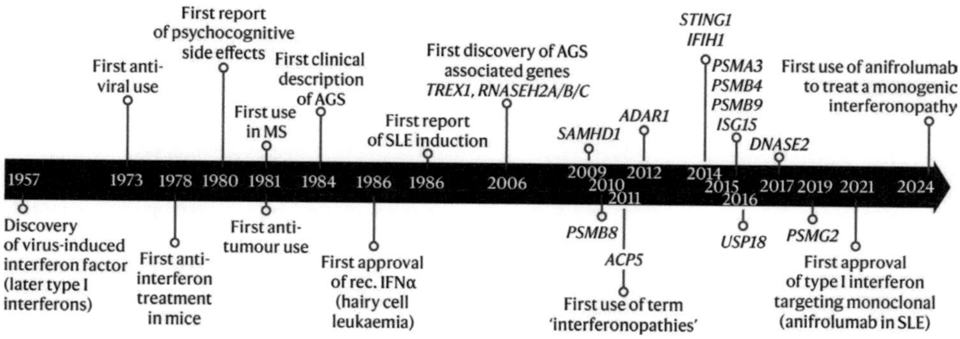

Figure 1.
Chronological overview of type I interferon-related discoveries. From the discovery of the virus-induced "interference" factors in 1957, type I interferons have been centre-stage for therapeutic development, both as exogenous administration, as disease biomarker, and ultimately as anti-cytokine therapy. From the first in human use of interferons first as an antiviral in 1973 and later for the treatment of MS and tumours in 1981, to the first approval of recombinant IFNα in 1986, type I interferons have provided numerous clinical benefits for patients across different disease areas. In the space of 16 years, interferons had gone from discovery to clinical use, a remarkable achievement for the time. Concurrently, reports of psychocognitive side effects were starting to appear from 1980 onwards, a testament to the immediacy of the effect in the CNS of these highly bioactive cytokines. It quickly became apparent that interferon therapy could lead to numerous other side effects such as SLE, and its involvement in autoinflammatory and autoimmune diseases was thereby discovered. The first description of Aicardi-Goutières Syndrome 1984, prior to the genomics revolution of the 2000s, would lead to the discovery of a new and expanding disease family called "interferonopathies". Despite the first preclinical evidence of the benefits of anti-interferon biologic use in 1978, it would take 43 years to the first approval of an anti-interferon signalling therapy, a full 28 years after the first anti-cytokine biologic therapy. The list of potential indications that could benefit from targeted inhibition of the type I interferon pathway is still being determined with ongoing clinical trials and case studies across different autoinflammatory and autoimmune diseases.

Family	Disease	Genes affected	Clinical characteristics	Neurologic symptoms
Classical interferonopathies	AGS	*TREX1, RNASEH2A, RNASEH2B, RNASEH2C, SAMHD1, ADAR1, IFIH1, DNASE2, RNU7-1, LSM11*	Intracranial calcification, skin inflammation, hepatosplenomegaly, thrombocytopenia, elevated liver enzymes, cerebrospinal fluid lymphocytosis	Progressive encephalopathy, microcephaly, spasticity, dystonia, seizures, cognitive impairment, white matter abnormalities
	USP18 loss of function	*USP18*	AGS, pseudo-TORCH syndrome	Microcephaly, intracranial calcifications, brain atrophy, seizures, developmental delay, hearing loss
	ISG15 loss of function	*ISG15*	AGS, dermatologic symptoms, increased susceptibility to mycobacterial infections	Seizures, developmental delay, microcephaly, ataxia, hypotonia, dystonia, spasticity, leukoencephalopathy
	SPENCD	*ACP5*	Short stature, spinal involvement, dermatologic manifestations	Intracranial calcifications, spasticity, developmental delay
	PRAAS	*PSMB4, PSMB8, PSMB9, PSMB10, PSMB12, PSMA3, PSMG2, POMP*	Recurrent fevers, nodular erythema, pernio-like rash, joint contractures, severe inflammation	Brain atrophy, encephalopathy, basal ganglia calcification
	SAVI	*STING1*	Skin lesions, interstitial lung disease, pulmonary hypertension	Cerebral vasculitis, ischemic stroke, intracranial hemorrhage
	SMS	*RIGI, IFIH1*	Aortic and mitral valve calcifications, dental dysplasia, osteoporosis, muscle weakness, delayed growth	Headache, mood disorders, psychosis, seizures, stroke, neuropathy, myelopathy
Brain vasculopathies	RVCL	*TREX1*	Vision loss, neurological involvement, kidney, liver, gastrointestinal, thyroid, and bone disease	Brain lesions, strokes, brain atrophy, dementia, headache, dizziness, seizures, paralysis of cranial nerves, cerebral infarcts and haemorrhage
	Interferon-associated TMA	Unknown	Endothelial dysfunction, microangiopathic hemolytic anemia, microvascular ischemia, kidney injury, hypertension	Headache, mental confusion, loss of cognitive function, loss of memory, slowing of speech, hemiparesis
	Kohlmeier Degos disease	Unknown	Papules with porcelain-white center and red border, gastrointestinal complications, neurological symptoms	Headache, vision loss, diplopia, papilledema, partial loss of vision, shortness of breath, chest pain, epilepsy, thickening of pericardium

Family	Disease	Genes affected	Clinical characteristics	Neurologic symptoms
Autoimmune diseases	SLE	*TREX1, DNASE1, DNASE1L3, PRDM1, IRF5, IRF7, STAT4, TNFAIP3, TNFSF4, C1QA, C1QB, C1QC*	Fever, rash, arthritis, serositis, nephritis, cytopenias, antinuclear antibodies	Neuropsychiatric manifestations, such as headache, mood disorders, psychosis, seizures, stroke, neuropathy, myelopathy2

AGS: Aicardi-Goutières Syndrome; USP18: Ubiquitin specific peptidase 18; ISG15: Interferon-stimulated gene 15; SPENCD: Spondyloenchondrodysplasia; PRAAS: Proteasome-associated autoinflammatory syndromes; SAVI: STING-associated vasculopathy with onset in infancy; SMS: Singleton-Merten syndrome; RVCL: Retinal vasculopathy with cerebral leukodystrophy; TMA: thrombotic microangiopathy; SLE: Systemic lupus erythematosus.

Table 1.
Type I interferonopathies associated with neurological dysfunction.

which bind to their receptors on the cell surface and initiate a signalling cascade that involves the phosphorylation and nuclear translocation of transcription factors. They thereby activate expression of hundreds of interferon-stimulated genes (ISGs), which mediate the antiviral, immunomodulatory, and inflammatory effects of type I interferons.

Interferonopathies can be classified into six main diseases, based on the clinical presentation and the genetic defect: (1) Aicardi-Goutières syndrome (AGS), (2) USP18 and ISG15 loss-of-function diseases, (3) spondyloenchondrodysplasia (SPENCD), (4) proteasome-associated autoinflammatory syndromes (PRAAS), (5) STING-associated vasculopathy with onset in infancy (SAVI), and (6) Singleton-Merten syndrome (SMS).

AGS is the most common among type I interferonopathies and is characterised by early-onset encephalopathy, calcification of the basal ganglia, leukodystrophy, skin lesions, and systemic inflammation. It is caused by mutations in genes encoding nucleases, such as *TREX1*, *RNASEH2A*, *RNASEH2B*, *RNASEH2C*, *SAMHD1*, and *ADAR1*, or genes involved in nucleic acid metabolism, such as *RNASEH2*, *IFIH1*, and *ADAR2*. These mutations impair the degradation or editing of endogenous nucleic acids, leading to the accumulation of self-DNA or RNA, which activate the cGAS-STING or RIG-I-MDA5 pathways, respectively. Gain-of-function mutations in STAT2 have also been identified [20–23], bypassing nucleic acid metabolism steps and highlighting the complexity of AGS. USP18 and ISG15 loss-of-function diseases share important similarities and display neuropathology similar to AGS. SPENCD and PRAAS are less well studied, and the mechanism by which type I interferons are induced is undefined, though patients also display basal ganglia calcifications.

Among the typically non encephalitogenic type I interferonopathies, SAVI is perhaps the better studied. It is caused by gain-of-function mutations in *STING1* (previously *TMEM173*), encoding the stimulator of interferon genes (STING) protein. STING is a key adaptor protein that activates type I interferon signalling in response to cytosolic DNA. It is diagnosed by genetic testing and by blood measurements of interferon response. Unlike AGS, systemic, rather than principally CNS-centred, symptoms are more pronounced, and often quite disparate. Early-onset systemic inflammation, skin vasculopathy, and interstitial lung disease have been described, with rare cases of accompanying alopecia [24]. The skin lesions typically affect the fingers, toes, ears, and nose and can lead to ulceration, necrosis, and sometimes amputation. The lung disease manifests as progressive fibrosis, respiratory failure, and pulmonary hypertension. What is surprising is that, often these symptoms can occur without simultaneous involvement of both skin and lungs. Yet, upon imaging, occasionally intracerebral calcifications are also observed and can aid diagnosis. Only a handful of cases have been reported so far; thus, many questions remain as to the differential clinical signs. SMS, while also a classical interferonopathy, presents with a yet different array of symptoms, including skin inflammation, calcifications of the aorta, and progressive osteoporosis. Neurologic symptoms have also been reported though they are not thought as the main clinical sign.

With more attentive clinical investigations, additional rare type I interferonopathies are being discovered. It is important to note that not all of them present with overt neurological signs and often certain subtypes will include patients with severe psychocognitive disease while others display only systemic signs of disease. The underlying cause for this is largely unknown. Throughout the rest of the chapter, special emphasis will be put on encephalopathic diseases.

1.3 Overview of type I interferon pathway

Being a complex and tightly regulated network of molecular interactions, this pathway mediates cellular responses to infections, as well as endogenous nucleic acids when recognised as danger signals. The pathway can be divided into three overarching stages: (1) sensing, (2) signalling, and (3) feedback regulation (**Figure 2**).

Sensing refers to the recognition of pathogen-associated molecular patterns (PAMPs) or danger-associated molecular patterns (DAMPs) by pattern recognition receptors (PRRs), such as Toll-like receptors (TLRs), RIG-I-like receptors (RLRs), and

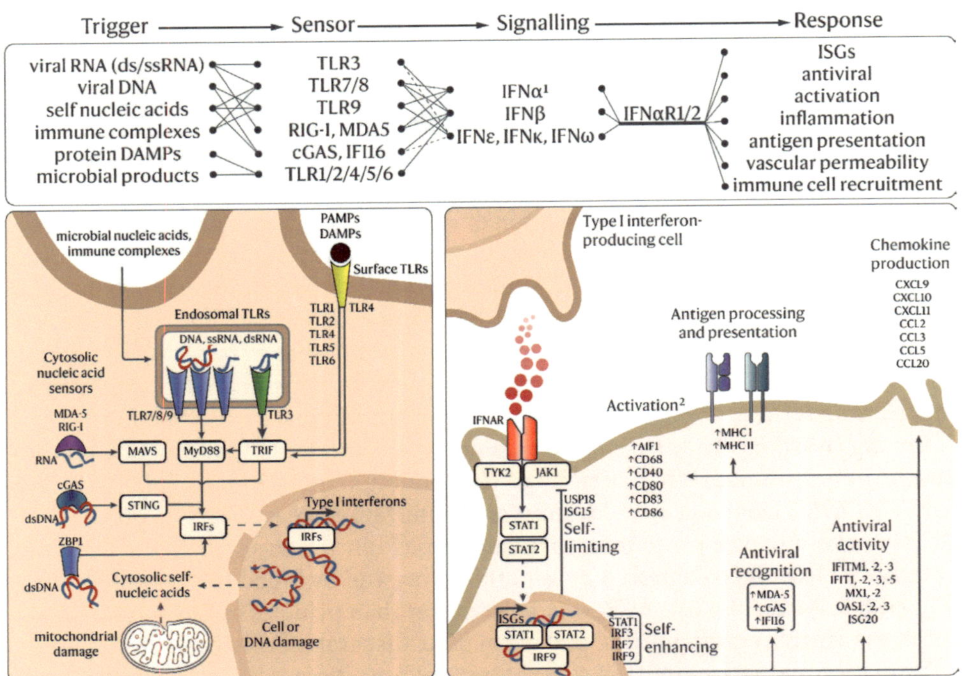

[1]Includes IFNα1, IFNα2, IFNα4, IFNα5, IFNα6, IFNα7, IFNα8, IFNα10, IFNα13, IFNα14, IFNα16, IFNα17, IFNα21
[2]Markers enumerated mostly associated with microglia

Figure 2.
Type I interferon signalling regulation and pathway. Simplified summary of triggering molecules, associated sensors, type I interferons produced, receptor-mediated signalling, and generic interferon-responses.

cGAS-STING. These receptors are expressed in different cellular compartments, such as the plasma membrane (TLR1, -2, -4, -5, -6), endosomes (TLR3, -7, -8, -9), cytosol (MDA-5, RIG-I, cGAS-STING, ZBP1, etc.), or nucleus (IFI16, hnRNPA2B1, cGAS in some contexts, etc.), and can detect different types of nucleic acids, such as viral or bacterial DNA or RNA, or self-DNA or RNA. Upon ligand binding, these receptors activate downstream signalling pathways that converge on the activation of interferon regulatory transcription factor 3 (IRF3) and 7 (IRF7), the master transcription factors of type I interferons [25].

Signalling initiates when binding to its cognate receptor is achieved, triggering the induction of downstream pathways and amplification of type I interferon production. IRF3 and IRF7 translocate to the nucleus and bind to the interferon-stimulated response elements (ISREs) in the promoters of type I interferon genes, such as *IFNA1*, *IFNA2*, and *IFNB1*, and induce their transcription, translation, and secretion. They then bind to their receptor, the interferon α/β receptor (IFNAR) formed of two chains: IFNAR1 and IFNAR2. This signalling can take place on the same or neighbouring cells and activate the Janus kinase (JAK) signal transducer and activator of transcription (STAT) pathway, which involves the phosphorylation and nuclear translocation of STAT1 and -2. These STATs form a complex with IRF9, called ISGF3, which binds to the ISREs in the promoters of ISGs, such as MX1, OAS1, and ISG15, and induce their transcription and expression. ISGs mediate the antiviral, immunomodulatory, and inflammatory effects of type I interferons. Other non-canonical pathways independent of JAK-STAT are also known to be activated in a cell- or context-specific manner, and signalling is mediated through PI3K-mTOR, NF-κB, and MAPK and can have broad outcomes [26–28].

Feedback regulation is initiated simultaneously following signalling, triggering both positive and negative modulation mechanisms for the pathway. Positive feedback loops involve the induction of IRF7, which enhances the expression of more type I interferons and ISGs, creating a feedforward loop that amplifies the response. Negative feedback loops involve the induction of suppressors of cytokine signalling (SOCS), protein inhibitors of activated STATs (PIAS), and ubiquitin-specific proteases (USPs), which inhibit the JAK-STAT pathway, or the induction of tripartite motif-containing proteins (TRIMs), which degrade IRF3 and IRF7, or the induction of microRNAs, such as miR-146a and miR-155, which silence certain mRNAs which are key components of the pathway. Ultimately, type I interferons are cytokines that play a crucial role in the innate immune response, but also act at the interface of adaptive immunity [29–31] and, as such, need to be tightly regulated. When its signalling is aberrantly activated or sustained, it can lead to a variety of clinical manifestations, ranging from autoinflammatory syndromes to autoimmune disorders.

2. Neurologic disease in type I interferonopathies

Type I interferonopathies are a group of rare monogenic disorders characterised by constitutive activation of type I interferon signalling, leading to chronic inflammation and multiorgan damage. Severe interferonopathies, and typically the most frequent ones, are first and foremost neuroinflammatory disorders. The most common clinical signs of type I interferonopathies are neurological, affecting the central and peripheral nervous systems. These include developmental delay, intellectual disability, seizures, spasticity, ataxia, dystonia, neuropathy, and hearing loss. The exact incidence and prevalence of type I interferonopathies are for the most part unknown, but estimates place incidence between 1:10,000 and 1:1,000,000 [32–34]. While the exact percentage of each type I interferonopathy among the total cases is also uncertain, the most common is Aicardi-Goutières syndrome (AGS).

2.1 Aicardi-Goutières syndrome

AGS is an interferonopathy, typically exemplified as a neuroinflammatory encephalopathy resembling congenital viral infection. By most accounts, AGS is the most common of the interferonopathies, and the better studied [34]. Clinically, AGS can present as neonatal-onset AGS or late-onset. Neonatal-onset can often be mistaken for a transplacental-acquired infection. When evidence for an obvious infection is lacking, common practice is that AGS should be considered. Symptoms during the first few weeks of life include slowed cognitive growth, abnormal movements, ataxia, and epileptic seizures, as well as systemic signs of infection including persistent fever. Late-onset AGS is challenging as symptoms may occur several months later alongside otherwise normal infantile development. Slowed growth of head circumference, spasticity, and weakness may sometimes be readily apparent. Imaging in both early and late onset forms often reveals microcephaly, intracranial calcification, leukoencephalopathy, necrosis, vasculopathy with aneurysms, infarcts, and sometimes discernible haemorrhage [35]. On a histopathological level, acute demyelinating lesions reveal the extent of neurological damage, especially in late-onset patients, with diffuse demyelination reminiscent of acute demyelinating encephalomyelitis [36]. Microangiopathy is also a common occurrence [37–40]. Calcium deposits form around the blood vessels, and it is thought that this is attributed to excessive cell senescence and apoptosis [41].

Type I interferons are found consistently in CSF and serum at the neonatal stage [17, 42]. As interferons display high bioactivity reflected by a short half-life, they are notoriously difficult to detect, and in the early days, cytopathic protection assays were performed. Simply, CSF from patients was found to contain sufficient interferons to avert toxicity associated with vesicular stomatitis virus challenge in a recipient cell line. Simple experiments first gave clues as to which interferon subtypes were present in patients with AGS, pinpointing IFNα as the principal culprit. Leaps in bioassay technologies have allowed detection down to 0.1 femtograms, confirming on average 1000-fold increase in IFNα compared to healthy individuals [42, 43]. Analysis of the largest AGS cohort to date reveals that significantly higher levels of IFNα in CSF are consistently found in earlier onset, more severe, disease supporting the notion of a detrimental role of type I interferons that is dose dependent [44]. Intriguingly, this is not observed consistently in serum [44] which supports that the production is central rather than systemic in AGS. Importantly, interferon-response gene expression has allowed the definition of an interferon-score, which is now a widely used, highly sensitive, rapid, cheap, and specific interferon metric [42, 45–50].

Mutations in nine genes have been identified to this day, all of which are involved in nucleic acid detection and metabolism. Overall, loss-of-function mutations lead to deficiencies in the clearance of nucleic acids, while the gain-of-function mutations cause overt sensing of nucleic acids. Mutations in *TREX1* [18], *RNASEH2A*, *RNASEH2B*, *RNASEH2C* [19], *SAMHD1* [51], and *ADAR1* [52] result in the accumulation of nucleic acids, sometimes derived from endogenous retroviral elements, which result in potent activation of nucleic acid sensors. In particular, *TREX1* is an important exonuclease, whose inactivation leads to accumulated DNAs in the cytoplasm that trigger overexpression of type I interferons [18] through the cGAS-STING pathway [53, 54]. Beyond AGS, mutations have been described in systemic lupus erythematosus (SLE) [55] and familial chilblain lupus (FCL) [56], linking together AGS and lupus. Similarly, mutations in RNASEH2A/B/C, which form a protein complex that degrades RNA:DNA hybrids and excises incorrectly inserted ribonucleotide monophosphates during DNA replication, lead to DNA damage and enhanced generation of byproducts of DNA repair [57]. Accumulated DNA repair metabolites in the cytoplasm caused by RNASEH2 mutants stimulate the cGAS-STING pathway, resulting in AGS [58]. Lastly, mutations in LSM11 and RNU7-1, which encode two components of the canonical replication-dependent histone pre-mRNA processing complex, cause impaired processing of mRNAs [59]. This leads to the release of cGAS from nucleosomes, thus binding to proximal nuclear DNA, and activates the cGAS-STING-TBK1 pathway inducing the expression of type I interferons [59]. Lastly, mutations in *ADAR1* cause aberrant activation of nucleic acid sensors MDA5 and ZBP1 through enhancement of recognition of endogenous retroviral elements and causing uncontrolled type I interferon production [60–62]. These mechanisms exemplify the importance of accurate regulation of endogenous nucleic acid sensing and how their loss-of-function inevitably results in overt type I interferon production. Similar aberrant responses can also happen with gain-of-function mutations. Mutations in *IFIH1* have resulted in overactivity of its gene product, MDA5, causing it to bind to RNA more avidly [63, 64]. This mimics excessive nucleic acid sensing and also results in type I interferon overproduction. While the genetic mutations and genes affected are numerous, mechanisms of AGS are related to aberrant nucleic acid sensing and defective DNA or RNA degradation. Mutations that cause dysfunctional negative regulation also exist, leading to other encephalopathic interferonopathies with substantial clinical overlap.

2.2 Other encephalopathic interferonopathies

Though rare, many other encephalopathic type I interferonopathies have been identified. Loss-of-function mutations in *ISG15* cause disease similar to AGS and SPENCD including calcifications of the cerebral basal ganglia and type I interferon signatures [65] but can also cause dermatologic disease as often seen with interferonopathies [66]. It is recognised that ISG15, itself an interferon-response gene, is important for limiting type I interferon production, and that disease in ISG15 deficiency is systemic, but the exact contribution to disease from within the brain is undetermined. Interestingly, it is through its interaction with USP18, mutations of which are also associated with AGS [67], that ISG15 can limit type I interferon signalling by displacing JAK1 from IFNAR [68, 69]. Importantly, in vivo loss of USP18 has been studied in rodents, and it was found to cause unabated – of otherwise tonic self-limiting – type I interferon signalling and to lead to the generation of over phagocytic microglia causing white matter damage and neurodegeneration [70].

Rare mutations in a lysosomal protein encoded by *ACP5*, also cause a type I interferonopathy called Spondyloenchondrodysplasia (SPENCD). It is characterised by skeletal dysplasia typified by vertebral abnormalities and metaphyseal lesions of the long bones. Concurrently, brain calcifications with neurological impairment, and high type I interferon signatures, reminiscent of classical AGS, are also observed [71, 72]. Little is known about the pathological mechanism, yet these mutations result in a highly penetrant monogenic systemic lupus erythematosus (SLE) manifestation [73–75], suggestive of a broader relationship between type I interferonopathies and lupus.

3. Encephalopathic non-monogenic type I interferonopathies

Systemic lupus erythematosus (SLE) is a disease driven by type I interferons and characterised by neuropsychiatric involvement. Interestingly, many overlapping psychocognitive disturbances are also observed as side effects from exogenous interferon therapies.

3.1 Neuropsychiatric involvement in lupus

Systemic lupus erythematosus is the historical and immunological archetype autoimmune disease, affecting multiple systems including the CNS. It is estimated that almost four million people worldwide live with SLE [76]. More than half of SLE patients exhibit some neuropsychiatric manifestation [77, 78] though the exact prevalence and list of symptoms describing it are debatable [79, 80]. It is associated with more severe cases as demonstrated by a threefold higher mortality rate than SLE patients without obvious neuropsychiatric affliction [78, 79]. Confusional state, anxiety, cognitive dysfunction, mood disorder, and psychosis are some common manifestations of neuropsychiatric lupus, delineating a group of syndromes [81]. Further evidence of neuronal involvement in lupus comes from increased neurofilament light (NfL) in both plasma and CSF [82–84]. NfL is a bonafide marker of neuronal damage that gets released and drained into the CSF, which pours out to the circulation, proportionally to the extent of axonal damage [85]. In SLE, NfL is further increased in patients with obvious neuropsychiatric involvement [83, 84] and correlates to neurocognitive and motor function [86].

SLE and AGS display some important commonalities that ultimately define both diseases as interferonopathies. Variants in *TREX1*, which cause AGS, also increase the risk of SLE [55, 87, 88], and particularly neuropsychiatric lupus [87]. Therefore, it is not surprising that type I interferons are strongly implicated in SLE [42, 89] and have been found to be pathogenic since targeting either IFNα [90, 91] or IFNAR signalling [92, 93] ameliorates disease progression. Higher IFNα in serum is also a strong predictor of mortality and correlates with neurological manifestations [94]. IFNα is also highly produced in CSF [43, 95–97], though it is unclear whether higher production in serum or CSF could inform on the central versus systemic source of type I interferon production [42, 43, 96]. As of yet, it is unknown whether targeting this pathway will be beneficial for neuropsychiatric lupus, but preclinical evidence suggests this.

Studying neuropsychiatric symptoms in mouse models of lupus is possible. However, similar to human studies, this aspect has been less investigated than its systemic disease counterpart. A lupus-prone mouse model overexpressing *Tlr7* among other genes and exhibiting high peripheral type I interferon signatures [98, 99], also develop strikingly elevated interferon signatures in CNS [100]. Importantly, these mice exhibit anxiety and fatigue similar to clinical symptoms in humans. The response seems spatially restricted in high intensity patches across the entire brain, affecting predominantly microglia but also neurons and oligodendrocytes [100]. This is also seen in a different lupus-prone mouse model, where induced interferon-responses accompanying microglial activation [101] suggest conserved pathology affecting the CNS. Additionally, exogenous administration of IFNα precipitates lupus pathology [102, 103] and neurologic disorder including anxiety, depression, and cognitive impairment.

The mechanisms by which type I interferons cause or aggravate development of neuropsychiatric symptoms in SLE have not been exhaustively investigated. One proposed mechanism is through modulation of neuroactive metabolites. SLE patients with cognitive dysfunction are found to have increased quinolinic acid [104–106], to kynurenic acid ratios [107]. Quinolinic acid is an NMDAR agonist causing glutamatergic excitotoxicity [108, 109] and more so when favoured over kynurenic acid [110]. This metabolite balance dysregulation concurrently correlates significantly with type I interferon-response [111]. Quinolinic acid is metabolised from tryptophan and through indoleamine 2,3-dioxygenase (IDO) [112], an interferon-inducible enzyme known to mediate neurobehavioural alterations [113]. In SLE patients, IDO is induced in a type I interferon-specific manner [114]. This is paralleled by an increase in kynureine to tryptophan ratio in the circulation as IDO metabolises tryptophan into kynureine [107, 111, 114]. Loss of serotonin is also reasoned to be affected in a similar way. Serotonin is an important neurotransmitter that is also metabolised from tryptophan [115] and which is deregulated in human SLE [114, 116] and in the hippocampus of lupus-prone mice [117]. Increased IDO in SLE can explain the reduction of serotonin observed in the periphery [114], and it is arguable that a similar mechanism may take place in the CNS though this has yet to be demonstrated in SLE.

Overall, while a lot of what is known about the pathological mechanisms of neuropsychiatric SLE are inspired from findings from AGS, clinical evidence is highly suggestive that the type I interferon pathway may be therapeutically relevant for the neuropsychiatric manifestations as well as well as for systemic disease. The associations between neuropsychiatric lupus and AGS, and the teachings it has provided, are a testament to how rare monogenic neuroinflammatory disorders can provide aetiological insights into the pathogenesis of more common polygenic disorders. Importantly, more learnings can also be achieved from clinical experience with exogenous IFNα and IFNβ therapies.

3.2 Exogenous interferon treatment

Type I interferons have been used in the clinics to treat different diseases for many years, including hairy cell leukaemia, chronic myeloid leukaemia, hepatitis C virus infection, melanoma, multiple sclerosis, systemic mastocytosis, chronic hepatitis B virus infection renal cell carcinoma, and Kaposi's sarcoma. Despite being used at refined therapeutic doses, psychocognitive side effects are common and have been well documented from 40 years of clinical experience with these cytokines [118–134]. Common side-effects in the short term include confusion, headaches, fatigue, myalgia, flu-like symptoms, and psycho-emotional disturbance. Longer treatment regimens often result in dementia-like outcomes [135–140]. Furthermore, high dose versus low dose IFNα therapy much exacerbated signs and incidence rates [141], indicative of a dose-dependent effect.

Depression is the most common occurrence. Incidence among both IFNα- or IFNβ-treated patients is estimated to be 50%, even with optimised dosages, and prophylactic antidepressant therapy is often initiated pre-emptively [123, 128] though its true efficacy is still debated [142, 143]. Major depressive episodes are also commonplace and have been reported in as many as 30% of HCV patients treated [126, 133]. Resting state fMRI performed in a cohort of 22 patients with hepatitis C infection pre- and post-peripheral therapeutic dosing of IFNα revealed rapid and profound changes in the brain [144]. The altered brain functional network and reduced global connectivity efficiency correlated well with changes in anxiety, fatigue, confusion, and mood, reinforcing the immediateness of changes to neuronal networks. Importantly, while the majority of cases of IFNα-induced depression will achieve remission following discontinuation or end of therapy, this can take up to 3 years [125, 130, 133] indicating long-lasting neural changes. These figures may be underestimated due to the lack of long-term follow-up after treatment cessation [130, 133].

Assessing the adverse impact of IFNβ therapy on multiple sclerosis (MS) has been challenging, as MS itself leads to cognitive dysfunction [145]. Cognitive dysfunction in MS also correlates with depression and fatigue [146, 147], adding a further layer of complexity. In comparison, fingolimod is a superior therapy for MS, providing better outcomes for cognitive decline compared to IFNβ [148–153]. Fingolimod causes immunosuppression as well as neuroprotection [154], an advantage over IFNβ which, specifically in MS, only exerts immunosuppression. It is therefore challenging to separate any neurotoxic effects associated with IFNβ. As new therapies are slowly making their way to more common clinical use in MS [155], more careful personalised medicine approaches can be achieved reducing long-term sequelae for patients.

The impact of type I interferons on psychocognitive states involves a complex, understudied, and multifactorial process involving changes in neuroactive metabolite balance, potentially hormonal dysfunction, brain microvascular dysfunction, and induction of psychoactive chemokines. As previously discussed, they potently induce IDO, which catalyses a key metabolic reaction that leads to the loss of serotonin and kynurenic acid, favouring the excitotoxic quinolinic acid [107, 113, 156]. Interferon therapies have also been found to induce thyroid dysfunction, ranging the entire spectrum of hypothyroidism, hyperthyroidism, and thyroiditis. Clinical thyroid disorders are frequently associated with psychiatric symptomatology [157–160]. The exact prevalence is difficult to determine as few studies evaluate thyroid status, but it may be as low as 11% and high as 45% [161–165]. While thyroid hormones are known to exert biochemical effects on the brain, the bulk of the research conducted is descriptive rather than mechanistic. No significant correlation could be easily discerned between thyroid hormones and development of major depression induced by IFNα [161], perhaps suggesting parallel pathways. Nevertheless, given the systematic thyroid hormone imbalance induction by IFNα therapy, perhaps some degree of mood dysfunction may be attributable to it, though research is for now lacking.

Interferons can also directly act on the brain. In mice, it was found that peripherally administered IFNβ was sufficient to induce depressive symptoms [166], and that IFNAR activation on brain endothelial cells was responsible for the depressive symptoms. Activation of the BBB's endothelial cell IFNAR pathway results in downregulation of adherens and tight junction transcripts causing endothelial dysfunction and exemplified by BBB leakage. Evidence of this is also perhaps apparent from the clinics. Thrombotic microangiopathy (TMA) is another serious side effect of interferon therapies [167–169] requiring immediate discontinuation and critical care. These events are associated with higher dose interferon therapy, and to result in leaky microvasculature accompanied by perivascular immune cell infiltration and narrowing of the endothelial cell lumen in human patients and in mice [168]. Chemokines CCL2 and CXCL10 are strongly induced by interferons in brain endothelial cells [166], providing a plausible explanation for the microvascular changes and infiltration. Of note, it is the microangiopathy that is the dominant brain characteristic, as also observed in neuropsychiatric lupus [170], and thrombosis is instead a far less prominent feature [168]. As not all microvessel damage is visible by MRI, it is unclear whether subclinical cerebral vascular damage is happening throughout all interferon-treated patients, thus widely contributing to the psychocognitive dysfunction induced by type I interferons. Lastly, activation of CXCR3 signalling in neurons by brain endothelial cell-derived CXCL10 elicits changes in synaptic plasticity responsible for the depressive phenotype in vivo and in vitro causing weakened synaptic long-term potentiation in hippocampus [166, 171].

Genetic associations between type I interferon-induced depression and gene variants exist, but knowledge is for now limited. One study linked polymorphisms in cyclooxygenase 2 (COX2) or phospholipase A2 (PLA2) with a more than three-fold increased risk of developing depression [172]. Intriguingly, an association in patients with major depression not induced by interferon therapy could also be made, suggesting some similar underlying mechanisms [172]. In line with this observation, IFNα-induced depressive symptoms could be mitigated in mice treated with non-steroidal anti-inflammatory drugs (NSAIDs) inhibiting COX1/COX2 [173]. This is an important consideration in light of reported anti-depressive effects of NSAIDs [174, 175] and of enhanced efficacy when used in combination with anti-depressants [176].

Interestingly, type I interferon signatures can also be found in major depression not induced by interferon therapy [177, 178]. Prototypical ISGs such as MXs, OASs, IFITs, ADAR, and CXCL10 [179] are found upregulated in the circulation of patients. It is unclear whether type I interferons might be causative; however, this would argue for a detrimental role in major depression. Depression is also suggested as a trigger for Alzheimer's disease and cognitive decline [180], raising important additional implications. In one study, an association was found between the Apolipoprotein E ε4 (APOE4) allele, which confers greater risk of Alzheimer's, and higher incidence of interferon-induced neuropsychiatric symptoms [181], suggesting a link between type I interferons, depression, and Alzheimer's disease.

The neurocognitive impact of exogenous therapy with type I interferons is well-recognised, and despite systemic administration routes and refined dosages, patients exhibit often debilitating and dangerous psychocognitive side-effects. While anxiety and depression can be partially mitigated, psychomotor dysfunction, fatigue, and confusion are difficult to alleviate [140]. Over the years, the standard of care for many of these indications is moving away from IFNα an IFNβ therapies, both as first-line therapy and often entirely. The advent of more efficacious, and safer direct-acting and all-oral antivirals [182, 183], checkpoint blockade inhibitors [184], and immunomodulating therapies [155, 185] has allowed a consistent phasing out of interferons in clinical care.

4. Translation to more common neurodegenerative diseases

There is growing interest in understanding neuroinflammation in rare diseases because it represents a promising and translatable therapeutic target, also for more common neurodegenerative disorders. Neuroinflammation is recognised as a key hallmark of diseases such as Alzheimer's and Parkinson's disease. While the role of type I interferons in these diseases remains to be fully understood, several lines of evidence suggest their implication in their disease process.

4.1 Alzheimer's disease

Alzheimer's disease (AD) is the most common cause of dementia, affecting more than 50 million individuals worldwide. It is characterised by gradual cognitive decline and behavioural changes due to chronic neurodegeneration, and predominant impairment of anterograde episodic memory. Individuals over the age of 65 are most commonly affected, representing 90 to 95% of all AD cases. Overall, age is the strongest risk factor for AD suggesting that the ageing process is strongly implicated [186]. Early-onset AD (EOAD) affects individuals below the age of 65 and is known to be caused by one of a handful mutations. The discovery that certain mutations in the amyloid precursor protein *APP* gene [187, 188] or the presenilin 1 [189] and 2 [189, 190] (*PSEN1* and *PSEN2*) genes, encoding the enzymes cleaving amyloid peptides, cause EOAD has galvanised the field and concomitantly allowed headway in the understanding of late-onset AD (LOAD). As aggregated misfolded amyloid β-containing extracellular plaques are a major pathologic hallmark of AD, the understanding of the amyloid misfolding and aggregation processes have led to major strides for elucidating the pathology. This is also thanks to the generation of mouse models with abnormalities in APP processing mimicking human EOAD [191]. After decades of therapeutics research, and at the time of writing, two biologics targeting amyloid deposits have been approved for therapy following modest but positive trial outcomes [192, 193]: aducanumab and lecanemab.

Subsequent work has identified and proposed many other components importantly implicated in AD. One such component is the protein tau. Tau, like Aβ, has a propensity to misfold, aggregate, and spread, and mutations in its gene, *MAPT*, have been identified in familial inherited tauopathies such as frontotemporal lobar degeneration with tau inclusions (FTLD-tau) [194]. Hyperphosphorylation is another key feature of tau and a marker of severity of neuronal pathology [195, 196]. Intracellular tau protein-containing neurofibrillary tangles are found in brain regions related to clinical symptoms and to better correlate with pathology than amyloid burden [197, 198], leading to believe that it may be directly implicated in the pathogenesis [199].

Aside from *APP*, *PSEN1* and *PSEN2*, and *MAPT*, APOE is the most important risk factor for AD [200–202]. Certain alleles substantially increase risk (E4/E4: 12-fold increase) while others confer resistance (E2/E2: 2.5-fold decrease), while others are the common variants (E3/E3: no impact). The impact that APOE has on AD is likely even more intricate. An R136 mutation was identified in an individual carrying an autosomal dominant mutation in *PSEN1*, but which was protected from developing EOAD [203]. Named after the city in New Zealand where it was discovered, the Christchurch mutation confers resistance to AD by reducing tau pathology [204]. The genetics of EOAD are complex, but they have allowed many advances in our understanding of AD. Genetic research of LOAD also revealed new facets of AD, especially the involvement of the immune system.

Neuroinflammation is increasingly being recognised as an important component in the pathogenesis of AD. Genome-wide association studies performed on LOAD have implicated the immune system. Loci mapped to genes hypothesised to carry out immune, or at least microglial, function-related roles have been proposed such as *ABI2, ACE, ADAM10, ADAMTS1, BIN1, CD2AP, CD33, CLU, CR1, HLA-DRB1, HLA-DRB5, IL34, MEF2C, MINK1, MTHFR, PCG2, PILRA, SHARPIN, SPI1, SORL1, TOMM40,* and *TREM2* [205–209]. Although more than 84 loci have been identified, they may not represent the full spectrum of risk variants for LOAD. As studies become larger and better powered for discovery of subtle associations, more are likely to be added to this list [209]. TREM2 is an important risk variant [210, 211] with consistently strong association and susceptibility risk, currently estimated to three- to four-fold increase [212]. One heterozygous R47H variant represents the highest risk for AD aside from familial mutations and APOE alleles, and has therefore been studied extensively despite sometimes contradictory results [213, 214].

AD is a multifactorial disease with complex cellular interactions that culminate in neuronal cell death. Numerous mouse models have allowed studying the pathogenesis of AD at the molecular and cellular level. Coupled with the advent of single-cell transcriptomic technologies [215], they have permitted a better understanding of the cellular states during AD and have allowed characterisation of virtually all brain cell types. Across AD models, microglia cell types have been identified and characterised according to their transcriptomes and consistently classified as "homeostatic", "disease associated microglia" or "DAM", and "type I interferon-responsive microglia" or "IRM" [216–221]. A lot of excitement was generated from research performed describing the DAM subsets in mice as they are believed to define a distinctive neurodegeneration microglial cluster [222, 223]. However, a clear and consistent DAM cluster has been difficult to pinpoint in humans [224]. IRM have been described in human AD, and the subset is found to be associated to microglia exhibiting endolysosomal dysfunction, cytoplasmic dsDNA, and activated morphology [224]. This same IRM subset also carries significant differential expression of genes associated with genetic risk for AD, such as *APP*, *APOE*, *GRN*, *CD33*, and *C4A* and hence is reasoned to be a putative target for therapeutic intervention [224]. While it is now clear that clues relating to presence of type I interferons are seen throughout human AD [224–229], its role can only be studied using mouse models.

Similar to human AD, type I interferon signatures can be found across different AD models of either amyloidosis, tauopathy, or combinations of the two [217, 220, 228–238] and despite differences in affected brain areas, temporal and cognitive pathology evolution, and disease mechanisms, suggesting conserved induction pathways. Importantly, genetic loss of IFNAR or targeting via monoclonal antibody is protective for the overall progression [228, 229, 232]. In an APP/PS1 mouse model, loss of IFNAR signalling leads to significant amelioration of the spatial memory deficits, and inhibition of inflammation and microgliosis markers, while astrocytes exhibit activation potentially as a compensatory mechanism [232]. These observations were accompanied by complete loss of interferon-signalling, as expected, but also of IFNα expression hinting at a potentially self-sustained pathway in AD [232]. Similarly, blockade of IFNAR signalling by delivery of a monoclonal antibody to the cerebral ventricles, thus bypassing the BBB, leads to significant reduction in microglial activation [228]. IFNAR signalling is similarly detrimental in tauopathy models [237]. Loss of IFNAR causes strikingly reduced tau hyperphosphorylation and inflammatory cytokine and chemokine production in vivo and in vitro stimulation of neurons with IFNα or IFNβ exacerbates tau hyperphosphorylation and seeded tau aggregation [237]. Furthermore, tau triggers the generation of interferon-responsive oligodendrocytes in vivo, as evidenced by single cell analyses [239], though their contribution to disease remains to be elucidated. Further evidence that tau drives disease through type I interferons comes from deeper investigations of the protective effects of the Christchurch APOE mutation [240]. Mice carrying tau mutations and the human E3/E3 Christchurch mutation were protected from tau pathology by loss of cGAS-STING-induced type I interferon production. While the complete mechanism is still unclear, microglia carrying the protective mutation had suppressed production interferons [240]. Other mutations commonly found in AD were also linked to type I interferons. Concurrent loss of function of TREM2 in tauopathy and amyloidosis AD-prone mice causes exacerbation of the type I interferon signatures, along with more pronounced tau aggregation, hyperphosphorylation, and neurodegeneration [220]. This is paralleled by findings in individuals carrying TREM2 variants R47H and R62H, which have a strongly increased AD risk, and concurrent enhancement of type I interferon signatures compared to TREM2 common variants [241, 242]. It is still not demonstrated whether these AD associated variants exacerbate pathology through IFNAR signalling, though mouse models of tau pathology with

TREM2 R47H-carrying variants recapitulate enhanced IRM [234], and this is through an increased responsiveness to triggers of type I interferon production [241].

The induction of type I interferons in AD is thought to be mediated by an amyloid-facilitated nucleic acid recognition process. Nucleic acids are found on and around amyloid plaques in human and mouse models [228, 243–246], which is probably linked to charge complementarity. Microglia, due to their phagocytic activity, actively take up oligomeric amyloids containing nucleic acids, which then signal to nucleic acid sensors leading to production of type I interferons [228]. Neurons are also capable of producing IFNα and IFNβ in response to Aβ peptide stimulation directly and without exogenous nucleic acids, and to do so via MyD88 and IRF7 [247], raising the prospect of a parallel pathway of mitochondrial or nuclear nucleic acid release following cell damage. cGAS-STING is also found to be expressed and induced in AD-prone mice across different neuronal cell types and is likely a key nucleic acid sensor mediating the production of type I interferons in response to amyloids [248, 249] but possibly not the only one.

Clearance of nucleic acids, whether following uptake or whether released subsequent to nuclear or mitochondrial damage, is an important process. Genetic loss of these mechanisms can result in severe diseases, including type I interferonopathies. Phospholipase D3 (PLD3) is an exonuclease that degrades mitochondrial DNA limiting exaggerated TLR9 [250, 251] and cGAS-STING [251, 252] responses which result in the induction of type I interferon production. Importantly, rare variants in PLD3 have been discovered to increase risk of AD [253, 254], and potentially in EOAD [255] suggesting that defective nucleic acid nuclease activity could be implicated in AD and cause aberrant triggering of type I interferons. PLD3 is indeed found deregulated in AD [256, 257] and accumulated in neuritic plaques [257], suggesting a defective intracellular exonuclease function. Another protein involved in clearance of nucleic acids is 2',5'-oligoadenylate synthetase 1 (OAS1). OAS1 is a type I interferon-inducible protein which, through its interaction with RNaseL, is known to degrade dsRNA and limit viral infection but to also limit sensing of intracellular RNAs [258, 259]. While the role of this interferon-inducible protein in the pathogenesis of AD still not known, risk variants have been identified suggesting that it may be implicated in the disease process [260, 261].

As for how type I interferons mediate neurodegeneration in AD, there are multiple mechanisms demonstrated so far. For one, Aβ stimulated IFNAR deficient glia produce significantly less or no inflammatory cytokines, including IFNα and IFNβ, compared to IFNAR sufficient glia, and transfer of conditioned media to neuronal cultures demonstrates a neurotoxic activity that requires IFNAR signalling [232, 262]. One way by which IFNβ has been proposed to be directly neurotoxic [263, 264] is through mitochondrial destabilisation [265]. Furthermore, IFNβ induced by nucleic acid recognition also cause further upregulation and hyperactivity of DNA sensors in microglia [266], suggestive of a self-propelled activation loop. Type I interferons also cause inhibition of Aβ peptide phagocytosis by microglia, suggesting that decreased clearance of reactive amyloid species could also exacerbate neuroinflammatory outcomes [262]. In vivo, IFNAR signalling activation leads to complement-driven elimination of synapses [228, 229], an effect that seems entirely driven by microglia, and likely mostly ones near plaques and co-expressing CLEC7 and AXL [229].

Ageing is the most important risk factor for AD. Type I interferons have been associated with brain ageing [267, 268] and are therefore thought to also impact AD through processes in common with ageing. One identified process is through inhibition of the transcription factor Myocyte-specific enhancer factor 2C (MEF2C)

[233, 249, 268]. MEF2C is involved in neuronal signalling, differentiation, and integrating memory formation [269–271]. Moreover, polymorphisms of the MEF2C locus have been identified in AD repeatedly across studies and cohorts [205, 272–274]. Type I interferons cause an inhibition of MEF2C during normal ageing which results in deteriorating cognitive function including learning and spatial memory and exacerbated neuroinflammation [268]. In AD-prone mouse models, both amyloid- [233] and tauopathy-based [249], type I interferons caused the downregulation of MEF2C leading to increased microglial activation, increased synaptic loss, and cognitive dysfunction.

However, the detrimental effects of IFNAR signalling in AD are likely not mediated solely by microglia. Neuronal, but not microglial, IFNAR signalling contributes to amyloid plaque formation in AD-prone mice, a mechanism suggested to be mediated by the interferon-induced transmembrane protein 3 (IFITM3) [229]. IFITM3 is an interferon-inducible protein that binds to the γ-secretase complex responsible for Aβ cleavage from APP and enhances its activity [275]. It is overexpressed in AD as well as mouse models, in line with the overexpression of other type I interferon stimulated genes, and loss of function leads to striking reduction in plaque density [275] supportive of the observation that IFNAR signalling in neurons participates in amyloid plaque deposition [229]. Certain variants of *IFITM3* are also significantly associated with cognitive decline, amyloid and tau burden and brain atrophy [276], though it remains to be demonstrated how these variants affect the amyloid processing-associated function of IFITM3. Neurons also respond directly Aβ by producing IFNα and IFNβ through MyD88-IRF7, a pathway which sensitised to concurrent neurotoxicity [247].

Evidence points to a predominantly detrimental role of type I interferons in BBB integrity. Interferon signatures in brain endothelial cells are elevated in AD-prone mice [277]. IFNβ directly increases endothelial cell permeability to large molecules, downregulating intercellular cadherins [277] and suggesting a direct consequence on BBB leakiness. Evidence is lacking in vivo, however, and it remains to be fully elucidated whether this can be replicated in endothelial cell targeted IFNAR-deficient AD-prone animals. This is especially important as there is contrasting evidence indicating that systemic IFNβ therapy in the context of MS participates in restoring BBB integrity [278]. It is unclear whether this is an indirect effect on the BBB via immunoregulation or a direct effect on endothelial cells. Different models of cerebrovascular damage [279, 280] and infection [281, 282], both of which trigger local type I interferon production by endothelial cells via cGAS-STING, demonstrate a detrimental role on BBB permeability. Thus, elucidating the role of type I interferon signalling according to the disease context and elucidating whether local and systemic effects may have opposing functions is important in understanding AD-associated BBB.

Type I interferon-induced CXCL10 has also been implicated in dementia associated with TAR DNA binding protein-43 (TDP-43) pathology. TDP-43 is an RNA interacting protein whose function is regulation of splicing, trafficking, and stabilisation of RNA [283]. Its normal function is lost in about 50% of frontotemporal dementia (FTD), a progressive neurodegenerative disease characterised by neuronal intranuclear and cytoplasmic inclusions [284, 285]. Loss of the normal function of TDP-43 triggers the production of type I interferons via dysregulation of normal RNA sequestration causing accumulation of dsRNA leading to activation of RIG-I [286] and by destabilisation of mitochondria causing mtDNA release and triggering of cGAS-STING [287]. This results in neurodegeneration in vitro and in vivo [286–288], and one proposed mechanism is through type I interferon-induction of CXCL10 and signalling to hippocampal presynaptic terminals overexpressing CXCR3 [288]. This triggers sustained neuronal hyperactivity and memory deficits in vivo [288]. It is not yet known what exactly causes upregulation of CXCR3 in neurons in the context of TDP-43 pathology, but clues of a TDP-43-type I interferon-CXCL10 pathway can be seen in human [287, 289–291]. It is noteworthy that TDP-43 pathology is also observed in about one-third of AD cases [292, 293] suggesting overlapping mechanisms with AD potentially via this identified axis.

Another CXCL10-driven mechanism involves CD8 T-cell infiltration [294–296]. In recent years, there has been new appreciation for the role of T cells in AD [297, 298]. Evidence now suggests that a CXCR3-CXCL10 axis exists for the recruitment of CD8 T cells, exacerbating neuronal damage and possibly also directly contribute to interferon signalling enhancement, and that this activity converges through the IFNAR1 [296]. The exact role of CD8 T cells in vivo in AD remains for now still elusive [296, 299], yet interferon-responsive CD8 T cells seem to be a common feature among amyloid [296] and tauopathy [300] models of AD. While microglia far outnumber CD8 T-cells in the brain, both in human AD and models, more work will be needed to discriminate between the type I interferon-driven recruitment and activation of CD8 T cells through CXCR3-CXCL10 mechanisms, and the type II interferon-mediated recruitment self-enhancement.

4.2 Down's syndrome

Down's syndrome (DS) occurs when an individual has an extra copy of chromosome 21, a phenomenon called trisomy 21. It is characterised by intellectual disability and developmental delay, and a striking incidence of early-onset AD (EOAD). The notable increase in life expectancy of individuals with DS has revealed dementia and other co-occurring neurological and immunological conditions. By age 40, half of the individuals develop AD, this increases to 77% by age 60, and virtually all develop AD by age 70 [301, 302]. Individuals also display important immune dysregulation [303, 304], with notable neuroinflammation [305] and resembling an interferonopathy [306, 307]. A higher prevalence of depression is also seen in DS, and this is associated more strongly with dementia [301, 302]. In addition, basal ganglia calcification is also found in 10–45% of individuals, [308–314] an observation that is not fully understood but thought to be attributed to an accelerated ageing process. While it was expected from a clinical perspective that DS ageing is accelerated, as evidenced by accelerated hair greying, decreased skin flexibility, and premature death among others, epigenetic age of both brain tissue and blood is confirmed from a molecular marker standpoint [315]. The epigenetic clock used to objectively assess ageing is based on a quantitative assessment of DNA methylation [316]. As a measure of ageing, it stands out among existing epigenetic clocks also because of its impressive predictive ability for time-to-death which further validates the approach [317, 318]. The ageing process is significantly accelerated circulating cells in DS, a process called immunosenescence [319], and this is further accentuated in brain [315].

Chromosome 21 carries ca. 200 genes, triplication of which causes DS and accompanying disease. Deconvolution of the specific role of each gene in DS is difficult. Triplication of *APP* gene is attributed as the main reason for EOAD, including accompanying senile plaque deposition paralleling genetic AD [320]. The *IFNAR1* and *IFNAR2* genes which form the two active chains of the functional IFNAR are also found on chromosome 21. Complicating interpretation, however, the interferon gamma receptor 2 (*IFNGR2*) chain and the interleukin 10 receptor beta subunit

(*IL10RB*) genes are also found on chromosome 21, one of the two heterodimers of the type II and type III receptors, respectively, and whose signalling overlaps substantially with type I interferon signalling. Nevertheless, much research has been carried out on the role of interferons in DS.

Firstly, cells isolated from DS individuals are more reactive to exogenous IFNα or IFNβ treatment demonstrating that the addition of an additional fully functional set of IFNAR receptors leads to an expected increased signalling [304, 306, 321, 322]. Remarkably, signalling downstream of IFNAR is not overcome by negative regulation, and no desensitisation is apparent [304]. However, it is argued that inappropriate and mistimed responses are likely to occur [322]. Importantly, IFNAR triplication also has consequences in vivo in patients. DS individuals display significant correlation between *IFNAR1* and inflammation markers including CRP and inflammatory gene signatures [323] as well as of the interferon-response signatures [307, 323]. Furthermore, systemic interferon signatures correlate with cardiovascular severity and depression [307] suggesting that increased interferon signalling associates with a more severe phenotype. While the increased interferon-response and dependence on JAK/STAT signalling seems obvious considering what precedes, the mechanism responsible for triggering of increased type I interferon production remains elusive. One hypothesis is that the aneuploidy state itself fundamentally triggers type I interferons via cGAS-STING signalling due to accumulation of dsDNA in the cytosol [324]. This provides a rationale for the mechanism of triggering type I interferon production in DS, though this remains to be specifically demonstrated.

To investigate mechanistically the role of type I interferons in DS much work has been performed using engineered mice that mimic the trisomy of chromosome 21. Early experiments showed overall amelioration of the phenotype by neutralisation of a cocktail of anti-interferon antibodies with DS mimicking mice available at the time [325]. Currently, numerous DS models exist, but the Dp16 model is often deemed superior. It is trisomic for the entire mouse chromosome 16 region, which includes approximately 113 orthologs found in human chromosome 21, and importantly excludes any orthologs of genes not found on human chromosome 21 [326]. While the same difficulty in distinguishing the contribution of each of type I, II, and III interferons exists in this DS mouse model as it does in human, it is found that the IFNAR receptor is overexpressed among all three interferon receptors and widely expressed in immune cells [323], mimicking the human condition [304]. Importantly, loss of the interferon receptor locus leads to spatial memory rescue and accompanying normalisation of synaptogenesis and dopamine receptor signalling [323].

Taken together, this research suggests a mild form of interferonopathy in DS [306]. It is important to better understand the clinical evolution of disease and define the pathogenic mechanisms to better guide clinical decisions. The predictable chronological sequence of DS allows for the rigorous investigation of the events preceding amyloid deposition and eventual neurodegeneration, making DS an important condition to further elucidate neurodegenerative diseases such as AD.

4.3 Inflammaging

Cell senescence is perhaps the most evident hallmark of ageing. Over the past 10 years, chronic low-grade inflammation has become recognised as an important addition to the hallmarks of ageing in a process dubbed "inflammaging" [327, 328]. Brain ageing, however, remains a challenging field and most research is performed using animal models.

To elucidate the molecular culprits of brain ageing, Michal Schwartz and colleagues performed transcriptomics profiling of various organs from aged mice and found selective upregulation of type I interferon signalling in the choroid plexus [267]. The choroid plexus is a critical structure in the brain that serves as a hub for neurovascular communication and as principal producer of CSF [329]. It would follow that consequences in the choroid plexus may affect wider brain activity. What the group found is that, not only are type I interferons overexpressed, they are also responsible for negatively affecting cognitive function and hippocampal neurogenesis during ageing. This was confirmed by other groups that found IFNα levels in CSF to significantly positively correlate with ageing-induced memory deficits in mice [231]. Blocking IFNAR signalling by delivering function-neutralising antibodies into the CSF via intracerebroventricular administration reduces interferon signalling in the choroid plexus. This leads to the restoration of brain-derived neurotrophic factor (BDNF) and insulin-like growth factor (IGF1). It also inhibits microgliosis and astrocytosis in the hippocampus, demonstrating the extensive harmful effects of ageing-induced type I interferons in the brain [267]. Importantly, type I interferons and interferon responses are also seen in human, in elderly individuals [267], but more research is needed to characterise the ageing responses in the choroid plexus and the consequences for neurocognitive and memory processes. Other lines of evidence suggest that interferon signalling in the choroid plexus has implications for neurodegeneration. During the COVID-19 pandemic it was noted that patients that exhibited severe respiratory symptoms also developed neuropsychiatric [330], neurocognitive [331, 332], and fatigue [333] symptoms at a significantly higher rate. It is suggested that cognitive dysfunction caused by COVID-19 may also be linked to aberrant type I interferon production in the choroid plexus [334] as evidenced by chronic interferon-responses during severe COVID-19 [335]. AD patients also exhibit ageing-related inflammation in the choroid plexus [336], which is also paralleled in a mouse model of AD [231], though more work is needed to define whether type I interferons are involved in ageing-associated AD changes in the choroid plexus.

Exactly how type I interferons participate in the aberrant process of inflammaging remains to be fully elucidated. One proposed mechanism is through suppression of anti-oxidative factors. In mice, mitochondrial instability due to old age leads to type I interferon responses via mitochondrial DNA release and activation of cGAS-STING [337–340]. The induced type I interferons then counteract NRF2, a potent antioxidant, leading to accumulated ROS and oxidative stress across different organs including heart, liver, kidney [339], and lung [341]. Although this mechanism has not been specifically demonstrated in the brain, studies in the retina and CNS indicate a similar ageing-related mechanism induced by interferons that leads to ROS [340]. Furthermore, cGAS-STING-type I interferon signalling also leads to anaemia by increasing inflammatory monocyte expansion and haemophagocytosis [339], something that could contribute to low grade chronic brain hypoxia [342].

Another mechanism proposed is linked to the senescence process. Senescence describes the abnormal state of permanent cell-cycle arrest, typically in response to stress or damage, and which is ultimately responsible for ageing [343]. Senescent cells also exhibit a senescence-associated secretory phenotype (SASP), releasing cytokines, chemokines and other molecules that can lead to tissue degeneration and a decline in organ function. Work performed to discover ageing-associated processes in the brain found that type I interferon signatures are specifically enriched across all neuronal cell types during ageing in mice, marking a unique signature capable of resolving chronological age [344]. This includes neural stem cells, a cell type vital for neuron renewal, maintenance, and repair, which also exhibited type I interferon signatures with its top gene being *Ifi27* [344]. Sophisticated work has been performed to understand how a senescent state occurs. Retrotransposable elements (RTEs), remnants from ancient retroviruses that have integrated permanently into the genome, become more active during cell senescence. This intriguing process is also believed to be a strong contributor to somatic retrotransposition in the brain, a process important for neuronal somatic mosaicism [345–347]. It is found that senescent cells downregulate TREX1, leading to accumulation of RTEs which then triggers cGAS-STING and strong induction of type I interferons [348, 349]. This explains the interferon signatures found in senescent cells and during ageing, and is therefore a great marker, but evidence suggests that they are also responsible for triggering senescence and ageing [268] through cGAS-STING [350]. Type I interferons are notorious for promoting cell cycle arrest and inhibit proliferation [258, 351], an antiviral tactic meant to slow down viral spread. They are also potent inducers of chemokines and other cytokines. Hence, it stands to reason that chronic overexposure may also itself participate in the senescence process. Indeed, microglia from DS have been found to enter a senescence programme along with type I interferon overexpression, and remarkably inhibition of this signalling prevents development of senescence [352]. Similar processes have been observed in the senescence of haematopoietic and germinal stem cells [353], as well as hepatic stellate cells [348], indicating a potential universal mechanism. In the brain, a mechanism whereby microglia are responsible for triggering senescence in neurons and other glial cells is now hypothesised to be a major driving force behind cognitive impairment both in ageing, AD, and during brain injury [354–356]. One proposed mechanism of type I interferon-driven ageing of microglia is through the downregulation of the protective and inflammation-limiting transcription factor MEF2C [268]. MEF2C is found to be implicated in brain development and neuropsychiatric disorders [357, 358]. Chronic production of IFNβ in the brain causes downregulation of MEF2C, as does ageing, and in so doing inhibits a resilience to ageing-induced [268] and disease-induced cognitive decline [249]. Lastly, two recognised pro-ageing SASPs which promote decreased hippocampal neurogenesis, synaptic plasticity, impaired learning and memory and increased microgliosis, are CCL11 and CCL2 [359, 360]. There is evidence demonstrating that type I interferons are inducers of CCL2 and CCL11 [166, 171, 361, 362], though it remains to be demonstrated whether type I interferons promote ageing and senescence also through CCL2 and CCL11.

4.4 Brain trauma

Traumatic brain injury (TBI) was once thought to cause static neurological damage. Yet, research now indicates that it can set off a chain reaction leading to ongoing neurodegeneration, widespread damage outside mechanically injured sites such as the hippocampus [363] and the onset of dementia. It is common for individuals to suffer prolonged cognitive deterioration, which can be attributed, to some extent, to the emergence of dementia and AD following concussive injury [364]. Large cohort and meta-analyses have attributed a 1.5-4 fold relative fold risk increase in dementia following TBI depending on number of concussive events, and time following the event [365, 366]. This effect is exacerbated in the elderly, as both functional outcome and survival are significantly worse in elderly individuals, making age one of the more reliable prognostic factor [367–369]. Older individuals also represent the highest proportion of TBI events [370], adding further credence to the need for enhanced care for the advanced age groups. Progressive neurodegeneration due to TBI may account for 5–15% of all cases [371], suggesting that understanding the pathological mechanism of TBI may lead to better treatments and a staggering reduction of incident neurodegenerative diseases.

Neuroinflammation is known to cause secondary injury progression following TBI, potentially leading to long-term sequelae and progressive neurodegeneration [372, 373]. Much effort has been made to characterise the inflammatory environment of TBI in carefully controlled conditions, and to investigate the contribution of identified pathways to the long-term outcomes. For this purpose, preclinical research in the mouse has been instrumental, providing a broadly homogenous induction and allowing for experimental therapies, a feat that is difficult to achieve in emergency medicine settings involving humans. Multiple lines of evidence have now identified the type I interferon pathway to be strongly implicated, both by spatial [374], single cell [375–379], microdissected tissue [380], as well as bulk [280, 381, 382] transcriptomic analyses. While expression of interferon-response genes is widespread across microglia, meningeal macrophages, astrocytes, and oligodendrocytes, most evidence points to microglia and macrophages as the main producer of type I interferons following injury. Importantly, activation of the type I interferon pathway is detrimental to the resolution process, as consistently evidenced across genetic ablation models and through intervention by monoclonal antibody treatments [382–384]. Pharmacologic inhibition or genetic ablation of cGAS-STING also cause abrogation of type I interferon signalling and confers neuroprotection and accelerated neurocognitive amelioration [379, 385–388] suggesting that aberrant DNA sensing through microglial STING may be a critical trigger for sustained and pathogenic inflammation following TBI. Activation of transposable elements as well as mitochondrial DNA release is found to trigger activation of cGAS-STING in this context [377, 389]. Other sources of nucleic acids, as well as nucleic acid sensors, are also likely to be involved. Neutrophil extracellular traps (NETs) have been found to be important in triggering neuroinflammation in TBI [390] and are triggers for TLR9 and type I interferon production [391].

Consistent evidence of the implication of this pathway is also seen during human TBI, despite high heterogeneity compared to preclinical models. Expression of *STING1* is significantly upregulated following trauma, both at the site of injury and at the contralateral side [385] confirming its potential implication in the detrimental neuroinflammatory process. Upregulation of IFNβ, but not IFNα, is also seen within the first 6 h post TBI in patients that succumbed to the trauma [383], though it remains to be determined whether this partiality for IFNβ is maintained during the secondary, chronic neuroinflammation. Furthermore, nucleic triggers for the cGAS-STING pathway and for other nucleic acid sensors are highly enriched following TBI. Cell-free nucleic acids have been found in enormous amounts in both CSF [392] and plasma [393], and correlate with severity of trauma and outcome following injury. The extent to which nucleic acids pour from the brain to the CSF and circulation is a testament to the excessive cell death and accompanying nucleic acid release, and highlights the quantities that must be present in parenchyma during the acute event and therafter. With such excess of type I interferon triggering molecules, it is not surprising that interferon responses are also apparent, evidenced from human single-nuclei transcriptional analyses [377]. Lastly, the more severe outcomes seen in elderly individuals may be paralleled by enhanced persistence of type I interferon signalling and worsened outcomes observed in aged mice [378, 380, 394] and may provide a model for uncovering age-related determinants of interferon-driven chronic neurodegeneration following TBI.

Mediating the pathogenic activities of the cGAS-STING-type I interferon pathway is likely to involve multiple downstream events. Evidence suggests that effector T-cell infiltration via CXCL10 is one important component, whereby infiltrating CXCR3+ Th1 cells cause white matter injury, promoting anxiety and depressive neurocognitive changes [395]. Neuron loss in the hippocampus could be attributed to sustained chronic IFNβ [384], yet exact mechanisms remain to be elucidated. NOX2, a subunit of NADPH important for the production of ROS, is highly neurotoxic during TBI [396–398] and particularly in the hippocampus. Loss of IFNβ significantly attenuates NOX2 [384], implicating the type I interferon pathway in pathogenic ROS production. Neutrophils, which are important producers of ROS, can in fact be instigated to produce ROS following IFNα stimulation [399]. One possibility is that type I interferons exert control over ROS production via infiltrating neutrophils, which are generally regarded as detrimental in a sterile injury context in the brain [400]. Adding further weight to this hypothesis is the observation that neutrophil infiltration is significantly decreased in microglial STING deficient animals during TBI [387]. However, neutrophil infiltration is thought to be a self-limiting event, which may not carry over during the secondary, chronic neurodegeneration phase. Thus, another possibility is that interferons carry ROS production over through chronic phases via exerted control over IDO [156]. IDO is known to be induced by type I interferons in microglia and to result in production of ROS in response to infection [156, 401]. Thus, in the context of unabated type I interferon signalling, microglial damage of neurons may be mediated by IDO-dependent ROS production.

TBI induces strong immediate damage and a neuroinflammatory response that is detrimental to the long-term recovery via secondary injury processes. Although complex and multifaceted, the neuroinflammatory response is characterised by type I interferon signalling, albeit not exclusively. Yet, blockade of the pathway in preclinical models and the parallels seen in human suggest that targeting this pathway in human may hamper the aberrant neuroinflammatory process and may improve neurocognitive outcomes by reducing neurodegenerative processes.

4.5 HIV/AIDS-associated neurocognitive disorders

Human Immunodeficiency Virus (HIV) is the devastating virus that causes acquired immunodeficiency syndrome (AIDS), and which affects an estimated 39 million people worldwide. HIV uses the CD4 surface protein and either the CXCR4 or CCR5 receptors to gain entry into cells, thereby infecting them, and killing them in the replication process [402, 403]. Over time, this causes systemic immunosuppression as CD4 T cells, dendritic cells, monocytes, and macrophages become depleted. Due to advancements in the standard of care, which relies on antiretroviral therapy (ART), AIDS has become a secondary concern as viral replication is inhibited and infected individuals live longer lives without developing immunosuppression. While viral replication is effectively hampered, infection persists.

HIV/AIDS-associated neurocognitive disorders (HAND) are a common occurrence among people with HIV. Meta-analyses suggest a combined prevalence of 50% among all infected individuals, presenting with at least one neurocognitive sign among all seropositive individuals. Of those, cognitive-motor disorder (60%), major depression (15-40%), and delirium (17%) [404] are some of the neurologic complications of HIV. The prevailing theory is that infected cells serve as a 'Trojan horse,' transporting HIV to the brain, and causing infection of microglia [405], and astrocytes by cell-to-cell transfer [406, 407]. Remarkably, while ART can reduce the prevalence of HAND, incidence remains abnormally high and a concern for virtually all HIV patients, a fact probably explained by increased longevity [408, 409]. This suggests that neurocognitive decline in HIV patients despite controlled viral load may have similar mechanisms as age-related cognitive decline.

A complete picture of the pathological mechanism behind neurocognitive disease in HIV is lacking. Its pathogenesis is attributed to persisting viral load in the brain, unabated neuroinflammation, and neuronal loss due to pro-inflammatory cytokines. Microglia and brain infiltrating macrophages serve as the main reservoirs following HIV neuroinvasion, typically within two weeks after infection. Gene expression profiling of brain samples from seropositive individuals that had neurocognitive impairment reveals strong type I interferon-response genes such as OASs, IFITs, IFITMs, and CXCL10 across multiple studies [410–414]. While this is not surprising for a viral infection, uncontrolled inflammation can become detrimental causing neuroinflammation and neurocognitive impairments [415]. This is exemplified in mice overexpressing IFNα in the brain, which are both protected from viral encephalitis, but also develop progressive neurodegeneration as a consequence of persistent neuroinflammation [416]. Importantly, IFNAR signalling is required for neurocognitive decline and neuroinflammation due to HIV, in vivo [417, 418]. Recognition is thought to occur via stimulation of nucleic acid sensors TLR7 and TLR9 [419], IFI16 and STING [420], RIG-I [421], all converging on type I interferon production. This is paralleled in HIV infected individuals as IFNα is detectable in CSF [422] and correlating with viral load [423, 424] as well as NfL [425] providing further credence to the neurotoxic effect of sustained type I interferon production in brain following HIV infection.

Evidence also exists that while ART may inhibit viral replication, neuroinflammation remains unabated. In a brain organoid model, HIV infection leads to upregulation of type I interferon, interferon-signatures, and of other inflammatory mediators in microglia, the main infected cell in brain, causing elevated inflammatory outcomes also in non-microglial cells [426]. This further reflects the extent of damaging responses to HIV in cells not directly infected. Importantly, while ART causes ablation of the expression of HIV proteins, microglia become a persistent reservoir of HIV [405] exemplified by continuous production of interferon-response CXCL10 and chemokine CCL2 despite ART [426] suggesting that intracellular viral recognition and response sustain a replication-independent inflammatory response. Consolidating the observation that ART does not abolish HAND incidence is the fact that, while it suppresses viral replication, it does not affect latent virus [427]. This is reflected by the persistence of interferon-response gene expression in patients undergoing ART [413]. Hence, it is reasoned that the microglial viral reservoir alone may be sufficient to perpetuate neuroinflammation and HAND, even at low or undetectable viraemic loads. It is important to note that not all ART display the same CNS penetrance. The structure of the BBB coupled with organised efflux mechanisms block or severely limit the access of ART to this reservoir and argues for the development of new generation ART with improved brain penetrance [428, 429].

Beyond HIV, there may be parallels to other viral infections. Cognitive deficits have been recorded in patients recovering from COVID-19 following SARS-CoV-2 infection [430–433]. The virus is known to infect the choroid plexus as viral entry factors including the receptor ACE2 are highly expressed by its epithelial cells [335, 434]. The interferon signatures [335] were found to parallel what is seen in neurodegenerative diseases [216–221] as well as choroid plexus during ageing [267], lending to the hypothesis of a type I interferon-associated cognitive dysfunction pathway in COVID-19 [334].

5. Mechanisms of neurologic dysfunction

Research on the rare type I interferonopathies, which typically present in infants, has been challenging. Case studies and small patient cohorts account for most of our knowledge of this family of diseases. Understanding the mechanisms by which type I interferon causes neurologic disease can have substantial impact on treatment of interferonopathies. Type I interferons are also implicated in other non-mendelian diseases which are often accompanied by a predominant neurological component. Therefore, a better mechanistic understanding could have important implications for more common neurological diseases. The following section describes some of the better-known effects in the brain, linking together different disorders and emerging concepts, and highlights some of the remaining open questions.

5.1 Local source of interferons in the brain

Type I interferons can be produced by almost every cell in the CNS, despite lacking dedicated – or "professional" – producers of these cytokines. Being most prominently produced in response to nucleic acids, expression patterns of nucleic acid sensors therefore dictate for the most part whether any specific cell type produces interferons. Some, basally express virtually all nucleic acid sensors, such as microglia, whereas others, such as astrocytes, express a more specialised subset of sensors.

Astrocytes have been proposed as a major producer and responder in AGS caused by *TREX1* or *RNASEH2* mutations [435–437]. Immunohistochemical staining of post-mortem brain sections revealed that astrocytes were the main producers of IFNα and CXCL10, a typically interferon-responsive chemokine. Mutations in the genes associated with AGS cause aberrant accumulation of DNA which becomes the trigger for production in astrocytes [438, 439]. Moreover, chronic exposure to IFNα was found to cause aberrant activation of astrocytes making them reactive, while simultaneously inducing gene expression changes reminiscent of AGS [436].

Microglia are thought of as the main producer in more common neurodegenerative diseases. In Alzheimer's disease, both Aβ oligomers [232, 247,] and amyloid-associated nucleic acids [228, 229], as well as soluble tau [237, 239, 240, 440] are capable of triggering production from microglia. This is also the case for HIV-associated neurocognitive disorders, which is less surprising given that microglia are the main CNS reservoir for HIV [405].

Neurons and oligodendrocytes can also produce type I interferons, albeit to a lesser extent than astrocytes and microglia. They have been found to express TLR3 and to be capable of producing IFNβ in response to dsRNAs [441, 442]. Neurons also express cGAS-STING and respond to mtDNA by triggering the production of IFNβ [287]. They are also found to express TLR9 [443, 444], TLR8 [445], TLR7 [446, 447], RIG-I [448], though evidence of their involvement in production of interferons remains for now limited.

Brain vascular endothelial cells form an important direct interface between the brain parenchyma and the circulation. The cGAS-STING pathway plays an important role in vascular endothelial cells, as exemplified by the observation that mutations in the *STING1* gene cause overt production of type I interferons leading to vasculopathy [449]. Brain endothelial cells produce type I interferons [282, 450] and they are known to be able to do so via STING [281, 451], via RIG-I [452, 453], or also in response to TNF through IRF1 [454]. While more research is needed on the endothelial cell contribution to type I interferon production specifically in the brain, convincing evidence exists that they are capable of it.

In addition to nucleic acid sensors, surface pattern recognition receptors are also expressed by cells in the brain. It is well-described that TLR2 and TLR4 respond to disparate triggers including viral proteins, protein aggregates, and bacterial lipids initiating production of pro-inflammatory cytokines. This includes type I interferons which are produced through TLR2-MyD88 and TLR4-TRIF [455, 456]. TLR2 and TLR4 are known to be expressed on microglia, astrocytes, and brain endothelial cells, and neurons are described to express TLR4. It is important to note that induction of type I interferons is also mediated through pathways other than nucleic acid sensing during neuroinflammation.

Direct evidence for type I interferon production in vivo is difficult to obtain. High, ubiquitous expression of the IFNAR causes low bioavailability of these cytokines, but also results in interferon-related signatures that are powerful surrogate markers. Despite this, technologies that allow the direct detection of IFNα and IFNβ have enabled the quantification of significant increases in the CSF of HAND, neurolupus, and AGS patients, suggesting high continuous CNS production. Ultimately, which cells in the CNS produce type I interferons is often context and disease dependent. Another important consideration is that some nucleic acid sensors can also be induced by type I interferons themselves, thereby initiating a chain reaction of production which can be self-sustained for as long as stimuli are present. In some cases, production is initiated in the periphery causing multiorgan diseases with sometimes prominent CNS involvement.

5.2 Systemic source of interferon

Interferons produce systemically are also capable of signalling to the brain [457]. In mice, it was demonstrated that delivery of systemic interferons stimulates the induction of interferon-response genes in brain parenchymal cells [458], and that microglia become strongly activated and to upregulate complement alongside classical pro-inflammatory interferon-responses [459].

The exact mechanisms by which peripheral type I interferons signal to the brain are not fully understood. From research on the cross-talk between peripheral inflammation and the CNS, it is reasoned this can happen in any of four different ways [460]: (1) passively across the BBB and through brain regions called circumventricular organs, which are devoid of a BBB and highly permeable to permit rapid communication between CNS and circulation [457, 458], (2) through induction of BBB leakiness via downregulation of adherens and tight junctions [166, 277, 450], (3) by active uptake through the choroid plexus endothelial cells [166, 267], or (4) through cell migration across the BBB, such as activated monocytes attracted to a microglial CCL2 gradient [361] which may carry type I interferon signalling. Though less is known about the latter mechanism, it is thought that this is a primary mechanism contributing to depression [460–462].

The most obvious example of systemic production of type I interferons is lupus. In SLE, plasmacytoid dendritic cells (pDCs) and monocytes are thought to be primary sources [463–467] however, despite being a systemic disease, it is difficult to posit that there is no production in the brain.

Type I interferons form an important innate immune defence barrier, and are, as such, capable of being produced by all cell types, depending on the inflammatory context. They can be produced in response to viral or bacterial infections, or in response to damage associated signals, either locally in the brain or systemically, and to freely traverse the BBB. It is probable that interferon production in both the circulation and the CNS concomitantly contribute to neuroinflammation, even when the source appears predominantly either systemic or central.

5.3 Cellular responses to interferon in the brain

While sources of interferon can be various, all type I interferon signalling converges through a single surface receptor, the IFNAR. This ubiquitously expressed dimeric receptor, formed of an IFNAR1 and an IFNAR2 chain, allows for a wide range of cellular responses, affecting various cell types. Microglia, astrocytes, neurons, and endothelial cells are known to respond strongly and in specific ways.

Microglia assume a hyper-ramified morphology [468], a typical change signifying activation and immune surveillance mechanisms. Microgliosis is strongly induced by type I interferons, and across neuroinflammation models, whether AD, AGS, or lupus, it is dependent on IFNAR signalling. Concurrently, increased processes and complexity are also induced, which typically signify increased synaptic pruning. Short-lived proliferation and apoptosis following long-term stimulation are also observed. Lastly, their antigen presentation capacities are enhanced by upregulation of MHC I and II genes and of activation markers CD68, CD40, CD80, and CD86 [228, 459, 468–470]. This is further exemplified in single cell studies across human AD and mouse models, where interferon-response signatures overlap with antigen processing and presentation genes.

Astrocytes also respond to type I interferons, though their interferon-response gene expression is less pronounced than that of microglia [469]. It also seems that, in AD models, astrocytosis is not dependent on interferons. This is in contrast to AGS, where astrocytes are thought of as the primary involved cell type [436]. Intriguingly, like microglia, they also upregulate genes related to the antigen presentation machinery, though they are not classically thought of as APCs. Yet, reactive astrocytes display antigen presentation characteristics, as well as astrocytic toxicity markers.

Endothelial cells of the brain vasculature are major responders to type I interferons. They respond by producing chemokines, allowing cell infiltration, and succumbing to apoptosis leading to vascular dysfunction. An AGS mouse model driven by astrocyte promoter-dependent production of IFNα recapitulates microangiopathy, perivascular T-cell infiltration, perivascular calcification, and capillary calibre and formation of aneurysms seen in human patients [44]. Importantly, endothelial cell-specific ablation of IFNAR causes near-complete rescue of cerebral vascular disease [44], suggesting that endothelial cells are the principal responders in AGS and a major target for type I interferon-driven neuroinflammation. Endothelial cells exposed to type I interferons display reduced mobility and invasion [471], in line with their cancer inhibiting properties [472]. In fact, IFNAR signalling inhibits vascular endothelial cell growth factor (VEGF)-induced proliferation [452] highlighting the anti-angiogenic potency of these cytokines. It was shown that CXCL10 can inhibit endothelial cell proliferation in a CXCR3-dependent [473] and -independent [474] pathway. Interferon-inducible IFI35 is also described as an important inhibitor of endothelial cell proliferation and migration [475], indicating that multiple parallel pathways exist. Further accentuating the importance of type I interferons in endothelial cell biology is the surprising discovery of basal interferon-response expressing endothelial cells across different organs including the brain [476] suggesting a regulatory and homeostatic role of tonic type I interferon signalling, though research is needed to characterise these cells and their roles.

5.4 Immune cell infiltration

Certain chemokines such as CXCL9, CXCL10, and CXCL11 are known to be preferentially interferon-inducible, while others, such as CCL2, CCL5, and CCL20, are also induced by interferons but not exclusively. While microglia also display important chemokine production in response to interferons, vascular endothelial cells are particularly suited to the task by virtue of their position at the interface between tissue and circulation. Chemokine gradients and presentation at the lumen side allows for efficient recruitment of immune cells expressing cognate chemokine receptors. In brain endothelial cells, IFNβ treatment causes upregulation and production of CXCL9, -10, -11, CCL2, and -5 which are also able to signal in the brain parenchyma [166]. They bind CXCR3, CCR2, and CCR5 which are predominantly expressed on T-cells, NK cells, monocytes, and dendritic cells, among others.

It has been reported that IFNβ can also inhibit monocyte infiltration by downregulation of adhesion molecules during experimental autoimmune encephalomyelitis (EAE) [477], a model of MS, supporting the anti-inflammatory characteristics observed in MS. It is unclear whether this is disease- or tissue-context specific, as subcutaneous administration of IFNβ in MS patients causes upregulation of the aforementioned chemokines accompanied by extensive T-cell and macrophage perivascular infiltrates [478]. IFNα overexpressing mice show extensive perivascular infiltrates in the brain [416, 479] which depend specifically on endothelial cell IFNAR signalling [44]. Despite having elevated interferon-responses, *ADAR1* mutation-carrying mice do not, display perivascular infiltrates [480], while a different nuclease deficiency, *RNASET2*, leads to IFNAR-driven T-cell and monocyte infiltration [481]. In the context of brain injury, IFNAR-signalling enhances T-cell and monocyte recruitment [382]. This suggests that type I interferon-driven immune cell infiltration is context dependent and requires more research to fully elucidate the underlying differences that set the final outcomes apart.

5.5 Vascular dysfunction

As a consequence of inhibition of normal endothelial cell proliferation and function, it is not surprising that type I interferons can also cause pathogenic vascular dysfunction. IFNAR signalling in endothelial cells specifically causes development of BBB disruption, microangiopathy, calcification, neuron loss and premature death in an AGS mouse model [45]. There is also clinical evidence supporting this observation. Exogenous interferon therapy has been associated with thrombotic microangiopathy in a dose dependent manner [168, 482]. Type I interferons cause abnormal brain vascular morphology, displaying smaller size microvasculature, sections of widened vessel formation, and microaneurysms. Specifically, vascular lumen narrowing is seen diffusely across the brain [168]. The interferon-inducible IFITM1 protein has been discovered to be implicated in the formation of stable vascular lumen during angiogenesis through stabilisation of endothelial cell-to-cell interactions [483]. While loss of IFITM1 leads to abnormal vessel formation, it is for now unknown whether upregulation can also disturb endothelial cell-to-cell contacts resulting in inappropriate vascular lumen formation and dysfunction.

Certain contexts, such as viral infection, can greatly inhibit normal function and healing until viral stimuli are cleared. In endothelial cells, it is found that viral sensing through MDA-5 triggers IFNβ production. This thereby blocks vascular repair, angiogenesis, and BBB restoration following injury, causing a failure to recover normal neurological function [280, 484]. It is likely that even milder neurovascular damage, in the presence of overactive interferon signalling, can cause similar outcomes. In a mouse model of AD, IFNβ correlates with BBB disruption and contributes to it by downregulating adherens junctions and tight junctions causing leakiness [277]. Both IFNβ and IFNAR1 expression is markedly increased in vascular endothelial cells in vivo compared to non-AD-prone mice, indicating an induced hyper-sensitivity to type I interferons which is likely caused in some form by amyloids. While Aβ can trigger microglia to produce type I interferons by multiple mechanisms, it is unknown whether similar mechanisms take place in endothelial cells. Importantly, upregulation of IFNAR can be a key sensitisation step that needs further research. Cerebral amyloid angiopathy (CAA) is a condition where amyloids deposit along the walls of cerebral blood vessels [485]. This causes microhaemorrhaging which further precipitates cognitive decline [486, 487]. Furthermore, current generation anti-amyloid therapies are known to cause amyloid-related imaging abnormalities (ARIA), essentially aggravated haemorrhaging induced by the amyloid targeting therapies. It is for now unknown whether there is a direct link between CAA and type I interferon signalling, and whether they participate in the induction of ARIA.

Following BBB disruption, leakage of blood products containing DAMPs of various sources gain access to the brain parenchyma and trigger damage sensors. One such activator is fibrin, a powerful trigger of CD11b/CD18 surface heterodimers expressed on microglia and which is gaining emerging interest as the full extent of its involvement in CNS diseases and neurodegeneration [488]. During AD progression, mice lacking fibrinogen, a plasma protein required to create fibrin, show reduced gliosis, neuronal damage and cognitive decline and suggest that vascular damage synergises with amyloid pathology [489]. The type I interferon pathway is found to be strongly triggered by fibrin [490] indicating that a leaky BBB can also directly trigger this neuroinflammatory pathway and suggesting a self-sustained feedforward mechanism of interferon-BBB leakage-interferon. The exact trigger for type I interferon production, whether indirect or direct, remains to be elucidated – whether indirectly through induction of DNA release following mitochondrial or cell damage, or directly through a potentially novel pathway. Yet, if not properly regulated, this is likely a mechanism through which neurodegeneration-inducing neuroinflammatory events can propagate throughout the brain.

As for how exactly type I interferons cause calcifying microangiopathy, this is still an open question. One hypothesis is that subclinical disruption of microvessels may be sufficient to cause continuous deposition of calcium along vessel walls. Evidence of direct induction of calcification also exists in vitro, as IFNα precipitates calcification at concentrations in the range found in CSF patients [491]. Finally, it is thought that cell senescence is linked to calcification, but it is unclear which one causes the other and how [41]. While type I interferons are known to cause both calcification and cell senescence, it remains to be discovered how this mechanism is mediated and whether through senescence.

5.6 Phagocytosis and synaptic pruning

Overall, type I interferons have been found to both inhibit appropriate microglial removal of aggregated proteins and debris, but also to enhance synaptic engulfment and neuronal elimination.

While in the context of AD it is still debated whether amyloid plaque formation is truly detrimental by enhancing neuronal network disruption or whether it renders reactive amyloid peptides unreactive in extracellular clumps, amyloid plaque deposition is generally accepted as a sign of exhausted phagocytosis. In vitro, both IFNα and IFNβ significantly reduce phagocytosis in a dose-dependent manner [262]. Furthermore, IFNAR signalling interferes with normal Aβ phagocytosis. This coincides with an increased pro-inflammatory state including increased cytokine production. This suggests that type I interferon drives mitochondria away from a phagocytic clean-up function towards a hyper-reactive pro-inflammatory state.

In vivo, there are some contradictory results, however [229, 262]. In APP/PS1 mice, plaque deposition seems grossly unaltered [262] whereas a different group could demonstrate decreased plaques [229]. Importantly, this was observed in mice lacking IFNAR specifically in non-microglial cells, but not in mice lacking microglial IFNAR. This seems to suggest that the phagocytic activity against plaques in microglia may be driven by unalterable genetic drivers which can, at best, be modulated by changes in neuronal interferon-inducible IFITM3. Likely, these results do not rule out clearance of reactive oligomeric amyloids, which may act by decreasing the overall inflammatory state. These results cannot rule out a possible effect in human LOAD where genetic drivers for amyloid deposition should be other than aberrant processing of amyloids.

Complicating matters further is the observation that type I interferons upregulate phagocytic markers [492] and promote synaptic pruning leading to neurodegeneration [228, 229, 233, 249, 352, 493]. Synapses are specialised junctions through which neurons signal to each other. They consist of three parts: the presynaptic terminal of the signalling neuron, the synaptic cleft, and the postsynaptic terminal of the target cell. Synaptophysin is a membrane glycoprotein present in presynaptic vesicles and is involved in the regulation of neurotransmitter release. Postsynaptic density protein 95 (PSD-95) is a scaffolding protein located in the postsynaptic density of excitatory synapses and it plays a critical role in anchoring and clustering neurotransmitter receptors and other signalling complexes at the synaptic membrane. Synaptic pruning mechanisms occur via phagocytic microglia and astrocytes in a complement-dependent mechanism [494, 495]. During synaptic pruning, certain synapses are tagged for removal by complement proteins such as C1q and C3. These proteins bind to the synapses and mark them for elimination. Microglia express complement receptors that recognise these tagged synapses. Once bound, microglia can engulf and digest the synaptic material, effectively pruning the synapse. This mechanism ensures the refinement of neural circuits and is essential for proper brain development and function. Dysregulation of this process leads, however, to neurodegenerative diseases. Type I interferons are found to induce complement-dependent synaptic pruning across multiple neurodegeneration models, but also in normal healthy development [496, 497] suggesting that this is a conserved mechanism and that it requires delicate regulation. Inducing the expression of complement components, such as C1q, C3, and C4, to mark synapses for elimination is perhaps only part of the mechanism, and it is still unclear whether interferons can also enhance the activity of complement receptors binding to complement-opsonized synapses, such as CR3 and CR4, and facilitate their engulfment.

Overall, type I interferons activate microglia to become reactive and pro-inflammatory, and to poise them for complement-driven synaptic pruning and neuronal engulfment, while rendering them unable to clean up reactive aggregated proteins. Whether this is a result of task overload, or a preferential outcome due to a switch in signalling remains to be determined and the underlying mechanisms discovered.

5.7 Mediating neuroinflammation-induced neurodegeneration

TBI is perhaps the most typical display of neuroinflammation features [498–500] which are associated with development of dementia [501, 502]. The neurodegeneration process persists long after the concussive event where reactive microglia morphology and upregulation of CD68 can be observed years after injury along with white matter atrophy [503]. Single nuclei RNA sequencing reveals an interferon signature in oligodendrocytes [377], the specialised glial cell type forming the myelin sheath typical of the white matter and allowing the efficacious saltatory nerve conduction between neurons.

These observations have been corroborated in bona fide mouse models of TBI which have been used to expand on the mechanistic link between brain injury, type I interferon signalling, reactive microglia, and neurodegeneration. Sustained type I interferon signatures are found strongly upregulated during TBI in both microglia and astrocytes, alongside genes related to glial reactivity [374]. Reactive microglia morphology and CD68 expression were also found to be induced by type I interferons directly in vivo [228]. Importantly, inactivation of IFNAR leads to reduced neuronal loss and protection of white matter resulting in improved neurocognitive function [382, 383]. STING-deficient animals lose most of the type I interferon signatures [385], hence the trigger itself can be speculated to be massive release of nucleic acids from damaged cells. Remarkably, neuronal STING-derived IFNβ alone is sufficient for promoting neuroinflammation [384, 395], in part through a decrease in NOX2, an important inflammatory mediator of post-traumatic neurodegeneration [396, 398]. IFNβ also initiates a CXCL10-driven white matter injury process, through CXCR3-dependent and -independent neurotoxic activities, and through induction of Th1 cell infiltration [395]. Yet, this does not account for the sustained interferon production succeeding acute trauma. Perhaps type I interferons cause a feed-forward loop of aberrant neuronal engulfment as explored in the previous section: nucleic acid sensing, accrued interferon production, more neuronal engulfment – rinse and repeat. While this remains to be demonstrated, an immune cell infiltration feed-forward loop exists which explains the self-sustained pathogenic interferon signatures [362, 378]. Monocytes in the meninges are found to produce CCL2 and to strongly upregulate interferon signatures [378]. That causes a CCR2-dependent recruitment process which is also remarkably required to propagate the type I interferon signatures during TBI [362], thus together suggesting a feed-forward loop of unabated interferon-response and immune cell infiltration.

Type I interferon initiates a potent neuroinflammatory response to brain injury, causing direct neuron and oligodendrocyte damage, and instigating monocyte and T-cell infiltration that potentiates and prolongs detrimental responses. The mechanisms identified validate targeting type I interferon or its downstream effectors as a therapeutic strategy in TBI. Inhibiting type I interferons leads to an ordered conclusion of the self-sustained inflammatory process, thereby promoting favourable neurocognitive outcomes.

Put together, the mechanisms by which type I interferons are known to affect the brain are numerous and act by perturbing multiple key processes required for neuronal function. From promoting neurodegeneration, to causing microangiopathy, to precipitating premature ageing, to promoting depressive states, type I interferons are an important neuroinflammatory target (**Figure 3**).

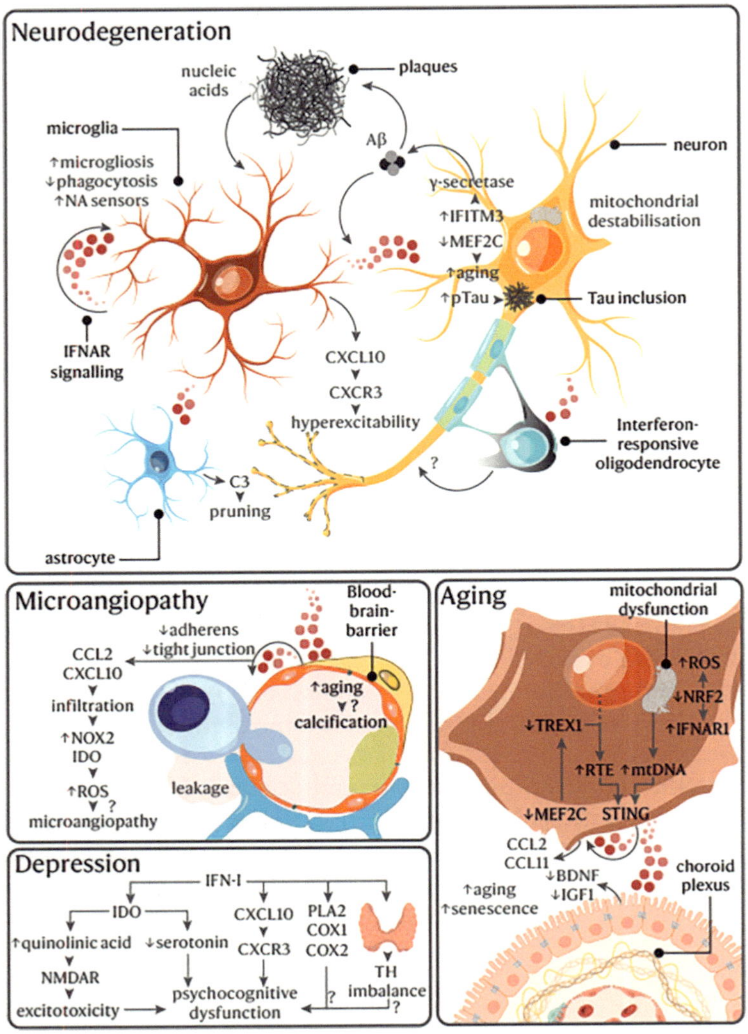

Figure 3.
Putative mechanisms of concerted psychocognitive disturbance by pathogenic type I interferon dysregulation. Neurodegeneration *in the context of Alzheimer's disease-related proteinopathies implicates type I interferon at multiple levels. DNA associated with amyloid plaques triggers the production of type I interferons by microglia, which become reactive in response to paracrine IFNAR signalling [228, 229]. Activation of IFNAR signalling in microglia causes upregulation of DNA sensors amplifying the response and promoting self-sustained activation [266]. CXCL10, produced in response to type I interferons, signals to CXCR3-expressing neuronal presynaptic terminals. This causes hyperexcitability and initiates chronic responses, leading to the impairment of new memory formation [286, 288, 504]. Interferon also activates complement driven neuronal synapse pruning by astrocytes contributing to loss of existing memory networks and cognitive decline [228, 229, 352]. They also induce direct effects on neurons. Neurons upregulate IFITM3, which enhances γ-secretase activity, increasing APP processing, and Aβ production [229, 275]. Aβ triggers type I interferon production by microglia [228] and neurons [247] while contributing to amyloid plaque formation when coupled with interferon-induced defective phagocytosis from microglia [262]. MEF2C, a cognitive resilience transcription factor, is downregulated in microglia and neurons. This leads to dysfunctional pro-inflammatory responses in microglia and the initiation of a premature cell senescence programme, promoting neuronal loss [233, 249, 268]. Interferons trigger mitochondrial destabilisation in neurons, contributing to neuronal cell death [263–265] and through concurrent activation of upregulated nucleic acid sensors [266] and mitochondrial DNA release, they cause neuronal type I interferon production [505–507]. Signalling to oligodendrocytes [239] leads to as yet undefined consequences, and in neurons promotes neuronal tau hyperphosphorylation and seeded aggregation [237] further contributing to the neurodegeneration process. Type I interferons also contribute to significant changes in the blood-brain barrier. Endothelial cells respond to type I interferons by producing chemokines CCL2 and CXCL10 which mediate perivascular immune cell infiltration [166, 168, 171, 294–296]. Recruited immune cells are activated by interferons*

to upregulate ROS via NOX2 and IDO1, contributing to neuronal and BBB damage [156, 384, 387, 396–399, 401]. Vascular endothelial cells from the BBB are concurrently activated by IFNAR-induced mediators CXCL10 and CCL2 to downregulate adherens and tight junctions, resulting in a leaky barrier and promoting microangiopathy [279–282, 300]. The mechanism by which type I interferons cause calcification of vessels in the systemic circulation and basal ganglia is unknown, but it is thought to be related to premature ageing. MEF2-family of transcription factors are gatekeepers of cellular senescence. Cognitive resilience-associated MEF2C is downregulated by IFNAR signalling, precipitating loss of endogenous retroviral element regulators such as TREX1, thereby inducing aberrant triggering of nucleic acid sensors and leading to self-amplified type I interferon production associated with the senescence-associated secretory phenotype (SASP) [258, 268, 348–352] as is the loss of MEF2A which also causes unabated IFNβ production through increased DNA:RNA hybrid accumulation [508]. Type I interferon-induced CCL2 and CCL11 are thought to be linked to induction of cell senescence [166, 171, 359–362] though the exact mechanisms remain to be fully elucidated. Finally, inhibition of NRF2 by IFNAR signalling leads to increased ROS which exacerbates the inflammaging process [339–341]. Put together, these mechanisms are responsible for ageing-related cognitive decline. These outcomes are overly apparent at the choroid plexus and likely take place diffusely across the brain parenchyma. Type I interferon is also well known to be an inducer of depression through metabolite, inflammatory, and hormonal mechanisms. IDO is induced in response to interferon and perturbs the balance between the excitotoxic quinolinic acid metabolite and the neuron protective kynurenic acid and serotonin, causing excessive NMDAR agonism [104–114, 156]. Cyclooxygenase inhibition via NSAIDs also attenuates IFNα-induced depression through undescribed mechanisms [173]. Concurrently, the interferon-inducible CXCL10 is also known to lead to weakened synaptic long-term potentiation in the hippocampus, resulting in a depressive phenotype [166, 171]. It remains to be elucidated whether the protective effects of COX1, -2, and PLA2 inhibition are acting through inhibition of the interferon-induced synaptic CXCL10-CXCR3 signalling. Together, all these mechanisms likely act in concert to cause the detrimental neuropsychiatric effects caused by type I interferons.

6. Therapeutic approaches

There are numerous existing approaches for targeting type I interferons and their downstream signalling, with great therapeutic application potential.

6.1 Targeting the receptor

The entire type I interferon pathway is dependent on a single juncture point, the IFNAR. This effectively acts as a central hub controlling all its downstream signalling. The advantage of targeting IFNAR over individually targeting any of its 13 IFNα subtypes, IFNβ, IFNε, IFNκ or IFNω, or combinations thereof, is evident. The generation of a mouse anti-IFNAR1 blocking monoclonal antibody [509] was a turning point for the field and for the pharmaceutical industry, both by facilitating research in vivo and elucidating the role of the pathway outside of genetic manipulation, and by providing a surrogate for the potential of therapeutic targeting in human. A fully human monoclonal IgG1κ antibody targets IFNAR1 with high affinity and specificity, neutralising its receptor activity [510]. Anifrolumab is now approved in most countries for the treatment of SLE following breakthrough improvement in disease scores, higher rate of achievement of remission, high retention rate and low immunogenicity and side effects [92, 93, 511–514]. It is important to note that the percentage of herpes zoster reactivation was increased by anifrolumab compared to placebo, surprisingly no other notable adverse events were seen up to 3-years after treatment initiation [512, 515]. Furthermore, an indirect analysis of results from the TULIP-1 and TULIP-2 phase III trials of anifrolumab, and BLISS-52 and BLISS-76 trials, two phase III trials randomised, double-blind, placebo-controlled tials of belimumab, an anti-BAFF monoclonal antibody, reveals that treatment with anifrolumab was associated with significantly greater benefits [516]. Belimumab had been a revolution in the treatment of SLE [517, 518], and is the only other and first approved biologic for SLE. Its potent B-cell survival inhibitory effect is being leveraged in combination therapies with tacrolimus [519] and rituximab [520, 521]. While no head-to-head comparisons have been made between anifrolumab and belimumab, warranting caution on conclusions drawn, anifrolumab far exceeds the efficacy outlook for the current approved treatment landscape for SLE. That includes sifalimumab and rontalizumab, two anti-IFNα monoclonal antibodies, which have shown efficacy and good tolerability profiles [90, 522–524], but which lack the broad efficacy achieved by the complete blockade of type I interferon signalling.

The approval of anifrolumab, only the second biologic for lupus, reinvigorated the field and validated a long-known central role of type I interferons in SLE. This created excitement beyond the lupus field, as trials are being conducted for other indications including for Rheumatoid Arthritis (NCT03435601), Primary Sjögren's Syndrome (NCT05383677), Systemic Sclerosis (NCT05925803), Progressive Vitiligo (NCT05917561), and Hidradenitis Suppurativa (NCT06374212). Regarding monogenic type I interferonopathies, as of yet, only one single patient carrying a *DNASE2* mutation has received anifrolumab, with remarkable amelioration [525]. While neurological involvement is frequent in *DNASE2* loss-of-function interferonopathies, this patient had normal neurologic status at the time of their treatment, thus it is not known whether this approach may be useful for treating psychocognitive symptoms.

6.2 JAK inhibitors

Inhibitors targeting the JAK/STAT signalling pathway have shown efficacy and promising results in various diseases. JAK inhibitors like tofacitinib, filgotinib, and upadacitinib have been approved for use in multiple disorders, modifying treatment algorithms across a range of disease states, including myeloproliferative neoplasms, rheumatoid arthritis, and various inflammatory dermatological disorders. The rapid and broad bench-to-bedside translation is a testament to the importance of this pathway to different disease mechanisms. For neurological diseases, however, there has been slower adoption, despite promising preclinical results. Notably, inhibition of JAK/STAT signalling in mouse models of DS resulted in attenuated interferon-response signatures [307]. Dp16 mice, which harbour a duplication of murine chromosome 16 and which is orthologous to human chromosome 21, show upregulation of inflammatory and interferon responses in brain, along with other tissues [307]. Treatment with the JAK1/2 inhibitor baricitinib caused attenuation of many dysregulated signatures of Dp16, including of interferon-response genes, and including in the brain. Importantly, a patient treated with tofacitinib for an underlying alopecia areata [526] displayed marked inhibition of interferon-response signatures in the circulation to levels similar to euploid and healthy individuals, including abrogation of the major signalling chemokines CXCL9 and CXCL10 [307]. Beyond neuroinflammation due to genomic aberrations specifically associated with DS, JAK/STAT signalling inhibition using ruxolitinib was also capable of inhibiting type I interferon-driven neurodegeneration in a model of ALS-FTD [527]. Specifically, C9orf72-mutation associated FTD and ALS are found to accumulate cytoplasmic dsRNAs which trigger production of type I interferons, and culminate in JAK/STAT-mediated neuronal cell death. Proof-of-concept evidence exists that the interferonopathy in DS and nucleic acid accumulation in FTD and ALS can be modulated pharmacologically by JAK/STAT inhibitors, and taken together with the mouse model assessments suggests that neurocognitive protection may be possible.

There are still questions about the efficacy of JAK/STAT inhibition for neurological disease. In both AGS [528–532], SPENCD [533], and SAVI [530] JAK1/2 inhibitors caused systemic amelioration of dermatologic or pulmonary disease, including of systemic type I interferon signatures, but neurological improvement was limited or absent. Frequent infections are also seen, as essentially all cytokine signalling is inhibited, and is an important consideration especially for paediatric patients lacking fully developed adaptive immunity relying on innate immunity. Often, this has led to transient discontinuation of therapy, which may have impacted outcomes. This suggests that targeted therapy, particularly one specifically targeting type I interferons, may be more efficacious. A handful of case studies have reported better success for neurologic signs in AGS [534–536], of which one demonstrated reduced type I interferon in CSF for one patient [534], arguing perhaps in favour of early and uninterrupted therapy. Assessment of CSF exposure of the inhibitors reveals levels below 10% that of plasma, which is reflected by poor biomarker responses in CSF compared to circulation [531] indicating a need for brain penetrant molecules for consistent responses.

6.3 Experimental therapeutic approaches

Few other interferon-targeting treatment approaches exist, and most remain for now experimental. Reverse-transcriptase inhibitors were found to strongly inhibit interferon-responses in circulation and in CSF in AGS [537]. It is thought that repressing expression of otherwise uncontrolled endogenous retroelements may be sufficient to regulate type I interferons, but perhaps not all patients may benefit similarly. These changes were most efficacious in patients carrying mutations in components of the RNASEH2 complex, and signatures were reversed upon discontinuation indicating specificity of the signal to the treatment. It is unclear if this treatment approach could be used for lasting responses with favourable clinical outcome, especially in the brain. It is also difficult to extrapolate from the clinical course of HAND where, despite anti-retroviral therapy, neurocognitive deterioration continues, as pathological mechanisms are different. Interestingly, trials are being conducted in Alzheimer's disease (NCT04552795) which may yield better understanding of how retroelements are implicated in neuroinflammation [538].

Synthetic nucleotides for gene silencing are being intensely researched for drug development [539]. Antisense oligonucleotides (ASOs) hybridise cellular RNA and modulate processing, splicing, cause competitive inhibition, block the translational machinery, or degrade the bound target mRNAs. Treatments based on ASOs have already reached the clinic for genetic disorders such as Duchenne muscular dystrophy [540] and SOD1 mutation-associated ALS [541]. In a type I interferonopathy mouse model, intrathecal delivery of ASOs targeting the *Ifnar1* gene rescued neuropathological phenotypes by reducing type I interferon-responses, which led to reduced gliosis, immune cell infiltration in brain, reduced neuronal death and tissue destruction, and prevention of BBB leakage [542]. Such an approach lends itself well to monogenic type I interferonopathies and, coupled with a rationale-driven administration method, may benefit patients based on their personalised symptomatology.

7. Conclusion and future directions

7.1 Summary and implications

Type I interferons are cytokines that play a crucial role in the innate immune response against viral infections and in anti-tumour activities within the CNS. Overactivity of this pathway, however, results in aberrant responses that cause neurodegeneration. Concrete examples of this are persistent viral infections of the brain causing HAND, neurocognitive symptoms in archetypically type I interferon-driven diseases such as SLE and AGS, and the profound psychocognitive effects of therapies with IFNα and IFNβ. Type I interferons are also found aberrantly overexpressed in more common diseases such as major depression, AD and dementia attributed to TBI, DS, and ageing, giving rise to the hypothesis that they may be detrimental more widely across neurodegeneration. With compelling evidence from preclinical models in all aforementioned disorders, there is interest in further developing therapeutics that target this pathway.

This also has implications for current clinical practice. The historical significance, extensive clinical experience, and diverse applications of IFNα and IFNβ therapies contribute to their sustained use in treatment practices. These once pioneering biologics remain relevant due to their foundational role in immunology and their proven benefits in some clinical indications. However, their long-lasting effects on the brain are an important consideration, and perhaps even more so due to their seeming implication in natural and disease-associated cognitive decline.

7.2 Limitations, challenges, and open questions

Open questions remain on the therapeutic potential of targeting type I interferon signalling for neurological disorders. SLE, a disease caused by systemic type I interferons, leads to neuropsychiatric symptoms, including depression, in a substantial proportion of patients, mirroring exogenous therapy with IFNα or IFNβ. It will therefore be important to evaluate if blockade of type I interferon signalling affects neuropsychiatric outcomes in lupus. The most direct evidence for this may come with the now marketed IFNAR1-targeting anifrolumab. Though trials performed to date were not powered for addressing this, long-term follow-up and more extensive clinical experience should clarify this. Also, it is unclear whether targeting the IFNAR systemically will be sufficient to influence the CNS. This may depend on the CNS-penetrance of anifrolumab, which has not been evaluated. Typical CNS penetrance of antibodies is 0.1%, so for a dose of 300 mg it may be conceivable that sufficient antibody reaches the brain parenchyma, but not necessarily that sufficient target is neutralised. High, ubiquitous, target expression explains a short half-life of the antibody, meaning lower amounts of free antibody capable of reaching the brain. PK/PD relationship studies from the TULIP-1 trial reveal that only the 300 mg dosing schedule allowed for approximately IC_{90} inhibition of interferon-response [513]. The lower dose group receiving 150 mg had sub-optimal or no inhibition of the systemic 21-IFNGS when the C average concentration in plasma was below 11.5 μg/mL, and at least 32 μg/mL plasma exposure was necessary to consistently and durably achieve IC_{90} [513]. This indicates that the current 300 mg IV Q4W regimen, while sufficient to block type I interferon signalling in circulation, may not be sufficient to achieve an effect in brain, and higher doses may be needed. Importantly, this problem applies to all neurologic and neurodegenerative diseases caused by type I interferons, so it remains to be determined whether anifrolumab in its current format may be sufficient to treat type I interferonopathies, AD, TBI, or depression.

Delivery of antibodies across the BBB is a hot research topic and remains a current challenge. Brain shuttling technologies are being developed [543], and higher brain penetrance is being achieved by adding shuttle peptides [544], receptor-mediated transcytosis mechanisms [545], and exosome [546] or viral [547] vector-mediated expression. Developing brain-penetrant IFNAR-inhibiting therapeutic compounds may be required to achieve neuropsychiatric or neurodegenerative improvement in type I interferon-driven diseases. Small molecules targeting upstream or downstream elements of the type I interferon pathway exist, and may be easier to be made brain penetrant.

Achieving clinical efficacy for neurologic disorders often requires long trials because of the inherent complexity of the nervous system and length of disease progression. Trials with anifrolumab have confirmed the importance of the type I interferon pathway in viral defence. Thus, further safety considerations may need to be addressed by future type I interferon-directed therapies, especially if made brain-targeting. Herpes zoster screening and patient selection may be needed to stave off serious adverse events, particularly in long trials. From a personalised medicine perspective, it may also become important to evaluate whether wider viral screening could inform response rates and side effects, as other immunological mechanisms may take over antiviral function.

In recent years there has been enormous advance in the use of neurological biomarkers, particularly NfL, following regulatory approval by the FDA as a surrogate marker of neurodegeneration in ALS [548, 549]. Unsurprisingly, the number of clinical trials of CNS diseases utilising this biomarker has been steadily increasing [548]. Broadened clinical use may also give further clues about the relationship with type I interferons and whether interferon-targeting therapies lead to any meaningful change in plasma or CSF NfL. NfL has already been shown to be correlated with IFNα in HAND [425]. It is unknown whether type I interferonopathies – archetypical neuroinflammatory diseases – display NfL release in plasma or CSF. This assessment could allow a better understanding of the mechanisms of neurodegeneration in a purely type I interferon-driven group of diseases In SLE, a disease characterised by systemic type I interferons, elevated NfL levels, particularly in patients with neuropsychiatric symptoms [83, 84, 86], may correlate with CSF or plasma IFNα or interferon-response signatures. As neuropsychiatric amelioration has for the most part not correlated well with general disease response, another interesting metric will be the assessment of NfL during therapy, and especially with the IFNAR pathway targeting therapies.

An important current consideration is whether it will be feasible to move away entirely from IFNα and IFNβ therapies. For MS, emerging treatments are proving to be more effective than IFNβ therapy, indicating a potential shift in therapeutic approaches [550]. In the context of chronic HCV, patients report better quality of life with oral antivirals than antivirals plus IFNα [551]. Newer generation antivirals may slowly phase out the need for interferons in viral infection [182, 183]. For cancer, new interest in the tumour microenvironment has created excitement leading to reticence in phasing out interferons from clinical care [552]. Some use may still remain for exogenous interferon therapies, particularly for high-risk patients in low-survivable diseases [553] where long-term neurocognitive effects may be less relevant or managed for the survival duration. Nevertheless, checkpoint blockade inhibitors [184], and immunomodulating therapies [155, 185] have allowed for advances in our understanding of cancer biology, and the creation of new classes of therapeutics.

Rare diseases can often inform findings relevant to more common diseases. Neurologic disorders are no exception. A prominent example is the role that early onset familial Alzheimer's disease, a very rare monogenic form of Alzheimer's, has had on shaping the understanding of sporadic disease. Perhaps the most important open question is whether our understanding of these relatively newly discovered type I interferonopathies may help develop therapeutics for more common, or equally devastating, neurologic diseases.

Acknowledgements

The author wishes to acknowledge the helpful editing, discussion, and scientific literature knowledge and contributions of Dr. Morgan Le Roux-Bourdieu and Rosaria Luongo. The author apologises for not being able to include the many other important articles that have contributed to the development of the type I interferon field.

Conflict of interest

A.M. is a full-time employee of AC Immune SA, a for-profit clinical-stage biotech. Other than salary, A.M. holds no equity, shares or financial conflicts of interest to disclose. The views expressed in this chapter are solely those of the author and the company had no role in the writing or editing of this chapter. At the time of writing, AC Immune SA is not pursuing any commercial interests related to interferons or their clinical use.

Author details

Alessio Mylonas[1,2]

1 Swiss Federal Institute of Technology Lausanne (EPFL), Lausanne, Switzerland

2 AC Immune SA, EPFL Innovation Park, Lausanne, Switzerland

*Address all correspondence to: alessio.mylonas@epfl.ch

References

[1] Crow YJ. Type I interferonopathies: A novel set of inborn errors of immunity. Annals of the New York Academy of Sciences. 2011;**1238**:91-98

[2] Isaacs A, Lindenmann J. Virus interference. I. The interferon. Proceedings of the Royal Society of London. Series B, Biological Sciences. 1957;**147**:258-267

[3] Isaacs A, Lindenmann J, Valentine RC. Virus interference. II. Some properties of interferon. Proceedings of the Royal Society B: Biological Sciences. 1957;**147**:268-273

[4] Merigan TC, Reed SE, Hall TS, et al. Inhibition of respiratory virus infection by locally applied interferon. Lancet. 1973;**1**:563-567

[5] Gresser I, Bourali C, Lévy JP, et al. Increased survival in mice inoculated with tumor cells and treated with interferon preparations. Proceedings of the National Academy of Sciences of the United States of America. 1969;**63**:51-57

[6] Haglund S, Lundquist PG, Cantell K, et al. Interferon therapy in juvenile laryngeal papillomatosis. Archives of Otolaryngology. 1981;**107**:327-332

[7] Jacobs L, O'Malley J, Freeman A, et al. Intrathecal interferon reduces exacerbations of multiple sclerosis. Science. 1981;**214**:1026-1028

[8] Priestman TJ. Initial evaluation of human lymphoblastoid interferon in patients with advanced malignant disease. Lancet. 1980;**2**:113-118

[9] Scott GM, Secher DS, Flowers D, et al. Toxicity of interferon. British Medical Journal (Clinical Research Ed.). 1981;**282**:1345-1348

[10] Smedley H, Katrak M, Sikora K, et al. Neurological effects of recombinant human interferon. British Medical Journal (Clinical Research Ed.). 1983;**286**:262-264

[11] Rönnblom LE, Alm GV, Oberg KE. Possible induction of systemic lupus erythematosus by interferon-alpha treatment in a patient with a malignant carcinoid tumor. Journal of Internal Medicine. 1990;**227**:207-210

[12] Gresser J, Morel-Maroger L, Verroust P, et al. Anti-interferon globulin inhibits the development of glomerulonephritis in mice infected at birth with lymphocytic choriomeningitis virus. Proceedings of the National Academy of Sciences of the United States of America. 1978;**75**:3413-3416

[13] Gresser I. On the varied biologic effects of interferon. Cellular Immunology. 1977;**34**:406-415

[14] Elliott MJ, Maini RN, Feldmann M, et al. Treatment of rheumatoid arthritis with chimeric monoclonal antibodies to tumor necrosis factor alpha. Arthritis and Rheumatism. 1993;**58**:S92-S101

[15] Loncharich MF, Anderson CW. Interferon inhibition for lupus with anifrolumab: Critical appraisal of the evidence leading to FDA approval. ACR Open Rheumatology. 2022. pp. 486-491. DOI: 10.1002/acr2.11414

[16] Aicardi J, Goutières F. A progressive familial encephalopathy in infancy with calcifications of the basal ganglia and chronic cerebrospinal fluid lymphocytosis. Annals of Neurology. 1984;**15**:49-54

[17] Lebon P, Badoual J, Ponsot G, et al. Intrathecal synthesis of interferon-alpha

in infants with progressive familial encephalopathy. Journal of the Neurological Sciences. 1988;**84**:201-208

[18] Crow YJ, Hayward BE, Parmar R, et al. Mutations in the gene encoding the 3′-5′ DNA exonuclease TREX1 cause Aicardi-Goutières syndrome at the AGS1 locus. Nature Genetics. 2006;**38**:917-920

[19] Crow YJ, Leitch A, Hayward BE, et al. Mutations in genes encoding ribonuclease H2 subunits cause Aicardi-Goutières syndrome and mimic congenital viral brain infection. Nature Genetics. 2006;**38**:910-916

[20] Duncan CJA, Thompson BJ, Chen R, et al. Severe type I interferonopathy and unrestrained interferon signaling due to a homozygous germline mutation in STAT2. Science Immunology. 2019;**4**. DOI: 10.1126/sciimmunol.aav7501

[21] Duncan CJA, Hambleton S. Human disease phenotypes associated with loss and gain of function mutations in STAT2: Viral susceptibility and type I interferonopathy. Journal of Clinical Immunology. 2021;**41**:1446-1456

[22] Kozlova AL, Leonteva ME, Burlakov VI, et al. Clinical case of type I interferonopathy: Homozygous STAT2 gain-of-function mutation. Voprosy Gematologii/onkologii i Immunopatologii v Pediatrii. 2021;**20**:132-139

[23] Zhu G, Badonyi M, Franklin L, et al. Type I interferonopathy due to a homozygous loss-of-inhibitory function mutation in STAT2. Journal of Clinical Immunology. 2023;**43**:808-818

[24] Weidler S, Koss S, Wolf C, et al. A rare manifestation of STING-associated vasculopathy with onset in infancy: A case report. Pediatric Rheumatology Online Journal. 2024;**22**:9

[25] Schlee M, Hartmann G. Discriminating self from non-self in nucleic acid sensing. Nature Reviews. Immunology. 2016;**16**:566-580

[26] Platanias LC. Introduction: Interferon signals: What is classical and what is nonclassical? Journal of Interferon & Cytokine Research. 2005;**25**:732

[27] Majoros A, Platanitis E, Kernbauer-Hölzl E, et al. Canonical and non-canonical aspects of JAK–STAT signaling: Lessons from interferons for cytokine responses. Frontiers in Immunology. 2017;**8**:29

[28] Mazewski C, Perez RE, Fish EN, et al. Type I interferon (IFN)-regulated activation of canonical and non-canonical signaling pathways. Frontiers in Immunology. 2020;**11**:606456

[29] Kadowaki N, Antonenko S, Lau JY, et al. Natural interferon alpha/beta-producing cells link innate and adaptive immunity. The Journal of Experimental Medicine. 2000;**192**:219-226

[30] Hoebe K, Janssen E, Beutler B. The interface between innate and adaptive immunity. Nature Immunology. 2004;**5**:971-974

[31] Hertzog PJ. Overview. Type I interferons as primers, activators and inhibitors of innate and adaptive immune responses. Immunology and Cell Biology. 2012;**90**:471-473

[32] Nesterova IV, Kovaleva SV, Malinovskaya VV, et al. Congenital and acquired interferonopathies: Differentiated approaches to interferon therapy. In: Innate Immunity in Health and Disease. London, UK: IntechOpen; 2020. Epub ahead of print 2020. DOI: 10.5772/intechopen.91723

[33] Møller RS, Zhao L, Shoaff JR, et al. Incidence of Aicardi-Goutières syndrome and KCNT1-related epilepsy in Denmark. Molecular Genetics and Metabolism Reports. 2022;**33**:100924

[34] Liu A, Ying S. Aicardi-Goutières syndrome: A monogenic type I interferonopathy. Scandinavian Journal of Immunology. 2023;**98**:e13314

[35] du Moulin M, Nürnberg P, Crow YJ, et al. Cerebral vasculopathy is a common feature in Aicardi-Goutieres syndrome associated with SAMHD1 mutations. Proceedings of the National Academy of Sciences of the United States of America. 2011;**108**:E232; author reply E233

[36] Piccoli C, Bronner N, Gavazzi F, et al. Late-onset Aicardi-Goutières syndrome: A characterization of presenting clinical features. Pediatric Neurology. 2021;**115**:1-6

[37] Barth PG, Walter A, van Gelderen I. Aicardi-Goutières syndrome: A genetic microangiopathy? Acta Neuropathologica. 1999;**98**:212-216

[38] Barth PG. The neuropathology of Aicardi-Goutières syndrome. European Journal of Pediatric Neurology. 2002;**6**(Suppl. A):A27-A31 discussion A37

[39] Østergaard JR, Christensen T. Aicardi-Goutières syndrome: Neuroradiological findings after nine years of follow-up. European Journal of Pediatric Neurology. 2004;**8**:243-246

[40] Rasmussen M, Skullerud K, Bakke SJ, et al. Cerebral thrombotic microangiopathy and antiphospholipid antibodies in Aicardi-Goutieres syndrome–report of two sisters. Neuropediatrics. 2005;**36**:40-44

[41] Maheshwari U, Huang S-F, Sridhar S, et al. The interplay between brain vascular calcification and microglia. Frontiers in Aging Neuroscience. 2022;**14**:848495

[42] Rodero MP, Decalf J, Bondet V, et al. Detection of interferon alpha protein reveals differential levels and cellular sources in disease. The Journal of Experimental Medicine. 2017;**214**:1547-1555

[43] Lodi L, Melki I, Bondet V, et al. Differential expression of interferon-alpha protein provides clues to tissue specificity across type I interferonopathies. Journal of Clinical Immunology. 2021;**41**:603-609

[44] Viengkhou B, Hayashida E, McGlasson S, et al. The brain microvasculature is a primary mediator of interferon-α neurotoxicity in human cerebral interferonopathies. Immunity. 2024;**57**:1696-1709.e10

[45] Rice GI, Forte GMA, Szynkiewicz M, et al. Assessment of interferon-related biomarkers in Aicardi-Goutières syndrome associated with mutations in TREX1, RNASEH2A, RNASEH2B, RNASEH2C, SAMHD1, and ADAR: A case–control study. Lancet Neurology. 2013;**12**:1159-1169

[46] Wang BX, Grover SA, Kannu P, et al. Interferon-stimulated gene expression as a preferred biomarker for disease activity in Aicardi-Goutières syndrome. Journal of Interferon & Cytokine Research. 2017;**37**:147-152

[47] Kim H, de Jesus AA, Brooks SR, et al. Development of a validated interferon score using nanostring technology. Journal of Interferon & Cytokine Research. 2018;**38**:171-185

[48] Pescarmona R, Belot A, Villard M, et al. Comparison of RT-qPCR and nanostring in the measurement of blood

interferon response for the diagnosis of type I interferonopathies. Cytokine. 2019;**113**:446-452

[49] de Jesus AA, Hou Y, Brooks S, et al. Distinct interferon signatures and cytokine patterns define additional systemic autoinflammatory diseases. The Journal of Clinical Investigation. 2020;**130**(4):1669-1682

[50] Demers-Mathieu V. Optimal selection of IFN-α-inducible genes to determine type I interferon signature improves the diagnosis of systemic lupus erythematosus. Biomedicine. 2023;**11**. DOI: 10.3390/biomedicines11030864

[51] Rice GI, Bond J, Asipu A, et al. Mutations involved in Aicardi-Goutières syndrome implicate SAMHD1 as regulator of the innate immune response. Nature Genetics. 2009;**41**:829-832

[52] Rice GI, Kasher PR, Forte GMA, et al. Mutations in ADAR1 cause Aicardi-Goutières syndrome associated with a type I interferon signature. Nature Genetics. 2012;**44**:1243-1248

[53] Gray EE, Treuting PM, Woodward JJ, et al. Cutting edge: cGAS is required for lethal autoimmune disease in the Trex1-deficient mouse model of Aicardi-Goutières syndrome. Journal of Immunology. 2015;**195**:1939-1943

[54] Ablasser A, Hemmerling I, Schmid-Burgk JL, et al. TREX1 deficiency triggers cell-autonomous immunity in a cGAS-dependent manner. Journal of Immunology. 2014;**192**:5993-5997

[55] Lee-Kirsch MA, Gong M, Chowdhury D, et al. Mutations in the gene encoding the 3′-5′ DNA exonuclease TREX1 are associated with systemic lupus erythematosus. Nature Genetics. 2007;**39**:1065-1067

[56] Rice G, Newman WG, Dean J, et al. Heterozygous mutations in TREX1 cause familial chilblain lupus and dominant Aicardi-Goutieres syndrome. American Journal of Human Genetics. 2007;**80**:811-815

[57] Günther C, Kind B, Reijns MAM, et al. Defective removal of ribonucleotides from DNA promotes systemic autoimmunity. The Journal of Clinical Investigation. 2015;**125**:413-424

[58] Pokatayev V, Hasin N, Chon H, et al. RNase H2 catalytic core Aicardi-Goutières syndrome-related mutant invokes cGAS-STING innate immune-sensing pathway in mice. The Journal of Experimental Medicine. 2016;**213**:329-336

[59] Uggenti C, Lepelley A, Depp M, et al. cGAS-mediated induction of type I interferon due to inborn errors of histone pre-mRNA processing. Nature Genetics. 2020;**52**:1364-1372

[60] Jiao H, Wachsmuth L, Wolf S, et al. ADAR1 averts fatal type I interferon induction by ZBP1. Nature. 2022;**607**:776-783

[61] Hubbard NW, Ames JM, Maurano M, et al. ADAR1 mutation causes ZBP1-dependent immunopathology. Nature. 2022;**607**:769-775

[62] de Reuver R, Verdonck S, Dierick E, et al. ADAR1 prevents autoinflammation by suppressing spontaneous ZBP1 activation. Nature. 2022;**607**:784-789

[63] Rice GI, Del Toro DY, Jenkinson EM, et al. Gain-of-function mutations in IFIH1 cause a spectrum of human disease phenotypes associated with upregulated

type I interferon signaling. Nature Genetics. 2014;**46**:503-509

[64] Oda H, Nakagawa K, Abe J, et al. Aicardi-Goutières syndrome is caused by IFIH1 mutations. American Journal of Human Genetics. 2014;**95**:121-125

[65] Zhang X, Bogunovic D, Payelle-Brogard B, et al. Human intracellular ISG15 prevents interferon-α/β over-amplification and auto-inflammation. Nature. 2015;**517**:89-93

[66] Martin-Fernandez M, Bravo García-Morato M, Gruber C, et al. Systemic type I IFN inflammation in human ISG15 deficiency leads to necrotizing skin lesions. Cell Reports. 2020;**31**:107633

[67] Meuwissen MEC, Schot R, Buta S, et al. Human USP18 deficiency underlies type 1 interferonopathy leading to severe pseudo-TORCH syndrome. The Journal of Experimental Medicine. 2016;**213**:1163-1174

[68] François-Newton V, de Freitas M, Almeida G, Payelle-Brogard B, et al. USP18-based negative feedback control is induced by type I and type III interferons and specifically inactivates interferon α response. PLoS One. 2011;**6**:e22200

[69] Francois-Newton V, Livingstone M, Payelle-Brogard B, et al. USP18 establishes the transcriptional and anti-proliferative interferon α/β differential. The Biochemical Journal. 2012;**446**:509-516

[70] Goldmann T, Zeller N, Raasch J, et al. USP18 lack in microglia causes destructive interferonopathy of the mouse brain. The EMBO Journal. 2015;**34**:1612-1629

[71] Girschick H, Wolf C, Morbach H, et al. Severe immune dysregulation with neurological impairment and minor bone changes in a child with spondyloenchondrodysplasia due to two novel mutations in the ACP5 gene. Pediatric Rheumatology Online Journal. 2015;**13**:37

[72] Briggs TA, Rice GI, Adib N, et al. Spondyloenchondrodysplasia due to mutations in ACP5: A comprehensive survey. Journal of Clinical Immunology. 2016;**36**:220-234

[73] Bilginer Y, Düzova A, Topaloğlu R, et al. Three cases of spondyloenchondrodysplasia (SPENCD) with systemic lupus erythematosus: A case series and review of the literature. Lupus. 2016;**25**:760-765

[74] Kim H, Sanchez GAM, Goldbach-Mansky R. Insights from mendelian interferonopathies: Comparison of CANDLE, SAVI with AGS, Monogenic Lupus. Journal of Molecular Medicine. 2016;**94**:1111-1127

[75] Demirkaya E, Sahin S, Romano M, et al. New horizons in the genetic etiology of systemic lupus erythematosus and lupus-like disease: Monogenic lupus and beyond. Journal of Clinical Medicine. 2020;**9**. DOI: 10.3390/jcm9030712

[76] Tian J, Zhang D, Yao X, et al. Global epidemiology of systemic lupus erythematosus: A comprehensive systematic analysis and modeling study. Annals of the Rheumatic Diseases. 2023;**82**:351-356

[77] Hanly JG, Li Q, Su L, et al. Psychosis in systemic lupus erythematosus: Results from an international inception cohort study. Arthritis & Rhematology. 2019;**71**:281-289

[78] Govoni M, Hanly JG. The management of neuropsychiatric

lupus in the 21st century: Still so many unmet needs? Rheumatology (Oxford). 2020;**59**:v52-v62

[79] Unterman A, Nolte JES, Boaz M, et al. Neuropsychiatric syndromes in systemic lupus erythematosus: A meta-analysis. Seminars in Arthritis and Rheumatism. 2011;**41**:1-11

[80] Sarwar S, Mohamed AS, Rogers S, et al. Neuropsychiatric systemic lupus erythematosus: A 2021 update on diagnosis, management, and current challenges. Cureus. 2021;**13**:e17969

[81] ACR Ad Hoc Committee on Neuropsychiatric Lupus Nomenclature. The American college of rheumatology nomenclature and case definitions for neuropsychiatric lupus syndromes. Arthritis and Rheumatism. 1999;**42**:599-608

[82] Tjensvoll AB, Lauvsnes MB, Zetterberg H, et al. Neurofilament light is a biomarker of brain involvement in lupus and primary Sjögren's syndrome. Journal of Neurology. 2021;**268**:1385-1394

[83] Engel S, Boedecker S, Marczynski P, et al. Association of serum neurofilament light chain levels and neuropsychiatric manifestations in systemic lupus erythematosus. Therapeutic Advances in Neurological Disorders. 2021;**14**:17562864211051496

[84] Zervides KA, Janelidze S, Nystedt J, et al. Plasma and cerebrospinal fluid neurofilament light concentrations reflect neuronal damage in systemic lupus erythematosus. BMC Neurology. 2022;**22**:467

[85] Gaetani L, Blennow K, Calabresi P, et al. Neurofilament light chain as a biomarker in neurological disorders. Journal of Neurology, Neurosurgery, and Psychiatry. 2019;**90**:870-881

[86] Lauvsnes MB, Zetterberg H, Blennow K, et al. Neurofilament light in plasma is a potential biomarker of central nervous system involvement in systemic lupus erythematosus. Journal of Neurology. 2022;**269**:3064-3074

[87] de Vries B, Steup-Beekman GM, Haan J, et al. TREX1 gene variant in neuropsychiatric systemic lupus erythematosus. Annals of the Rheumatic Diseases. 2010;**69**:1886-1887

[88] Namjou B, Kothari PH, Kelly JA, et al. Evaluation of the TREX1 gene in a large multi-ancestral lupus cohort. Genes and Immunity. 2011;**12**:270-279

[89] Labouret M, Costi S, Bondet V, et al. Juvenile neuropsychiatric systemic lupus erythematosus: Identification of novel central neuroinflammation biomarkers. Journal of Clinical Immunology. 2023;**43**:615-624

[90] Khamashta M, Merrill JT, Werth VP, et al. Sifalimumab, an anti-interferon-α monoclonal antibody, in moderate to severe systemic lupus erythematosus: A randomized, double-blind, placebo-controlled study. Annals of the Rheumatic Diseases. 2016;**75**:1909-1916

[91] Houssiau FA, Thanou A, Mazur M, et al. IFN-α kinoid in systemic lupus erythematosus: Results from a phase IIb, randomized, placebo-controlled study. Annals of the Rheumatic Diseases. 2020;**79**:347-355

[92] Vital EM, Merrill JT, Morand EF, et al. Anifrolumab efficacy and safety by type I interferon gene signature and clinical subgroups in patients with SLE: Post hoc analysis of pooled data from two phase III trials. Annals of the Rheumatic Diseases. 2022;**81**:951-961

[93] Kalunian KC, Furie R, Morand EF, et al. A randomized, placebo-controlled phase III extension trial of the long-term safety and tolerability of anifrolumab in active systemic lupus erythematosus. Arthritis & Rhematology. 2023;**75**:253-265

[94] Yerram KV, Baisya R, Kumar P, et al. Serum interferon-alpha predicts in-hospital mortality in patients hospitalized with acute severe lupus. Lupus Science & Medicine. 2023;**10**. DOI: 10.1136/lupus-2023-000933

[95] Lebon P, Lenoir GR, Fischer A, et al. Synthesis of intrathecal interferon in systemic lupus erythematosus with neurological complications. British Medical Journal (Clinical Research Edition). 1983;**287**:1165

[96] Shiozawa S, Kuroki Y, Kim M, et al. Interferon-alpha in lupus psychosis. Arthritis and Rheumatism. 1992;**35**:417-422

[97] Fragoso-Loyo H, Atisha-Fregoso Y, Núñez-Alvarez CA, et al. Utility of interferon-α as a biomarker in central neuropsychiatric involvement in systemic lupus erythematosus. The Journal of Rheumatology. 2012;**39**:504-509

[98] Deane JA, Pisitkun P, Barrett RS, et al. Control of toll-like receptor 7 expression is essential to restrict autoimmunity and dendritic cell proliferation. Immunity. 2007;**27**:801-810

[99] Richard ML, Gilkeson G. Mouse models of lupus: What they tell us and what they do not. Lupus Science & Medicine. 2018;**5**:e000199

[100] Aw E, Zhang Y, Yalcin E, et al. Spatial enrichment of the type 1 interferon signature in the brain of a neuropsychiatric lupus murine model. Brain, Behavior, and Immunity. 2023;**114**:511-522

[101] Nomura A, Noto D, Murayama G, et al. Unique primed status of microglia under the systemic autoimmune condition of lupus-prone mice. Arthritis Research & Therapy. 2019;**21**:303

[102] Ramanujam M, Kahn P, Huang W, et al. Interferon-alpha treatment of female (NZW x BXSB)F(1) mice mimics some but not all features associated with the Yaa mutation. Arthritis and Rheumatism. 2009;**60**:1096-1101

[103] Zeng J, Meng X, Zhou P, et al. Interferon-α exacerbates neuropsychiatric phenotypes in lupus-prone mice. Arthritis Research & Therapy. 2019;**21**:205

[104] Åkesson K, Pettersson S, Ståhl S, et al. Kynurenine pathway is altered in patients with SLE and associated with severe fatigue. Lupus Science & Medicine. 2018;**5**:e000254

[105] Vogelgesang SA, Heyes MP, West SG, et al. Quinolinic acid in patients with systemic lupus erythematosus and neuropsychiatric manifestations. The Journal of Rheumatology. 1996;**23**:850-855

[106] Eryavuz Onmaz D, Tezcan D, Yilmaz S, et al. Altered kynurenine pathway metabolism and association with disease activity in patients with systemic lupus. Amino Acids. 2023;**55**:1937-1947

[107] Anderson EW, Fishbein J, Hong J, et al. Quinolinic acid, a kynurenine/tryptophan pathway metabolite, associates with impaired cognitive test performance in systemic lupus erythematosus. Lupus Science & Medicine. 2021;**8**. DOI: 10.1136/lupus-2021-000559

[108] Yan EB, Frugier T, Lim CK, et al. Activation of the kynurenine pathway and increased production of the excitotoxin quinolinic acid following traumatic brain injury in humans. Journal of Neuroinflammation. 2015;**12**:110

[109] Pérez-De La Cruz V, Carrillo-Mora P, Santamaría A. Quinolinic acid, an endogenous molecule combining excitotoxicity, oxidative stress and other toxic mechanisms. International Journal of Tryptophan Research. 2012;**5**:1-8

[110] Latif-Hernandez A, Shah D, Ahmed T, et al. Quinolinic acid injection in mouse medial prefrontal cortex affects reversal learning abilities, cortical connectivity and hippocampal synaptic plasticity. Scientific Reports. 2016;**6**:36489

[111] Anderson EW, Jin Y, Shih A, et al. Associations between circulating interferon and kynurenine/tryptophan pathway metabolites: Support for a novel potential mechanism for cognitive dysfunction in SLE. Lupus Science & Medicine. 2022;**9**. DOI: 10.1136/lupus-2022-000808

[112] Hestad K, Alexander J, Rootwelt H, et al. The role of tryptophan dysmetabolism and quinolinic acid in depressive and neurodegenerative diseases. Biomolecules. 2022;**12**. DOI: 10.3390/biom12070998

[113] Wichers MC, Koek GH, Robaeys G, et al. IDO and interferon-alpha-induced depressive symptoms: A shift in hypothesis from tryptophan depletion to neurotoxicity. Molecular Psychiatry. 2005;**10**:538-544

[114] Lood C, Tydén H, Gullstrand B, et al. Type I interferon-mediated skewing of the serotonin synthesis is associated with severe disease in systemic lupus erythematosus. PLoS One. 2015;**10**:e0125109

[115] Müller N, Schwarz MJ. The immune-mediated alteration of serotonin and glutamate: Toward an integrated view of depression. Molecular Psychiatry. 2007;**12**:988-1000

[116] Meyerhoff J, Dorsch CA. Decreased platelet serotonin levels in systemic lupus erythematosus. Arthritis and Rheumatism. 1981;**24**:1495-1500

[117] Nikolopoulos D, Nakos-Bimpos M, Manolakou T, et al. Impaired serotonin synthesis in hippocampus of murine lupus represents an early neuropsychiatric event. Lupus. 2024;**33**:166-171

[118] Merimsky O, Reider-Groswasser I, Inbar M, et al. Interferon-related mental deterioration and behavioral changes in patients with renal cell carcinoma. European Journal of Cancer. 1990;**26**:596-600

[119] Poutiainen E, Hokkanen L, Niemi ML, et al. Reversible cognitive decline during high-dose alpha-interferon treatment. Pharmacology, Biochemistry, and Behavior. 1994;**47**:901-905

[120] Valentine AD, Meyers CA, Kling MA, et al. Mood and cognitive side effects of interferon-alpha therapy. Seminars in Oncology. 1998;**25**:39-47

[121] Capuron L, Ravaud A. Prediction of the depressive effects of interferon alfa therapy by the patient's initial affective state. The New England Journal of Medicine. 1999;**340**:1370-1370

[122] Dieperink E, Willenbring M, Ho SB. Neuropsychiatric symptoms associated

with hepatitis C and interferon alpha: A review. The American Journal of Psychiatry. 2000;**157**:867-876

[123] Musselman DL, Lawson DH, Gumnick JF, et al. Paroxetine for the prevention of depression induced by high-dose interferon alfa. The New England Journal of Medicine. 2001;**344**:961-966

[124] Hauser P, Khosla J, Aurora H, et al. A prospective study of the incidence and open-label treatment of interferon-induced major depressive disorder in patients with hepatitis C. Molecular Psychiatry. 2002;7:942-947

[125] Gohier B, Goeb J-L, Rannou-Dubas K, et al. Hepatitis C, alpha interferon, anxiety and depression disorders: A prospective study of 71 patients. The World Journal of Biological Psychiatry. 2003;**4**:115-118

[126] Reichenberg A, Gorman JM, Dieterich DT. Interferon-induced depression and cognitive impairment in hepatitis C virus patients: A 72 week prospective study. AIDS. 2005;**19**(Suppl. 3):S174-S178

[127] Heinze S, Egberts F, Rötzer S, et al. Depressive mood changes and psychiatric symptoms during 12-month low-dose interferon-alpha treatment in patients with malignant melanoma: Results from the multicenter DeCOG trial. Journal of Immunotherapy. 2010;**33**:106-114

[128] Udina M, Castellví P, Moreno-España J, et al. Interferon-induced depression in chronic hepatitis C: A systematic review and meta-analysis. The Journal of Clinical Psychiatry. 2012;**73**:1128-1138

[129] Baranyi A, Meinitzer A, Stepan A, et al. A biopsychosocial model of interferon-alpha-induced depression in patients with chronic hepatitis C infection. Psychotherapy and Psychosomatics. 2013;**82**:332-340

[130] Cattie JE, Letendre SL, Woods SP, et al. Persistent neurocognitive decline in a clinic sample of hepatitis C virus-infected persons receiving interferon and ribavirin treatment. Journal of Neurovirology. 2014;**20**:561-570

[131] Huckans M, Fuller B, Wheaton V, et al. A longitudinal study evaluating the effects of interferon-alpha therapy on cognitive and psychiatric function in adults with chronic hepatitis C. Journal of Psychosomatic Research. 2015;**78**:184-192

[132] Sarkar S, Sarkar R, Berg T, et al. Sadness and mild cognitive impairment as predictors for interferon-alpha-induced depression in patients with hepatitis C. The British Journal of Psychiatry. 2015;**206**:45-51

[133] Chiu WC, Su YP, Su KP, et al. Recurrence of depressive disorders after interferon-induced depression. Translational Psychiatry. 2017;7:e1026

[134] Jain KK. Drug-induced Neurological Disorders. Cham: Springer International Publishing; 2021. Epub ahead of print 2021. DOI: 10.1007/978-3-030-73503-6

[135] Meyers CA, Scheibel RS, Forman AD. Persistent neurotoxicity of systemically administered interferon-alpha. Neurology. 1991;**41**:672-676

[136] Pavol MA, Meyers CA, Rexer JL, et al. Pattern of neurobehavioral deficits associated with interferon alfa therapy for leukemia. Neurology. 1995;**45**:947-950

[137] Capuron L, Ravaud A, Dantzer R. Timing and specificity of the cognitive changes induced by interleukin-2 and

interferon-alpha treatments in cancer patients. Psychosomatic Medicine. 2001;**63**:376-386

[138] Capuron L, Gumnick JF, Musselman DL, et al. Neurobehavioral effects of interferon-alpha in cancer patients: Phenomenology and paroxetine responsiveness of symptom dimensions. Neuropsychopharmacology. 2002;**26**:643-652

[139] Wichers MC, Koek GH, Robaeys G, et al. Early increase in vegetative symptoms predicts IFN-alpha-induced cognitive-depressive changes. Psychological Medicine. 2005;**35**:433-441

[140] Raison CL, Demetrashvili M, Capuron L, et al. Neuropsychiatric adverse effects of interferon-alpha: Recognition and management. CNS Drugs. 2005;**19**:105-123

[141] Kluin-Nelemans HC, Buck G, le Cessie S, et al. Randomized comparison of low-dose versus high-dose interferon-Alfa in chronic myeloid leukemia: Prospective collaboration of 3 joint trials by the MRC and HOVON groups. Blood. 2004;**103**:4408-4415

[142] Morasco BJ, Loftis JM, Indest DW, et al. Prophylactic antidepressant treatment in patients with hepatitis C on antiviral therapy: A double-blind, placebo-controlled trial. Psychosomatics. 2010;**51**:401-408

[143] Diez-Quevedo C, Masnou H, Planas R, et al. Prophylactic treatment with escitalopram of pegylated interferon alfa-2a-induced depression in hepatitis C: A 12-week, randomized, double-blind, placebo-controlled trial. The Journal of Clinical Psychiatry. 2011;**72**:522-528

[144] Dipasquale O, Cooper EA, Tibble J, et al. Interferon-α acutely impairs whole-brain functional connectivity network architecture - A preliminary study. Brain, Behavior, and Immunity. 2016;**58**:31-39

[145] Højsgaard Chow H, Schreiber K, Magyari M, et al. Progressive multiple sclerosis, cognitive function, and quality of life. Brain and Behavior: A Cognitive Neuroscience Perspective. 2018;**8**:e00875

[146] Heesen C, Schulz KH, Fiehler J, et al. Correlates of cognitive dysfunction in multiple sclerosis. Brain, Behavior, and Immunity. 2010;**24**:1148-1155

[147] Rocca MA, Valsasina P, Hulst HE, et al. Functional correlates of cognitive dysfunction in multiple sclerosis: A multicenter fMRI Study. Human Brain Mapping. 2014;**35**:5799-5814

[148] Chiba K, Kataoka H, Seki N, et al. Fingolimod (FTY720), sphingosine 1-phosphate receptor modulator, shows superior efficacy as compared with interferon-β in mouse experimental autoimmune encephalomyelitis. International Immunopharmacology. 2011;**11**:366-372

[149] Pozzilli C, Prosperini L, Borriello G. Treating multiple sclerosis with fingolimod or intramuscular interferon. Expert Opinion on Pharmacotherapy. 2010;**11**:1957-1960

[150] Cohen JA, Barkhof F, Comi G, et al. Oral fingolimod or intramuscular interferon for relapsing multiple sclerosis. The New England Journal of Medicine. 2010;**362**:402-415

[151] Gasperini C, Ruggieri S. Development of oral agent in the treatment of multiple sclerosis: How the first available oral therapy, fingolimod will change therapeutic paradigm

approach. Drug Design, Development and Therapy. 2012;**6**:175-186

[152] El Ayoubi NK, Bou Reslan SW, Baalbaki MM, et al. Effect of fingolimod vs. interferon treatment on OCT measurements and cognitive function in RRMS. Multiple Sclerosis and Related Disorders. 2021;**53**:103041

[153] Krupp L, Banwell B, Chitnis T, et al. Effect of fingolimod on health-related quality of life in pediatric patients with multiple sclerosis: Results from the phase 3 PARADIGMS study. BMJ Neurology Open. 2022;**4**:e000215

[154] Bascuñana P, Möhle L, Brackhan M, et al. Fingolimod as a treatment in neurologic disorders beyond multiple sclerosis. Drugs in Research & Development. 2020;**20**:197-207

[155] Yang JH, Rempe T, Whitmire N, et al. Therapeutic advances in multiple sclerosis. Frontiers in Neurology. 2022;**13**:824926

[156] Wichers MC, Maes M. The role of indoleamine 2,3-dioxygenase (IDO) in the pathophysiology of interferon-alpha-induced depression. Journal of Psychiatry & Neuroscience. 2004;**29**:11-17

[157] Kirkegaard C, Faber J. The role of thyroid hormones in depression. European Journal of Endocrinology. 1998;**138**:1-9

[158] Hage M, Azar S. The link between thyroid function and depression. Journal of Thyroid Research. 2020;**2012**

[159] Thvilum M, Brandt F, Almind D, et al. Increased psychiatric morbidity before and after the diagnosis of hypothyroidism: A nationwide register study. Thyroid. 2014;**24**:802-808

[160] Bauer M, Whybrow PC. Role of thyroid hormone therapy in depressive disorders. Journal of Endocrinological Investigation. 2021;**44**:2341-2347

[161] Loftis JM, Wall JM, Linardatos E, et al. A quantitative assessment of depression and thyroid dysfunction secondary to interferon-alpha therapy in patients with hepatitis C. Journal of Endocrinological Investigation. 2004;**27**:RC16-20

[162] Carella C, Mazziotti G, Amato G, et al. Interferon-α-related thyroid disease: Pathophysiological, epidemiological, and clinical aspects. The Journal of Clinical Endocrinology & Metabolism. 2004;**89**:3656-3661

[163] Tran HA, Reeves GEM, Jones TL. The natural history of interferon-alpha2b-induced thyroiditis and its exclusivity in a cohort of patients with chronic hepatitis C infection. QJM. 2009;**102**:117-122

[164] Yan Z, Fan K, Fan Y, et al. Thyroid dysfunction in Chinese patients with chronic hepatitis C treated with interferon alpha: Incidence, long-term outcome and predictive factors. Hepatitis Monthly. 2012;**12**:e6390

[165] Nair Kesavachandran C, Haamann F, Nienhaus A. Frequency of thyroid dysfunctions during interferon alpha treatment of single and combination therapy in hepatitis C virus-infected patients: A systematic review based analysis. PLoS One. 2013;**8**:e55364

[166] Blank T, Detje CN, Spieß A, et al. Brain endothelial- and epithelial-specific interferon receptor chain 1 drives virus-induced sickness behavior and cognitive impairment. Immunity. 2016;**44**:901-912

[167] Hunt D, Kavanagh D, Drummond I, et al. Thrombotic microangiopathy

associated with interferon beta. The New England Journal of Medicine. 2014;**370**:1270-1271

[168] Kavanagh D, McGlasson S, Jury A, et al. Type I interferon causes thrombotic microangiopathy by a dose-dependent toxic effect on the microvasculature. Blood. 2016;**128**:2824-2833

[169] Wang C, Fang W, Sun W, et al. Clinical characteristics, treatments, and outcomes of interferon-beta-induced thrombotic microangiopathy: A literature-based retrospective analysis. Therapeutic Advances in Neurological Disorders. 2023;**16**:17562864231216634

[170] Sarbu N, Alobeidi F, Toledano P, et al. Brain abnormalities in newly diagnosed neuropsychiatric lupus: Systematic MRI approach and correlation with clinical and laboratory data in a large multicenter cohort. Autoimmunity Reviews. 2015;**14**:153-159

[171] Vlkolinský R, Siggins GR, Campbell IL, et al. Acute exposure to CXC chemokine ligand 10, but not its chronic astroglial production, alters synaptic plasticity in mouse hippocampal slices. Journal of Neuroimmunology. 2004;**150**:37-47

[172] Su K-P, Huang S-Y, Peng C-Y, et al. Phospholipase A2 and cyclooxygenase 2 genes influence the risk of interferon-alpha-induced depression by regulating polyunsaturated fatty acids levels. Biological Psychiatry. 2010;**67**:550-557

[173] Mesripour A, Shahnooshi S, Hajhashemi V. Celecoxib, ibuprofen, and indomethacin alleviate depression-like behavior induced by interferon-Alfa in mice. Journal of Complementary and Integrative Medicine. 2019;**17**. DOI: 10.1515/jcim-2019-0016

[174] Köhler O, Benros ME, Nordentoft M, et al. Effect of anti-inflammatory treatment on depression, depressive symptoms, and adverse effects: A systematic review and meta-analysis of randomized clinical trials. JAMA Psychiatry. 2014;**71**:1381-1391

[175] Bai S, Guo W, Feng Y, et al. Efficacy and safety of anti-inflammatory agents for the treatment of major depressive disorder: A systematic review and meta-analysis of randomized controlled trials. Journal of Neurology, Neurosurgery, and Psychiatry. 2020;**91**:21-32

[176] Husain MI, Chaudhry IB, Khoso AB, et al. Minocycline and celecoxib as adjunctive treatments for bipolar depression: A multicentre, factorial design randomized controlled trial. Lancet Psychiatry. 2020;7:515-527

[177] Hoyo-Becerra C, Huebener A, Trippler M, et al. Concomitant interferon alpha stimulation and TLR3 activation induces neuronal expression of depression-related genes that are elevated in the brain of suicidal persons. PLoS One. 2013;**8**:e83149

[178] Mostafavi S, Battle A, Zhu X, et al. Type I interferon signaling genes in recurrent major depression: Increased expression detected by whole-blood RNA sequencing. Molecular Psychiatry. 2014;**19**:1267-1274

[179] Wong ML, Dong C, Maestre-Mesa J, et al. Polymorphisms in inflammation-related genes are associated with susceptibility to major depression and antidepressant response. Molecular Psychiatry. 2008;**13**:800-812

[180] Wallensten J, Ljunggren G, Nager A, et al. Stress, depression, and risk of dementia - A cohort study in the total population between 18 and 65 years

old in region Stockholm. Alzheimer's Research & Therapy. 2023;**15**:161

[181] Gochee PA, Powell EE, Purdie DM, et al. Association between apolipoprotein E epsilon4 and neuropsychiatric symptoms during interferon alpha treatment for chronic hepatitis C. Psychosomatics. 2004;**45**:49-57

[182] Sperl J, Horvath G, Halota W, et al. Efficacy and safety of elbasvir/grazoprevir and sofosbuvir/pegylated interferon/ribavirin: A phase III randomized controlled trial. Journal of Hepatology. 2016;**65**:1112-1119

[183] Murira A, Lamarre A. Type-I interferon responses: From friend to FOE in the battle against chronic viral infection. Frontiers in Immunology. 2016;7:609

[184] Ribas A, Wolchok JD. Cancer immunotherapy using checkpoint blockade. Science. 2018;**359**:1350-1355

[185] Goldschmidt CH, Hua LH. Re-evaluating the use of IFN-β and relapsing multiple sclerosis: Safety, efficacy and place in therapy. Degenerative Neurological and Neuromuscular Disease. 2020;**10**:29-38

[186] Hou Y, Dan X, Babbar M, et al. Aging as a risk factor for neurodegenerative disease. Nature Reviews. Neurology. 2019;**15**:565-581

[187] Goate A, Chartier-Harlin MC, Mullan M, et al. Segregation of a missense mutation in the amyloid precursor protein gene with familial Alzheimer's disease. Nature. 1991;**349**:704-706

[188] Chartier-Harlin MC, Crawford F, Houlden H, et al. Early-onset alzheimer's disease caused by mutations at codon 717 of the beta-amyloid precursor protein gene. Nature. 1991;**353**:844-846

[189] Sherrington R, Rogaev EI, Liang Y, et al. Cloning of a gene bearing missense mutations in early-onset familial Alzheimer's disease. Nature. 1995;**375**:754-760

[190] Levy-Lahad E, Wasco W, Poorkaj P, et al. Candidate gene for the chromosome 1 familial Alzheimer's disease locus. Science. 1995;**269**:973-977

[191] Esquerda-Canals G, Montoliu-Gaya L, Güell-Bosch J, et al. Mouse models of Alzheimer's disease. Journal of Alzheimer's Disease. 2017;**57**:1171-1183

[192] Budd Haeberlein S, Aisen PS, Barkhof F, et al. Two randomized phase 3 studies of aducanumab in early Alzheimer's disease. The Journal of Prevention of Alzheimer's Disease. 2022;**9**:197-210

[193] van Dyck CH, Swanson CJ, Aisen P, et al. Lecanemab in early Alzheimer's disease. The New England Journal of Medicine. 2023;**388**:9-21

[194] Goedert M. Tau filaments in neurodegenerative diseases. FEBS Letters. 2018;**592**:2383-2391

[195] Augustinack JC, Schneider A, Mandelkow E-M, et al. Specific tau phosphorylation sites correlate with severity of neuronal cytopathology in Alzheimer's disease. Acta Neuropathologica. 2002;**103**:26-35

[196] Braak H, Alafuzoff I, Arzberger T, et al. Staging of Alzheimer disease-associated neurofibrillary pathology using paraffin sections and immunocytochemistry. Acta Neuropathologica. 2006;**112**:389-404

[197] Arriagada PV, Growdon JH, Hedley-Whyte ET, et al. Neurofibrillary tangles but not senile plaques parallel duration and severity of Alzheimer's disease. Neurology. 1992;**42**:631-639

[198] Dronse J, Fliessbach K, Bischof GN, et al. In vivo patterns of tau pathology, amyloid-β burden, and neuronal dysfunction in clinical variants of Alzheimer's disease. Journal of Alzheimer's Disease. 2017;**55**:465-471

[199] Congdon EE, Ji C, Tetlow AM, et al. Tau-targeting therapies for Alzheimer disease: Current status and future directions. Nature Reviews. Neurology. 2023;**19**:715-736

[200] Corder EH, Saunders AM, Strittmatter WJ, et al. Gene dose of apolipoprotein E type 4 allele and the risk of Alzheimer's disease in late onset families. Science. 1993;**261**:921-923

[201] Farrer LA, Cupples LA, Haines JL, et al. Effects of age, sex, and ethnicity on the association between apolipoprotein E genotype and Alzheimer disease. JAMA. 1997;**278**:1349

[202] Blumenfeld J, Yip O, Kim MJ, et al. Cell type-specific roles of APOE4 in Alzheimer disease. Nature Reviews. Neuroscience. 2024;**25**:91-110

[203] Arboleda-Velasquez JF, Lopera F, O'Hare M, et al. Resistance to autosomal dominant Alzheimer's disease in an APOE3 Christchurch homozygote: A case report. Nature Medicine. 2019;**25**:1680-1683

[204] Chen Y, Song S, Parhizkar S, et al. APOE3ch alters microglial response and suppresses Aβ-induced tau seeding and spread. Cell. 2024;**187**:428-445.e20

[205] Lambert JC, Ibrahim-Verbaas CA, Harold D, et al. Meta-analysis of 74,046 individuals identifies 11 new susceptibility loci for Alzheimer's disease. Nature Genetics. 2013;**45**:1452-1458

[206] Marioni RE, Harris SE, Zhang Q, et al. GWAS on family history of Alzheimer's disease. Translational Psychiatry. 2018;**8**:99

[207] Jansen IE, Savage JE, Watanabe K, et al. Genome-wide meta-analysis identifies new loci and functional pathways influencing Alzheimer's disease risk. Nature Genetics. 2019;**51**:404-413

[208] Kunkle BW, Grenier-Boley B, Sims R, et al. Genetic meta-analysis of diagnosed Alzheimer's disease identifies new risk loci and implicates Aβ, tau, immunity and lipid processing. Nature Genetics. 2019;**51**:414-430

[209] Wightman DP, Jansen IE, Savage JE, et al. Largest GWAS (N = 1,126,563) of Alzheimer's disease implicates microglia and immune cells. medRxiv. 2020. DOI: 10.1101/2020.11.20.20235275

[210] Guerreiro R, Wojtas A, Bras J, et al. TREM2 variants in Alzheimer's disease. The New England Journal of Medicine. 2013;**368**:117-127

[211] Jonsson T, Stefansson H, Steinberg S, et al. Variant of TREM2 associated with the risk of Alzheimer's disease. The New England Journal of Medicine. 2013;**368**:107-116

[212] Jin SC, Benitez BA, Karch CM, et al. Coding variants in TREM2 increase risk for Alzheimer's disease. Human Molecular Genetics. 2014;**23**:5838-5846

[213] Cheng-Hathaway PJ, Reed-Geaghan EG, Jay TR, et al. The Trem2 R47H variant confers loss-of-function-like phenotypes in Alzheimer's disease. Molecular Neurodegeneration. 2018;**13**:29

[214] Song WM, Joshita S, Zhou Y, et al. Humanized TREM2 mice reveal microglia-intrinsic and -extrinsic effects of R47H polymorphism. The Journal of Experimental Medicine. 2018;**215**:745-760

[215] Tang F, Barbacioru C, Wang Y, et al. mRNA-Seq whole-transcriptome analysis of a single cell. Nature Methods. 2009;**6**:377-382

[216] Mathys H, Adaikkan C, Gao F, et al. Temporal tracking of microglia activation in neurodegeneration at single-cell resolution. Cell Reports. 2017;**21**:366-380

[217] Friedman BA, Srinivasan K, Ayalon G, et al. Diverse brain myeloid expression profiles reveal distinct microglial activation states and aspects of Alzheimer's disease not evident in mouse models. Cell Reports. 2018;**22**:832-847

[218] Sala Frigerio C, Wolfs L, Fattorelli N, et al. The major risk factors for Alzheimer's disease: Age, sex, and genes modulate the microglia response to aβ plaques. Cell Reports. 2019;**27**:1293-1306.e6

[219] Rexach JE, Polioudakis D, Yin A, et al. Tau pathology drives dementia risk-associated gene networks toward chronic inflammatory states and immunosuppression. Cell Reports. 2020;**33**:108398

[220] Lee S-H, Meilandt WJ, Xie L, et al. Trem2 restrains the enhancement of tau accumulation and neurodegeneration by β-amyloid pathology. Neuron. 2021;**109**:1283-1301.e6

[221] Mancuso R, Fattorelli N, Martinez-Muriana A, et al. Xenografted human microglia display diverse transcriptomic states in response to Alzheimer's disease-related amyloid-β pathology. Nature Neuroscience. 2024;**27**:886-900

[222] Keren-Shaul H, Spinrad A, Weiner A, et al. A unique microglia type associated with restricting development of Alzheimer's disease. Cell. 2017;**169**:1276-1290.e17

[223] Deczkowska A, Keren-Shaul H, Weiner A, et al. Disease-associated microglia: A universal immune sensor of neurodegeneration. Cell. 2018;**173**:1073-1081

[224] Prater KE, Green KJ, Mamde S, et al. Human microglia show unique transcriptional changes in Alzheimer's disease. Nature Aging. 2023;**3**:894-907

[225] Yamada T, Horisberger MA, Kawaguchi N, et al. Immunohistochemistry using antibodies to alpha-interferon and its induced protein, MxA, in Alzheimer's and Parkinson's disease brain tissues. Neuroscience Letters. 1994;**181**:61-64

[226] Stopa EG, Tanis KQ, Miller MC, et al. Comparative transcriptomics of choroid plexus in Alzheimer's disease, frontotemporal dementia and Huntington's disease: Implications for CSF homeostasis. Fluids and Barriers of the CNS. 2018;**15**:18

[227] Li QS, De Muynck L. Differentially expressed genes in Alzheimer's disease highlighting the roles of microglia genes including OLR1 and astrocyte gene CDK2AP1. Brain, Behavior, and Immunity Health. 2021;**13**:100227

[228] Roy ER, Wang B, Wan Y-W, et al. Type I interferon response drives neuroinflammation and synapse loss in Alzheimer disease. The Journal of Clinical Investigation. 2020;**130**:1912-1930

[229] Roy ER, Chiu G, Li S, et al. Concerted type I interferon signaling in microglia and neural cells promotes memory impairment associated with amyloid β plaques. Immunity. 2022;**55**:879-894.e6

[230] Taylor JM, Minter MR, Newman AG, et al. Type-1 interferon signaling mediates neuro-inflammatory events in models of Alzheimer's disease. Neurobiology of Aging. 2014;**35**:1012-1023

[231] Mesquita SD, Ferreira AC, Gao F, et al. The choroid plexus transcriptome reveals changes in type I and II interferon responses in a mouse model of Alzheimer's disease. Brain, Behavior, and Immunity. 2015;**49**:280-292

[232] Minter MR, Moore Z, Zhang M, et al. Deletion of the type-1 interferon receptor in APPSWE/PS1ΔE9 mice preserves cognitive function and alters glial phenotype. Acta Neuropathologica Communications. 2016;**4**:72

[233] Xue F, Tian J, Yu C, et al. Type I interferon response-related microglial Mef2c deregulation at the onset of Alzheimer's pathology in 5 × FAD mice. Neurobiology of Disease. 2021;**152**:105272

[234] Sayed FA, Kodama L, Fan L, et al. AD-linked R47H-TREM2 mutation induces disease-enhancing microglial states via AKT hyperactivation. Science Translational Medicine. 2021;**13**:eabe3947

[235] Sanna PP, Cabrelle C, Kawamura T, et al. A history of repeated alcohol intoxication promotes cognitive impairment and gene expression signatures of disease progression in the 3xtg mouse model of Alzheimer's disease. eNeuro. 2023;**10**. DOI: 10.1523/ENEURO.0456-22.2023

[236] Shippy DC, Ulland TK. Genome-wide identification of murine interferon genes in microglial-mediated neuroinflammation in Alzheimer's disease. Journal of Neuroimmunology. 2023;**375**:578031

[237] Sanford SAI, Miller LVC, Vaysburd M, et al. The type-I interferon response potentiates seeded tau aggregation and exacerbates tau pathology. Alzheimer's and Dementia. 2023;**20**(2):1013-1025. DOI: 10.1002/alz.13493

[238] Carling GK, Fan L, Foxe NR, et al. Alzheimer's disease-linked risk alleles elevate microglial cGAS-associated senescence and neurodegeneration in a tauopathy model. BioRxiv. 2024. DOI: 10.1101/2024.01.24.577107

[239] Pandey S, Shen K, Lee S-H, et al. Disease-associated oligodendrocyte responses across neurodegenerative diseases. Cell Reports. 2022;**40**:111189

[240] Naguib S, Torres ER, Lopez-Lee C, et al. APOE3-R136S mutation confers resilience against tau pathology via cGAS-STING-IFN inhibition. BioRxiv. 2024. DOI: 10.1101/2024.04.25.591140

[241] Korvatska O, Kiianitsa K, Ratushny A, et al. Triggering receptor expressed on myeloid cell 2 R47H exacerbates immune response in Alzheimer's disease brain. Frontiers in Immunology. 2020;**11**:559342

[242] Fancy N, Willumsen N, Tsartsalis S, et al. Mechanisms contributing to differential genetic risks for TREM2 R47H and R62H variants in Alzheimer's disease. medRxiv. 2022. DOI: 10.1101/2022.07.12.22277509

[243] Ginsberg SD, Crino PB, Lee VM-Y, et al. Sequestration of RNA in

Alzheimer's disease neurofibrillary tangles and senile plaques. Annals of Neurology. 1997;**41**:200-209

[244] Ginsberg SD, Crino PB, Hemby SE, et al. Predominance of neuronal mRNAs in individual Alzheimer's disease senile plaques. Annals of Neurology. 1999;**45**:174-181

[245] Uchida Y, Takahashi H. Rapid detection of Abeta deposits in APP transgenic mice by Hoechst 33342. Neuroscience Letters. 2008;**448**:279-281

[246] Pensalfini A, Albay R, Rasool S, et al. Intracellular amyloid and the neuronal origin of Alzheimer neuritic plaques. Neurobiology of Disease. 2014;**71**:53-61

[247] Minter MR, Main BS, Brody KM, et al. Soluble amyloid triggers a myeloid differentiation factor 88 and interferon regulatory factor 7 dependent neuronal type-1 interferon response in vitro. Journal of Neuroinflammation. 2015;**12**:71

[248] Xie X, Ma G, Li X, et al. Activation of innate immune cGAS-STING pathway contributes to Alzheimer's pathogenesis in 5 × FAD mice. Nature Aging. 2023;**3**:202-212

[249] Udeochu JC, Amin S, Huang Y, et al. Tau activation of microglial cGAS-IFN reduces MEF2C-mediated cognitive resilience. Nature Neuroscience. 2023;**26**:737-750

[250] Gavin AL, Huang D, Huber C, et al. PLD3 and PLD4 are single-stranded acid exonucleases that regulate endosomal nucleic-acid sensing. Nature Immunology. 2018;**19**:942-953

[251] Gavin AL, Huang D, Blane TR, et al. Cleavage of DNA and RNA by PLD3 and PLD4 limits autoinflammatory triggering by multiple sensors. Nature Communications. 2021;**12**:5874

[252] Van Acker ZP, Perdok A, Hellemans R, et al. Phospholipase D3 degrades mitochondrial DNA to regulate nucleotide signaling and APP metabolism. Nature Communications. 2023;**14**:2847

[253] Cruchaga C, Karch CM, Jin SC, et al. Rare coding variants in the phospholipase D3 gene confer risk for Alzheimer's disease. Nature. 2014;**505**:550-554

[254] Zhang D-F, Fan Y, Wang D, et al. PLD3 in Alzheimer's disease: A modest effect as revealed by updated association and expression analyses. Molecular Neurobiology. 2016;**53**:4034-4045

[255] Zhang W, Jiao B, Xiao T, et al. Targeted sequencing on neurodegenerative genes identified novel causal and risk variants of familial Alzheimer's disease. 2020. DOI: 10.21203/rs.3.rs-24070/v1

[256] Wang J, Yu J-T, Tan L. PLD3 in Alzheimer's disease. Molecular Neurobiology. 2015;**51**:480-486

[257] Satoh J-I, Kino Y, Yamamoto Y, et al. PLD3 is accumulated on neuritic plaques in Alzheimer's disease brains. Alzheimer's Research & Therapy. 2014;**6**:70

[258] Sadler AJ, BRG W. Interferon-inducible antiviral effectors. Nature Reviews. Immunology. 2008;**8**:559-568

[259] Lee W-B, Choi WY, Lee D-H, et al. OAS1 and OAS3 negatively regulate the expression of chemokines and interferon-responsive genes in human macrophages. BMB Reports. 2019;**52**:133-138

[260] Salih DA, Bayram S, Guelfi S, et al. Genetic variability in response to amyloid beta deposition influences Alzheimer's disease risk. Brain Communications. 2019;**1**:fcz022

[261] Magusali N, Graham AC, Piers TM, et al. A genetic link between risk for Alzheimer's disease and severe COVID-19 outcomes via the OAS1 gene. Brain. 2021;**144**:3727-3741

[262] Moore Z, Mobilio F, Walker FR, et al. Abrogation of type-I interferon signaling alters the microglial response to Aβ1-42. Scientific Reports. 2020;**10**:3153

[263] Dedoni S, Olianas MC, Onali P. Interferon-β induces apoptosis in human SH-SY5Y neuroblastoma cells through activation of JAK–STAT signaling and down-regulation of PI3K/Akt pathway. Journal of Neurochemistry. 2010;**115**:1421-1433

[264] Dedoni S, Olianas MC, Ingianni A, et al. Type I interferons impair BDNF-induced cell signaling and neurotrophic activity in differentiated human SH-SY5Y neuroblastoma cells and mouse primary cortical neurons. Journal of Neurochemistry. 2012;**122**:58-71

[265] Olianas MC, Dedoni S, Onali P. Protection from interferon-β-induced neuronal apoptosis through stimulation of muscarinic acetylcholine receptors coupled to ERK1/2 activation. British Journal of Pharmacology. 2016;**173**:2910-2928

[266] Cox DJ, Field RH, Williams DG, et al. DNA sensors are expressed in astrocytes and microglia in vitro and are upregulated during gliosis in neurodegenerative disease. Glia. 2015;**63**:812-825

[267] Baruch K, Deczkowska A, David E, et al. Aging. Aging-induced type I interferon response at the choroid plexus negatively affects brain function. Science. 2014;**346**:89-93

[268] Deczkowska A, Matcovitch-Natan O, Tsitsou-Kampeli A, et al. Mef2C restrains microglial inflammatory response and is lost in brain aging in an IFN-I-dependent manner. Nature Communications. 2017;**8**:717

[269] Leifer D, Krainc D, Yu YT, et al. MEF2C, a MADS/MEF2-family transcription factor expressed in a laminar distribution in cerebral cortex. Proceedings of the National Academy of Sciences of the United States of America. 1993;**90**:1546-1550

[270] Li H, Radford JC, Ragusa MJ, et al. Transcription factor MEF2C influences neural stem/progenitor cell differentiation and maturation in vivo. Proceedings of the National Academy of Sciences of the United States of America. 2008;**105**:9397-9402

[271] Rashid AJ, Cole CJ, Josselyn SA. Emerging roles for MEF2 transcription factors in memory. Genes, Brain, and Behavior. 2014;**13**:118-125

[272] Ruiz A, Heilmann S, Becker T, et al. Follow-up of loci from the international genomics of Alzheimer's disease project identifies TRIP4 as a novel susceptibility gene. Translational Psychiatry. 2014;**4**:e358

[273] Tang S-S, Wang H-F, Zhang W, et al. MEF2C rs190982 polymorphism with late-onset alzheimer's disease in Han Chinese: A replication study and meta-analyses. Oncotarget. 2016;7:39136-39142

[274] Sunderaraman P, Cosentino S, Schupf N, et al. MEF2C common genetic variation is associated with different aspects of cognition in non-hispanic

white and Caribbean hispanic non-demented older adults. Frontiers in Genetics. 2021;**12**:642327

[275] Hur J-Y, Frost GR, Wu X, et al. The innate immunity protein IFITM3 modulates γ-secretase in Alzheimer's disease. Nature. 2020;**586**:735-740

[276] Pyun J-M, Park YH, Hodges A, et al. Immunity gene IFITM3 variant: Relation to cognition and Alzheimer's disease pathology. Alzheimer's & Dementia (Amsterdam, Netherlands). 2022;**14**:e12317

[277] Jana A, Wang X, Leasure JW, et al. Increased type I interferon signaling and brain endothelial barrier dysfunction in an experimental model of Alzheimer's disease. Scientific Reports. 2022;**12**:16488

[278] Stone LA, Frank JA, Albert PS, et al. The effect of interferon-beta on blood–brain barrier disruptions demonstrated by contrast-enhanced magnetic resonance imaging in relapsing–remitting multiple sclerosis. Annals of Neurology. 1995;**37**:611-619

[279] Rossi JL, Todd T, Daniels Z, et al. Interferon-stimulated gene 15 upregulation precedes the development of blood–brain barrier disruption and cerebral edema after traumatic brain injury in young mice. Journal of Neurotrauma. 2015;**32**:1101-1108

[280] Mastorakos P, Russo MV, Zhou T, et al. Antimicrobial immunity impedes CNS vascular repair following brain injury. Nature Immunology. 2021;**22**:1280-1293

[281] Pais TF, Ali H, Moreira da Silva J, et al. Brain endothelial STING1 activation by plasmodium-sequestered heme promotes cerebral malaria via type I IFN response. Proceedings of the National Academy of Sciences of the United States of America. 2022;**119**:e2206327119

[282] Shafi AM, Végvári Á, Zubarev RA, et al. Brain endothelial cells exposure to malaria parasites links type I interferon signaling to antigen presentation, immunoproteasome activation, endothelium disruption, and cellular metabolism. Frontiers in Immunology. 2023;**14**:1149107

[283] Tziortzouda P, Van Den Bosch L, Hirth F. Triad of TDP43 control in neurodegeneration: Autoregulation, localization and aggregation. Nature Reviews. Neuroscience. 2021;**22**:197-208

[284] Bright F, Werry EL, Dobson-Stone C, et al. Neuroinflammation in frontotemporal dementia. Nature Reviews. Neurology. 2019;**15**:540-555

[285] Grossman M, Seeley WW, Boxer AL, et al. Frontotemporal lobar degeneration. Nature Reviews. Disease Primers. 2023;**9**:40

[286] Dunker W, Ye X, Zhao Y, et al. TDP-43 prevents endogenous RNAs from triggering a lethal RIG-I-dependent interferon response. Cell Reports. 2021;**35**:108976

[287] Yu C-H, Davidson S, Harapas CR, et al. TDP-43 triggers mitochondrial DNA release via mPTP to activate cGAS/STING in ALS. Cell. 2020;**183**:636-649.e18

[288] Licht-Murava A, Meadows SM, Palaguachi F, et al. Astrocytic TDP-43 dysregulation impairs memory by modulating antiviral pathways and interferon-inducible chemokines. Science Advances. 2023;**9**:eade1282

[289] Galimberti D, Schoonenboom N, Scheltens P, et al. Intrathecal chemokine synthesis in mild cognitive impairment

and Alzheimer disease. Archives of Neurology. 2006;**63**:538-543

[290] Xia MQ, Bacskai BJ, Knowles RB, et al. Expression of the chemokine receptor CXCR3 on neurons and the elevated expression of its ligand IP-10 in reactive astrocytes: In vitro ERK1/2 activation and role in Alzheimer's disease. Journal of Neuroimmunology. 2000;**108**:227-235

[291] Galimberti D, Bonsi R, Fenoglio C, et al. Inflammatory molecules in frontotemporal dementia: Cerebrospinal fluid signature of progranulin mutation carriers. Brain, Behavior, and Immunity. 2015;**49**:182-187

[292] Davidson YS, Raby S, Foulds PG, et al. TDP-43 pathological changes in early onset familial and sporadic Alzheimer's disease, late onset alzheimer's disease and Down's syndrome: Association with age, hippocampal sclerosis and clinical phenotype. Acta Neuropathologica. 2011;**122**:703-713

[293] Buciuc M, Tosakulwong N, Machulda MM, et al. TAR DNA-binding protein 43 is associated with rate of memory, functional and global cognitive decline in the decade prior to death. Journal of Alzheimer's Disease. 2021;**80**:683-693

[294] Kaya T, Mattugini N, Liu L, et al. CD8+ T cells induce interferon-responsive oligodendrocytes and microglia in white matter aging. Nature Neuroscience. 2022;**25**:1446-1457

[295] Jorfi M, Park J, Hall CK, et al. Infiltrating CD8+ T cells exacerbate Alzheimer's disease pathology in a 3D human neuroimmune axis model. Nature Neuroscience. 2023;**26**:1489-1504

[296] Fernando N, Gopalakrishnan J, Behensky A, et al. Single-cell multiomic analysis reveals the involvement of type I interferon-responsive CD8+ T cells in amyloid beta-associated memory loss. BioRxiv. 2023. DOI: 10.1101/2023.03.18.533293

[297] Ferretti MT, Merlini M, Späni C, et al. T-cell brain infiltration and immature antigen-presenting cells in transgenic models of Alzheimer's disease-like cerebral amyloidosis. Brain, Behavior, and Immunity. 2016;**54**:211-225

[298] Gate D, Saligrama N, Leventhal O, et al. Clonally expanded CD8 T cells patrol the cerebrospinal fluid in Alzheimer's disease. Nature. 2020;**577**:399-404

[299] Unger MS, Li E, Scharnagl L, et al. CD8+ T-cells infiltrate Alzheimer's disease brains and regulate neuronal- and synapse-related gene expression in APP-PS1 transgenic mice. Brain, Behavior, and Immunity. 2020;**89**:67-86

[300] Chen X, Firulyova M, Manis M, et al. Microglia-mediated T cell infiltration drives neurodegeneration in tauopathy. Nature. 2023;**615**:668-677

[301] Ballard C, Mobley W, Hardy J, et al. Dementia in down's syndrome. Lancet Neurology. 2016;**15**:622-636

[302] Bayen E, Possin KL, Chen Y, et al. Prevalence of aging, dementia, and multimorbidity in older adults with down syndrome. JAMA Neurology. 2018;**75**:1399-1406

[303] Araya P, Waugh KA, Sullivan KD, et al. Trisomy 21 dysregulates T cell lineages toward an autoimmunity-prone state associated with interferon hyperactivity. Proceedings of the National Academy of Sciences of the United States of America. 2019;**116**:24231-24241

[304] Waugh KA, Araya P, Pandey A, et al. Mass cytometry reveals global immune remodeling with multi-lineage hypersensitivity to type I interferon in down syndrome. Cell Reports. 2019;**29**:1893-1908.e4

[305] Ahmed MM, Johnson NR, Boyd TD, et al. Innate immune system activation and neuroinflammation in down syndrome and neurodegeneration: Therapeutic targets or partners? Frontiers in Aging Neuroscience. 2021;**13**:718426

[306] Kong X-F, Worley L, Rinchai D, et al. Three copies of four interferon receptor genes underlie a mild type I interferonopathy in down syndrome. Journal of Clinical Immunology. 2020;**40**:807-819

[307] Galbraith MD, Rachubinski AL, Smith KP, et al. Multidimensional definition of the interferonopathy of down syndrome and its response to JAK inhibition. Science Advances. 2023;**9**:eadg6218

[308] Wisniewski KE, French JH, Rosen JF, et al. Basal ganglia calcification (BGC) in Down's syndrome (DS)– Another manifestation of premature aging. Annals of the New York Academy of Sciences. 1982;**396**:179-189

[309] Takashima S, Becker LE. Basal ganglia calcification in Down's syndrome. Journal of Neurology, Neurosurgery, and Psychiatry. 1985;**48**:61-64

[310] Ieshima A, Kisa T, Yoshino K, et al. A morphometric CT study of Down's syndrome showing small posterior fossa and calcification of basal ganglia. Neuroradiology. 1984;**26**:493-498

[311] Sadana KS, Goraya JS. Intracranial calcification in down syndrome. Journal of Pediatric Neurosciences. 2018;**13**:120-121

[312] Thoms L, Idowu A, Nehra A, et al. Significance of basal ganglia calcification in Down's syndrome. Advances in Mental Health and Intellectual Disabilities. 2020;**14**:103-110

[313] Panda PK, Elwadhi A, Sharawat IK. Intracranial calcification and seizures in Down syndrome. BML Case Reports. 2021;**14**. DOI: 10.1136/bcr-2021-243180

[314] Almudhry M, Prasad C, Tay K, et al. Progressive neurological decline associated with intracranial calcification in down syndrome; Fahr disease Mimic? The Canadian Journal of Neurological Sciences. 2023:1-2

[315] Horvath S, Garagnani P, Bacalini MG, et al. Accelerated epigenetic aging in Down syndrome. Aging Cell. 2015;**14**:491-495

[316] Horvath S. DNA methylation age of human tissues and cell types. Genome Biology. 2013;**14**:R115

[317] Chen BH, Marioni RE, Colicino E, et al. DNA methylation-based measures of biological age: Meta-analysis predicting time to death. Aging (Albany NY). 2016;**8**:1844-1865

[318] Lu AT, Quach A, Wilson JG, et al. DNA methylation GrimAge strongly predicts lifespan and healthspan. Aging (Albany NY). 2019;**11**:303-327

[319] Gensous N, Bacalini MG, Franceschi C, et al. Down syndrome, accelerated aging and immunosenescence. Seminars in Immunopathology. 2020;**42**:635-645

[320] Snyder HM, Bain LJ, Brickman AM, et al. Further understanding the connection between Alzheimer's disease and Down syndrome. Alzheimers Dement. 2020;**16**:1065-1077

[321] Sullivan KD, Lewis HC, Hill AA, et al. Trisomy 21 consistently activates the interferon response. eLife. 2016;**5**. DOI: 10.7554/eLife.16220

[322] Malle L, Martin-Fernandez M, Buta S, et al. Excessive negative regulation of type I interferon disrupts viral control in individuals with Down syndrome. Immunity. 2022;**55**:2074-2084.e5

[323] Waugh KA, Minter R, Baxter J, et al. Triplication of the interferon receptor locus contributes to hallmarks of Down syndrome in a mouse model. Nature Genetics. 2023;**55**:1034-1047

[324] Krivega M, Stiefel CM, Karbassi S, et al. Genotoxic stress in constitutive trisomies induces autophagy and the innate immune response via the cGAS-STING pathway. Communications Biology. 2021;**4**:831

[325] Maroun LE. Anti-interferon immunoglobulins can improve the trisomy 16 mouse phenotype. Teratology. 1995;**51**:329-335

[326] Gupta M, Dhanasekaran AR, Gardiner KJ. Mouse models of Down syndrome: Gene content and consequences. Mammalian Genome. 2016;**27**:538-555

[327] Franceschi C, Bonafè M, Valensin S, et al. Inflamm-aging. An evolutionary perspective on immunosenescence. Annals of the New York Academy of Sciences. 2000;**908**:244-254

[328] López-Otín C, Blasco MA, Partridge L, et al. Hallmarks of aging: An expanding universe. Cell. 2023;**186**:243-278

[329] MacAulay N, Keep RF, Zeuthen T. Cerebrospinal fluid production by the choroid plexus: A century of barrier research revisited. Fluids and Barriers of the CNS. 2022;**19**:26

[330] Boldrini M, Canoll PD, Klein RS. How COVID-19 affects the brain. JAMA Psychiatry. 2021;**78**:682-683

[331] Asadi-Pooya AA, Akbari A, Emami A, et al. Long COVID syndrome-associated brain fog. Journal of Medical Virology. 2022;**94**:979-984

[332] Xu Z, Wang H, Jiang S, et al. Brain pathology in COVID-19: Clinical manifestations and potential mechanisms. Neuroscience Bulletin. 2024;**40**:383-400

[333] Wulf Hanson S, Abbafati C, et al. Estimated global proportions of individuals with persistent fatigue, cognitive, and respiratory symptom clusters following symptomatic COVID-19 in 2020 and 2021. JAMA. 2022;**328**:1604-1615

[334] Suzzi S, Tsitsou-Kampeli A, Schwartz M. The type I interferon antiviral response in the choroid plexus and the cognitive risk in COVID-19. Nature Immunology. 2023;**24**:220-224

[335] Yang AC, Kern F, Losada PM, et al. Dysregulation of brain and choroid plexus cell types in severe COVID-19. Nature. 2021;**595**:565-571

[336] Čarna M, Onyango IG, Katina S, et al. Pathogenesis of Alzheimer's disease: Involvement of the choroid plexus. Alzheimers Dement. 2023;**19**:3537-3554

[337] West AP, Shadel GS. Mitochondrial DNA in innate immune responses and inflammatory pathology. Nature Reviews. Immunology. 2017;**17**:363-375

[338] Jauhari A, Baranov SV, Suofu Y, et al. Melatonin inhibits cytosolic mitochondrial DNA–induced neuroinflammatory signaling in accelerated aging and neurodegeneration. The Journal of Clinical Investigation. 2020;**130**(6):3124-3136

[339] Lei Y, Guerra Martinez C, Torres-Odio S, et al. Elevated type I interferon responses potentiate metabolic dysfunction, inflammation, and accelerated aging in mtDNA mutator mice. Science Advances. 2021;**7**. DOI: 10.1126/sciadv.abe7548

[340] Jiménez-Loygorri JI, Villarejo-Zori B, Viedma-Poyatos Á, et al. Mitophagy curtails cytosolic mtDNA-dependent activation of cGAS/STING inflammation during aging. Nature Communications. 2024;**15**:830

[341] Ansar M, Qu Y, Ivanciuc T, et al. Lack of type I interferon signaling ameliorates respiratory syncytial virus-induced lung inflammation and restores antioxidant defenses. Antioxidants (Basel). 2021;**11**. DOI: 10.3390/antiox11010067

[342] Wang X, Cui L, Ji X. Cognitive impairment caused by hypoxia: From clinical evidences to molecular mechanisms. Metabolic Brain Disease. 2022;**37**:51-66

[343] Huang W, Hickson LJ, Eirin A, et al. Cellular senescence: The good, the bad and the unknown. Nature Reviews. Nephrology. 2022;**18**:611-627

[344] Buckley MT, Sun ED, George BM, et al. Cell-type-specific aging clocks to quantify aging and rejuvenation in neurogenic regions of the brain. Nature Aging. 2023;**3**:121-137

[345] De Cecco M, Criscione SW, Peckham EJ, et al. Genomes of replicatively senescent cells undergo global epigenetic changes leading to gene silencing and activation of transposable elements. Aging Cell. 2013;**12**:247-256

[346] Muotri AR, Chu VT, Marchetto MCN, et al. Somatic mosaicism in neuronal precursor cells mediated by L1 retrotransposition. Nature. 2005;**435**:903-910

[347] Erwin JA, Marchetto MC, Gage FH. Mobile DNA elements in the generation of diversity and complexity in the brain. Nature Reviews. Neuroscience. 2014;**15**:497-506

[348] Takahashi A, Loo TM, Okada R, et al. Downregulation of cytoplasmic DNases is implicated in cytoplasmic DNA accumulation and SASP in senescent cells. Nature Communications. 2018;**9**:1249

[349] De Cecco M, Ito T, Petrashen AP, et al. L1 drives IFN in senescent cells and promotes age-associated inflammation. Nature. 2019;**566**:73-78

[350] Gulen MF, Samson N, Keller A, et al. cGAS-STING drives aging-related inflammation and neurodegeneration. Nature. 2023;**620**:374-380

[351] DeMaeyer EM, De Maeyer-Guignard J. Interferons and Other Regulatory Cytokines. illustrated ed. New York City, United States: Wiley; 1988

[352] Jin M, Xu R, Wang L, et al. Type-I-interferon signaling drives microglial dysfunction and senescence in human iPSC models of Down syndrome and Alzheimer's disease. Cell Stem Cell. 2022;**29**:1135-1153.e8

[353] Yu Q, Katlinskaya YV, Carbone CJ, et al. DNA-damage-induced type I interferon promotes senescence and

inhibits stem cell function. Cell Reports. 2015;**11**:785-797

[354] Lau V, Ramer L, Tremblay M-È. An aging, pathology burden, and glial senescence build-up hypothesis for late onset alzheimer's disease. Nature Communications. 2023;**14**:1670

[355] Ng PY, Zhang C, Li H, et al. Senescent microglia represent a subset of disease-associated microglia in P301S mice. Journal of Alzheimer's Disease. 2023;**95**:493-507

[356] Rim C, You M-J, Nahm M, et al. Emerging role of senescent microglia in brain aging-related neurodegenerative diseases. Translational Neurodegeneration. 2024;**13**:10

[357] Harrington A, Raissi AJ, Rajkovich K, et al. MEF2C regulates cortical inhibitory and excitatory synapses and behaviors relevant to neurodevelopmental disorders. eLife. 2016;**25**(5)

[358] Zhang L, Chen D, Song D, et al. Clinical and translational values of spatial transcriptomics. Signal Transduction and Targeted Therapy. 2022;**7**:111

[359] Villeda SA, Luo J, Mosher KI, et al. The aging systemic milieu negatively regulates neurogenesis and cognitive function. Nature. 2011;**477**:90-94

[360] Bieri G, Schroer AB, Villeda SA. Blood-to-brain communication in aging and rejuvenation. Nature Neuroscience. 2023;**26**:379-393

[361] D'Mello C, Le T, Swain MG. Cerebral microglia recruit monocytes into the brain in response to tumor necrosis factoralpha signaling during peripheral organ inflammation. The Journal of Neuroscience. 2009;**29**:2089-2102

[362] Somebang K, Rudolph J, Imhof I, et al. CCR2 deficiency alters activation of microglia subsets in traumatic brain injury. Cell Reports. 2021;**36**:109727

[363] Atkins CM. Decoding hippocampal signaling deficits after traumatic brain injury. Translational Stroke Research. 2011;**2**:546-555

[364] Smith DH, Johnson VE, Stewart W. Chronic neuropathologies of single and repetitive TBI: Substrates of dementia? Nature Reviews. Neurology. 2013;**9**:211-221

[365] Li Y, Li Y, Li X, et al. Head injury as a risk factor for dementia and Alzheimer's disease: A systematic review and meta-analysis of 32 observational studies. PLoS One. 2017;**12**:e0169650

[366] Fann JR, Ribe AR, Pedersen HS, et al. Long-term risk of dementia among people with traumatic brain injury in Denmark: A population-based observational cohort study. Lancet Psychiatry. 2018;**5**:424-431

[367] Gardner RC, Burke JF, Nettiksimmons J, et al. Dementia risk after traumatic brain injury vs. nonbrain trauma: The role of age and severity. JAMA Neurology. 2014;**71**:1490-1497

[368] Gardner RC, Burke JF, Nettiksimmons J, et al. Traumatic brain injury in later life increases risk for Parkinson disease. Annals of Neurology. 2015;**77**:987-995

[369] Herklots MW, Kroon M, Roks G, et al. Poor outcome in frail elderly patient after severe TBI. Brain Injury. 2022;**36**:1118-1122

[370] Albrecht JS. Impact of dementia on days at home after traumatic brain injury among older medicare beneficiaries.

Alzheimer's Dement. 2023;**19**. DOI: 10.1002/alz.075534

[371] Shively S, Scher AI, Perl DP, et al. Dementia resulting from traumatic brain injury: What is the pathology? Archives of Neurology. 2012;**69**:1245-1251

[372] Kuo YG, Tarzi FP, Louie S, et al. Neuroinflammation in traumatic brain injury. In: Lv X, Guo Y, Mao G, editors. Frontiers in traumatic Brain Injury. IntechOpen; 2022. Epub ahead of print November 30, 2022. DOI: 10.5772/intechopen.105178

[373] Shao F, Wang X, Wu H, et al. Microglia and neuroinflammation: Crucial pathological mechanisms in traumatic brain injury-induced neurodegeneration. Frontiers in Aging Neuroscience. 2022;**14**:825086

[374] Todd BP, Chimenti MS, Luo Z, et al. Traumatic brain injury results in unique microglial and astrocyte transcriptomes enriched for type I interferon response. Journal of Neuroinflammation. 2021;**18**:151

[375] Hammond TR, Dufort C, Dissing-Olesen L, et al. Single-cell RNA sequencing of microglia throughout the mouse lifespan and in the injured brain reveals complex cell-state changes. Immunity. 2019;**50**:253-271.e6

[376] Witcher KG, Bray CE, Chunchai T, et al. Traumatic brain injury causes chronic cortical inflammation and neuronal dysfunction mediated by microglia. The Journal of Neuroscience. 2021;**41**:1597-1616

[377] Garza R, Sharma Y, Atacho DAM, et al. Single-cell transcriptomics of human traumatic brain injury reveals activation of endogenous retroviruses in oligodendroglia. Cell Reports. 2023;**42**:113395

[378] Bolte AC, Shapiro DA, Dutta AB, et al. The meningeal transcriptional response to traumatic brain injury and aging. eLife. 2023;**12**. DOI: 10.7554/eLife.81154

[379] Packer JM, Bray CE, Beckman NB, et al. Impaired cortical neuronal homeostasis and cognition after diffuse traumatic brain injury are dependent on microglia and type I interferon responses. Glia. 2024;**72**:300-321

[380] Wangler LM, Bray CE, Packer JM, et al. Amplified gliosis and interferon-associated inflammation in the aging brain following diffuse traumatic brain injury. The Journal of Neuroscience. 2022;**42**:9082-9096

[381] Barrett JP, Knoblach SM, Bhattacharya S, et al. Traumatic brain injury induces cGAS activation and type I interferon signaling in aged mice. Frontiers in Immunology. 2021;**12**:710608

[382] Todd BP, Luo Z, Gilkes N, et al. Selective neuroimmune modulation by type I interferon drives neuropathology and neurologic dysfunction following traumatic brain injury. Acta Neuropathologica Communications. 2023;**11**:134

[383] Karve IP, Zhang M, Habgood M, et al. Ablation of type-1 IFN signaling in hematopoietic cells confers protection following traumatic brain injury. eNeuro. 2016;**3**. DOI: 10.1523/ENEURO.0128-15.2016

[384] Barrett JP, Henry RJ, Shirey KA, et al. Interferon-β plays a detrimental role in experimental traumatic brain injury by enhancing neuroinflammation that drives chronic neurodegeneration. The Journal of Neuroscience. 2020;**40**:2357-2370

[385] Abdullah A, Zhang M, Frugier T, et al. STING-mediated type-I interferons contribute to the neuroinflammatory process and detrimental effects following traumatic brain injury. Journal of Neuroinflammation. 2018;**15**:323

[386] Fritsch LE, Ju J, Gudenschwager Basso EK, et al. Type I interferon response is mediated by NLRX1-cGAS-STING signaling in brain injury. Frontiers in Molecular Neuroscience. 2022;**15**:852243

[387] Fritsch LE, Kelly C, Leonard J, et al. STING-dependent signaling in microglia or peripheral immune cells orchestrates the early inflammatory response and influences brain injury outcome. The Journal of Neuroscience. 2024;**44**. DOI: 10.1523/JNEUROSCI.0191-23.2024

[388] Fryer AL, Abdullah A, Mobilio F, et al. Pharmacological inhibition of STING reduces neuroinflammation-mediated damage post-traumatic brain injury. British Journal of Pharmacology. 2024. pp. 1-18. DOI: 10.1111/bph.16347

[389] Saleh A, Macia A, Muotri AR. Transposable elements, inflammation, and neurological disease. Frontiers in Neurology. 2019;**10**:894

[390] Vaibhav K, Braun M, Alverson K, et al. Neutrophil extracellular traps exacerbate neurological deficits after traumatic brain injury. Science Advances. 2020;**6**:eaax8847

[391] Mi L, Min X, Shi M, et al. Neutrophil extracellular traps aggravate neuronal endoplasmic reticulum stress and apoptosis via TLR9 after traumatic brain injury. Cell Death & Disease. 2023;**14**:374

[392] Walko TD, Bola RA, Hong JD, et al. Cerebrospinal fluid mitochondrial DNA: A novel DAMP in pediatric traumatic brain injury. Shock. 2014;**41**:499-503

[393] Rodrigues Filho EM, Simon D, Ikuta N, et al. Elevated cell-free plasma DNA level as an independent predictor of mortality in patients with severe traumatic brain injury. Journal of Neurotrauma. 2014;**31**:1639-1646

[394] Ritzel RM, Li Y, Lei Z, et al. Functional and transcriptional profiling of microglial activation during the chronic phase of TBI identifies an age-related driver of poor outcome in old mice. Geroscience. 2022;**44**:1407-1440

[395] Sen T, Saha P, Gupta R, et al. Aberrant ER stress induced neuronal-IFNβ elicits white matter injury due to microglial activation and T-cell infiltration after TBI. The Journal of Neuroscience. 2020;**40**:424-446

[396] Dohi K, Ohtaki H, Nakamachi T, et al. Gp91phox (NOX2) in classically activated microglia exacerbates traumatic brain injury. Journal of Neuroinflammation. 2010;7:41

[397] Zhang Q-G, Laird MD, Han D, et al. Critical role of NADPH oxidase in neuronal oxidative damage and microglia activation following traumatic brain injury. PLoS One. 2012;7:e34504

[398] Kumar A, Barrett JP, Alvarez-Croda D-M, et al. NOX2 drives M1-like microglial/macrophage activation and neurodegeneration following experimental traumatic brain injury. Brain, Behavior, and Immunity. 2016;**58**:291-309

[399] Glennon-Alty L, Moots RJ, Edwards SW, et al. Type I interferon regulates cytokine-delayed neutrophil apoptosis, reactive oxygen species production and chemokine expression.

Clinical and Experimental Immunology. 2021;**203**:151-159

[400] Huber-Lang M, Lambris JD, Ward PA. Innate immune responses to trauma. Nature Immunology. 2018;**19**:327-341

[401] Kwidzinski E, Bechmann I. IDO expression in the brain: A double-edged sword. Journal of Molecular Medicine. 2007;**85**:1351-1359

[402] Berger EA, Murphy PM, Farber JM. Chemokine receptors as HIV-1 coreceptors: Roles in viral entry, tropism, and disease. Annual Review of Immunology. 1999;**17**:657-700

[403] Bekker L-G, Beyrer C, Mgodi N, et al. HIV infection. Nature Reviews. Disease Primers. 2023;**9**:42

[404] Day C, Manning K, Abdullah F, et al. Delirium in HIV-infected patients admitted to acute medical wards post universal access to antiretrovirals in South Africa. South African Medical Journal. 2021;**111**:974-980

[405] Tang Y, Chaillon A, Gianella S, et al. Brain microglia serve as a persistent HIV reservoir despite durable antiretroviral therapy. The Journal of Clinical Investigation. 2023;**133**. DOI: 10.1172/JCI167417

[406] Luo X, He JJ. Cell–cell contact viral transfer contributes to HIV infection and persistence in astrocytes. Journal of Neurovirology. 2015;**21**:66-80

[407] Wahl A, Al-Harthi L. HIV infection of non-classical cells in the brain. Retrovirology. 2023;**20**:1

[408] Bandera A, Taramasso L, Bozzi G, et al. HIV-associated neurocognitive impairment in the modern ART era: Are we close to discovering reliable biomarkers in the setting of virological suppression? Frontiers in Aging Neuroscience. 2019;**11**:187

[409] Mastrorosa I, Pinnetti C, Brita AC, et al. Declining prevalence of human immunodeficiency virus (HIV)-associated neurocognitive disorders in recent years and associated factors in a large cohort of antiretroviral therapy-treated individuals with HIV. Clinical Infectious Diseases. 2023;**76**:e629-e637

[410] Borjabad A, Morgello S, Chao W, et al. Significant effects of antiretroviral therapy on global gene expression in brain tissues of patients with HIV-1-associated neurocognitive disorders. PLoS Pathogens. 2011;**7**:e1002213

[411] Shityakov S, Dandekar T, Förster C. Gene expression profiles and protein–protein interaction network analysis in AIDS patients with HIV-associated encephalitis and dementia. HIV/AIDS (Auckland, N.Z.). 2015;**7**:265-276

[412] Solomon IH, De Girolami U, Chettimada S, et al. Brain and liver pathology, amyloid deposition, and interferon responses among older HIV-positive patients in the late HAART era. BMC Infectious Diseases. 2017;**17**:151

[413] Sanfilippo C, Pinzone MR, Cambria D, et al. OAS gene family expression is associated with HIV-related neurocognitive disorders. Molecular Neurobiology. 2018;**55**:1905-1914

[414] Garces A, Martinez B, De La Garza R, et al. Differential expression of interferon-induced protein with tetratricopeptide repeats 3 (IFIT3) in Alzheimer's disease and HIV-1 associated neurocognitive disorders. Scientific Reports. 2023;**13**:3276

[415] Tavazzi E, Morrison D, Sullivan P, et al. Brain inflammation is a common

feature of HIV-infected patients without HIV encephalitis or productive brain infection. Current HIV Research. 2014;**12**:97-110

[416] Akwa Y, Hassett DE, Eloranta ML, et al. Transgenic expression of IFN-alpha in the central nervous system of mice protects against lethal neurotropic viral infection but induces inflammation and neurodegeneration. Journal of Immunology. 1998;**161**:5016-5026

[417] Sas AR, Bimonte-Nelson H, Smothers CT, et al. Interferon-alpha causes neuronal dysfunction in encephalitis. The Journal of Neuroscience. 2009;**29**:3948-3955

[418] Singh H, Ojeda-Juárez D, Maung R, et al. A pivotal role for Interferon-α receptor-1 in neuronal injury induced by HIV-1. Journal of Neuroinflammation. 2020;**17**:226

[419] Mandl JN, Barry AP, Vanderford TH, et al. Divergent TLR7 and TLR9 signaling and type I interferon production distinguish pathogenic and nonpathogenic AIDS virus infections. Nature Medicine. 2008;**14**:1077-1087

[420] Jakobsen MR, Bak RO, Andersen A, et al. IFI16 senses DNA forms of the lentiviral replication cycle and controls HIV-1 replication. Proceedings of the National Academy of Sciences of the United States of America. 2013;**110**:E4571-E4580

[421] Wang MQ, Huang YL, Huang J, et al. RIG-I detects HIV-1 infection and mediates type I interferon response in human macrophages from patients with HIV-1-associated neurocognitive disorders. Genetics and Molecular Research. 2015;**14**:13799-13811

[422] Rho MB, Wesselingh S, Glass JD, et al. A potential role for interferon-alpha in the pathogenesis of HIV-associated dementia. Brain, Behavior, and Immunity. 1995;**9**:366-377

[423] Krivine A, Force G, Servan J, et al. Measuring HIV-1 RNA and interferon-alpha in the cerebrospinal fluid of AIDS patients: Insights into the pathogenesis of AIDS Dementia Complex. Journal of Neurovirology. 1999;**5**:500-506

[424] Perrella O, Carreiri PB, Perrella A, et al. Transforming growth factor beta-1 and interferon-alpha in the AIDS dementia complex (ADC): Possible relationship with cerebral viral load? European Cytokine Network. 2001;**12**:51-55

[425] Anderson AM, Lennox JL, Mulligan MM, et al. Cerebrospinal fluid interferon alpha levels correlate with neurocognitive impairment in ambulatory HIV-Infected individuals. Journal of Neurovirology. 2017;**23**:106-112

[426] Kong W, Frouard J, Xie G, et al. Neuroinflammation generated by HIV-infected microglia promotes dysfunction and death of neurons in human brain organoids. PNAS Nexus. 2024;**3**:pgae179

[427] Lamers SL, Rose R, Maidji E, et al. HIV DNA is frequently present within pathologic tissues evaluated at autopsy from combined antiretroviral therapy-treated patients with undetectable viral loads. Journal of Virology. 2016;**90**:8968-8983

[428] Osborne O, Peyravian N, Nair M, et al. The paradox of HIV blood–brain barrier penetrance and antiretroviral drug delivery deficiencies. Trends in Neurosciences. 2020;**43**:695-708

[429] Ene L, Duiculescu D, Ruta SM. How much do antiretroviral drugs penetrate

into the central nervous system? Journal of Medicine and Life. 2011;**4**:432-439

[430] Helms J, Kremer S, Merdji H, et al. Neurologic features in severe SARS-CoV-2 Infection. The New England Journal of Medicine. 2020;**382**:2268-2270

[431] Mao L, Jin H, Wang M, et al. Neurologic manifestations of hospitalized patients with coronavirus disease 2019 in Wuhan, China. JAMA Neurology. 2020. pp. 683-690. DOI: 10.1001/jamaneurol.2020.1127

[432] Hampshire A, Trender W, Chamberlain SR, et al. Cognitive deficits in people who have recovered from COVID-19. EClinicalMedicine. 2021;**39**:101044

[433] Liu Y-H, Chen Y, Wang Q-H, et al. One-year trajectory of cognitive changes in older survivors of COVID-19 in Wuhan, China: A longitudinal cohort study. JAMA Neurology. 2022;**79**:509-517

[434] Pellegrini L, Albecka A, Mallery DL, et al. SARS-CoV-2 infects the brain choroid plexus and disrupts the blood-CSF barrier in human brain organoids. Cell Stem Cell. 2020;**27**:951-961.e5

[435] van Heteren JT, Rozenberg F, Aronica E, et al. Astrocytes produce interferon-alpha and CXCL10, but not IL-6 or CXCL8, in Aicardi-Goutières syndrome. Glia. 2008;**56**:568-578

[436] Cuadrado E, Jansen MH, Anink J, et al. Chronic exposure of astrocytes to interferon-α reveals molecular changes related to Aicardi-Goutieres syndrome. Brain. 2013;**136**:245-258

[437] Sase S, Takanohashi A, Vanderver A, et al. Astrocytes, an active player in Aicardi-Goutières syndrome. Brain Pathology. 2018;**28**:399-407

[438] Cuadrado E, Michailidou I, van Bodegraven EJ, et al. Phenotypic variation in Aicardi-Goutières syndrome explained by cell-specific IFN-stimulated gene response and cytokine release. Journal of Immunology. 2015;**194**:3623-3633

[439] Giordano AMS, Luciani M, Gatto F, et al. DNA damage contributes to neurotoxic inflammation in Aicardi-Goutières syndrome astrocytes. The Journal of Experimental Medicine. 2022;**219**. DOI: 10.1084/jem.20211121

[440] Jin M, Shiwaku H, Tanaka H, et al. Tau activates microglia via the PQBP1-cGAS-STING pathway to promote brain inflammation. Nature Communications. 2021;**12**:6565

[441] Préhaud C, Mégret F, Lafage M, et al. Virus infection switches TLR-3-positive human neurons to become strong producers of beta interferon. Journal of Virology. 2005;**79**:12893-12904

[442] Lafaille FG, Pessach IM, Zhang S-Y, et al. Impaired intrinsic immunity to HSV-1 in human iPSC-derived TLR3-deficient CNS cells. Nature. 2012;**491**:769-773

[443] Tang S-C, Arumugam TV, Xu X, et al. Pivotal role for neuronal toll-like receptors in ischemic brain injury and functional deficits. Proceedings of the National Academy of Sciences of the United States of America. 2007;**104**:13798-13803

[444] Jovasevic V, Wood EM, Cicvaric A, et al. Formation of memory assemblies through the DNA-sensing TLR9 pathway. Nature. 2024;**628**:145-153

[445] Ma Y, Haynes RL, Sidman RL, et al. TLR8: An innate immune receptor in brain, neurons and axons. Cell Cycle. 2007;**6**:2859-2868

[446] Liu T, Xu Z-Z, Park C-K, et al. Toll-like receptor 7 mediates pruritus. Nature Neuroscience. 2010;**13**:1460-1462

[447] Lehmann SM, Krüger C, Park B, et al. An unconventional role for miRNA: Let-7 activates toll-like receptor 7 and causes neurodegeneration. Nature Neuroscience. 2012;**15**:827-835

[448] Nazmi A, Dutta K, Basu A. RIG-I mediates innate immune response in mouse neurons following Japanese encephalitis virus infection. PLoS One. 2011;**6**:e21761

[449] Liu Y, Jesus AA, Marrero B, et al. Activated STING in a vascular and pulmonary syndrome. The New England Journal of Medicine. 2014;**371**:507-518

[450] Chaudhuri A, Duan F, Morsey B, et al. HIV-1 activates proinflammatory and interferon-inducible genes in human brain microvascular endothelial cells: Putative mechanisms of blood–brain barrier dysfunction. Journal of Cerebral Blood Flow and Metabolism. 2008;**28**:697-711

[451] Kang L, Yu H, Yang X, et al. Neutrophil extracellular traps released by neutrophils impair revascularization and vascular remodeling after stroke. Nature Communications. 2020;**11**:2488

[452] Ma B, Dela Cruz CS, Hartl D, et al. RIG-like helicase innate immunity inhibits vascular endothelial growth factor tissue responses via a type I IFN-dependent mechanism. American Journal of Respiratory and Critical Care Medicine. 2011;**183**:1322-1335

[453] Sprokholt JK, Kaptein TM, van Hamme JL, et al. RIG-I-like receptor triggering by dengue virus drives dendritic cell immune activation and TH1 differentiation. Journal of Immunology. 2017;**198**:4764-4771

[454] Venkatesh D, Ernandez T, Rosetti F, et al. Endothelial TNF receptor 2 induces IRF1 transcription factor-dependent interferon-β autocrine signaling to promote monocyte recruitment. Immunity. 2013;**38**:1025-1037

[455] Kim H-J, Kim H, Lee J-H, et al. Toll-like receptor 4 (TLR4): New insight immune and aging. Immunity & Ageing. 2023;**20**:67

[456] Colleselli K, Stierschneider A, Wiesner C. An update on Toll-like receptor 2, its function and dimerization in pro- and anti-inflammatory processes. International Journal of Molecular Sciences. 2023;**24**. DOI: 10.3390/ijms241512464

[457] Pan W, Banks WA, Kastin AJ. Permeability of the blood–brain and blood-spinal cord barriers to interferons. Journal of Neuroimmunology. 1997;**76**:105-111

[458] Wang J, Campbell IL, Zhang H. Systemic interferon-alpha regulates interferon-stimulated genes in the central nervous system. Molecular Psychiatry. 2008;**13**:293-301

[459] Aw E, Zhang Y, Carroll M. Microglial responses to peripheral type 1 interferon. Journal of Neuroinflammation. 2020;**17**:340

[460] Felger JC. Role of inflammation in depression and treatment implications. Handbook of Experimental Pharmacology. 2019;**250**:255-286

[461] Torres-Platas SG, Cruceanu C, Chen GG, et al. Evidence for increased microglial priming and macrophage recruitment in the dorsal anterior cingulate white matter of depressed suicides. Brain, Behavior, and Immunity. 2014;**42**:50-59

[462] Curzytek K, Leśkiewicz M. Targeting the CCL2-CCR2 axis in depressive disorders. Pharmacological Reports. 2021;**73**:1052-1062

[463] Blomberg S, Eloranta M-L, Magnusson M, et al. Expression of the markers BDCA-2 and BDCA-4 and production of interferon-alpha by plasmacytoid dendritic cells in systemic lupus erythematosus. Arthritis and Rheumatism. 2003;**48**:2524-2532

[464] Rönnblom L, Pascual V. The innate immune system in SLE: Type I interferons and dendritic cells. Lupus. 2008;**17**:394-399

[465] Lindau D, Mussard J, Rabsteyn A, et al. TLR9 independent interferon α production by neutrophils on NETosis in response to circulating chromatin, a key lupus autoantigen. Annals of the Rheumatic Diseases. 2014;**73**:2199-2207

[466] Nehar-Belaid D, Hong S, Marches R, et al. Mapping systemic lupus erythematosus heterogeneity at the single-cell level. Nature Immunology. 2020;**21**:1094-1106

[467] Karnell JL, Wu Y, Mittereder N, et al. Depleting plasmacytoid dendritic cells reduces local type I interferon responses and disease activity in patients with cutaneous lupus. Science Translational Medicine. 2021;**13**. DOI: 10.1126/scitranslmed.abf8442

[468] West PK, McCorkindale AN, Guennewig B, et al. The cytokines interleukin-6 and interferon-α induce distinct microglia phenotypes. Journal of Neuroinflammation. 2022;**19**:96

[469] Li W, Viengkhou B, Denyer G, et al. Microglia have a more extensive and divergent response to interferon-α compared with astrocytes. Glia. 2018;**66**:2058-2078

[470] Qin H, Wilson CA, Lee SJ, et al. IFN-beta-induced SOCS-1 negatively regulates CD40 gene expression in macrophages and microglia. The FASEB Journal. 2006;**20**:985-987

[471] Albini A, Marchisone C, Del Grosso F, et al. Inhibition of angiogenesis and vascular tumor growth by interferon-producing cells: A gene therapy approach. The American Journal of Pathology. 2000;**156**:1381-1393

[472] Indraccolo S. Interferon-alpha as angiogenesis inhibitor: Learning from tumor models. Autoimmunity. 2010;**43**:244-247

[473] Romagnani P, Annunziato F, Lasagni L, et al. Cell cycle-dependent expression of CXC chemokine receptor 3 by endothelial cells mediates angiostatic activity. The Journal of Clinical Investigation. 2001;**107**:53-63

[474] Campanella GSV, Colvin RA, Luster AD. CXCL10 can inhibit endothelial cell proliferation independently of CXCR3. PLoS One. 2010;**5**:e12700

[475] Jian D, Wang W, Zhou X, et al. Interferon-induced protein 35 inhibits endothelial cell proliferation, migration and re-endothelialization of injured arteries by inhibiting the nuclear factor-kappa B pathway. Acta Physiologica (Oxford, England). 2018;**223**:e13037

[476] Kalucka J, de Rooij LPMH, Goveia J, et al. Single-cell transcriptome atlas of murine endothelial cells. Cell. 2020;**180**:764-779.e20

[477] Floris S, Ruuls SR, Wierinckx A, et al. Interferon-beta directly influences monocyte infiltration into the central nervous system. Journal of Neuroimmunology. 2002;**127**:69-79

[478] Buttmann M, Goebeler M, Toksoy A, et al. Subcutaneous interferon-beta injections in patients with multiple sclerosis initiate inflammatory skin reactions by local chemokine induction. Journal of Neuroimmunology. 2005;**168**:175-182

[479] Campbell IL, Krucker T, Steffensen S, et al. Structural and functional neuropathology in transgenic mice with CNS expression of IFN-alpha. Brain Research. 1999;**835**:46-61

[480] Wiley CA, Steinman RA, Wang Q. Innate immune activation without immune cell infiltration in brains of murine models of Aicardi-Goutières syndrome. Brain Pathology. 2023;**33**:e13118

[481] Kettwig M, Ternka K, Wendland K, et al. Interferon-driven brain phenotype in a mouse model of RNaseT2 deficient leukoencephalopathy. Nature Communications. 2021;**12**:6530

[482] Larochelle C, Grand'maison F, Bernier GP, et al. Thrombotic thrombocytopenic purpura-hemolytic uremic syndrome in relapsing–remitting multiple sclerosis patients on high-dose interferon β. Multiple Sclerosis. 2014;**20**:1783-1787

[483] Popson SA, Ziegler ME, Chen X, et al. Interferon-induced transmembrane protein 1 regulates endothelial lumen formation during angiogenesis. Arteriosclerosis, Thrombosis, and Vascular Biology. 2014;**34**:1011-1019

[484] Herrmann JR, Simon DW. Interfer(on)-ing with vascular repair after acute brain injury. Nature Immunology. 2021;**22**:1205-1206

[485] Weller RO, Boche D, Nicoll JAR. Microvasculature changes and cerebral amyloid angiopathy in Alzheimer's disease and their potential impact on therapy. Acta Neuropathologica. 2009;**118**:87-102

[486] Charidimou A, Boulouis G, Gurol ME, et al. Emerging concepts in sporadic cerebral amyloid angiopathy. Brain. 2017;**140**:1829-1850

[487] Greenberg SM, Bacskai BJ, Hernandez-Guillamon M, et al. Cerebral amyloid angiopathy and Alzheimer disease - One peptide, two pathways. Nature Reviews. Neurology. 2020;**16**:30-42

[488] Petersen MA, Ryu JK, Akassoglou K. Fibrinogen in neurological diseases: Mechanisms, imaging and therapeutics. Nature Reviews. Neuroscience. 2018;**19**:283-301

[489] Merlini M, Rafalski VA, Rios Coronado PE, et al. Fibrinogen induces microglia-mediated spine elimination and cognitive impairment in an Alzheimer's disease model. Neuron. 2019;**101**:1099-1108.e6

[490] Mendiola AS, Yan Z, Dixit K, et al. Defining blood-induced microglia functions in neurodegeneration through multiomic profiling. Nature Immunology. 2023;**24**:1173-1187

[491] Klok MD, Bakels HS, Postma NL, et al. Interferon-α and the calcifying microangiopathy in Aicardi-Goutières syndrome. Annals of Clinical Translational Neurology. 2015;**2**:774-779

[492] Nazmi A, Field RH, Griffin EW, et al. Chronic neurodegeneration induces type I interferon synthesis via STING, shaping microglial phenotype and accelerating disease progression. Glia. 2019;**67**:1254-1276

[493] Lall D, Lorenzini I, Mota TA, et al. C9orf72 deficiency promotes microglial-mediated synaptic loss in aging and

amyloid accumulation. Neuron. 2021;**109**:2275-2291.e8

[494] Stevens B, Allen NJ, Vazquez LE, et al. The classical complement cascade mediates CNS synapse elimination. Cell. 2007;**131**:1164-1178

[495] Stevens B, Johnson MB. The complement cascade repurposed in the brain. Nature Reviews. Immunology. 2021;**21**:624-625

[496] Escoubas CC, Dorman LC, Nguyen PT, et al. Type-I-interferon-responsive microglia shape cortical development and behavior. Cell. 2024;**187**:1936-1954.e24

[497] Baker CA, Iwasaki A. Beyond antiviral: Role of IFN-I in brain development. Trends in Immunology. 2024. pp. 322-324. DOI: 10.1016/j.it.2024.04.004

[498] Ramlackhansingh AF, Brooks DJ, Greenwood RJ, et al. Inflammation after trauma: Microglial activation and traumatic brain injury. Annals of Neurology. 2011;**70**:374-383

[499] Smith C, Gentleman SM, Leclercq PD, et al. The neuroinflammatory response in humans after traumatic brain injury. Neuropathology and Applied Neurobiology. 2013;**39**:654-666

[500] Kou Z, VandeVord PJ. Traumatic white matter injury and glial activation: From basic science to clinics. Glia. 2014;**62**:1831-1855

[501] Graham NSN, Jolly A, Zimmerman K, et al. Diffuse axonal injury predicts neurodegeneration after moderate–severe traumatic brain injury. Brain. 2020;**143**:3685-3698

[502] Raj R, Kaprio J, Jousilahti P, et al. Risk of dementia after hospitalization due to traumatic brain injury: A longitudinal population-based study. Neurology. 2022;**98**:e2377-e2386

[503] Johnson VE, Stewart JE, Begbie FD, et al. Inflammation and white matter degeneration persist for years after a single traumatic brain injury. Brain. 2013;**136**:28-42

[504] Krauthausen M, Kummer MP, Zimmermann J, et al. CXCR3 promotes plaque formation and behavioral deficits in an Alzheimer's disease model. The Journal of Clinical Investigation. 2015;**125**:365-378

[505] Yu Z-X, Song H-M. Toward a better understanding of type I interferonopathies: A brief summary, update and beyond. World Journal of Pediatrics. 2020;**16**:44-51

[506] Matsui H, Ito J, Matsui N, et al. Cytosolic dsDNA of mitochondrial origin induces cytotoxicity and neurodegeneration in cellular and zebrafish models of Parkinson's disease. Nature Communications. 2021;**12**:3101

[507] Yoshimoto N, Nakamura Y, Hisaoka-Nakashima K, et al. Mitochondrial dysfunction and type I interferon signaling induce anxiodepressive-like behaviors in mice with neuropathic pain. Experimental Neurology. 2023;**367**:114470

[508] Smith JR, Dowling JW, McFadden MI, et al. MEF2A suppresses stress responses that trigger DDX41-dependent IFN production. Cell Reports. 2023;**42**:112805

[509] Sheehan KCF, Lai KS, Dunn GP, et al. Blocking monoclonal antibodies specific for mouse IFN-alpha/beta receptor subunit 1 (IFNAR-1) from mice immunized by in vivo hydrodynamic transfection. Journal

of Interferon & Cytokine Research. 2006;**26**:804-819

[510] Peng L, Oganesyan V, Wu H, et al. Molecular basis for antagonistic activity of anifrolumab, an anti-interferon-α receptor 1 antibody. MAbs. 2015;7:428-439

[511] Furie R, Khamashta M, Merrill JT, et al. Anifrolumab, an anti-interferon-α receptor monoclonal antibody, in moderate-to-severe systemic lupus erythematosus. Arthritis & Rhematology. 2017;**69**:376-386

[512] Morand EF, Furie R, Tanaka Y, et al. Trial of anifrolumab in active systemic lupus erythematosus. The New England Journal of Medicine. 2020;**382**:211-221

[513] Tang W, Tummala R, Almquist J, et al. Clinical pharmacokinetics, pharmacodynamics, and immunogenicity of anifrolumab. Clinical Pharmacokinetics. 2023;**62**:655-671

[514] Tanaka Y. Viewpoint on anifrolumab in patients with systemic lupus erythematosus and a high unmet need in clinical practice. RMD Open. 2023;**9**. DOI: 10.1136/rmdopen-2023-003270

[515] Chatham WW, Furie R, Saxena A, et al. Long-term safety and efficacy of anifrolumab in adults with systemic lupus erythematosus: Results of a phase II open-label extension study. Arthritis & Rhematology. 2021;**73**:816-825

[516] Bruce IN, Golam S, Steenkamp J, et al. Indirect treatment comparison of anifrolumab efficacy versus belimumab in adults with systemic lupus erythematosus. Journal of Comparative Effectiveness Research. 2022;**11**:765-777

[517] Furie R, Rovin BH, Houssiau F, et al. Two-year, randomized, controlled trial of belimumab in lupus nephritis. The New England Journal of Medicine. 2020;**383**:1117-1128

[518] Brunner HI, Abud-Mendoza C, Viola DO, et al. Safety and efficacy of intravenous belimumab in children with systemic lupus erythematosus: Results from a randomized, placebo-controlled trial. Annals of the Rheumatic Diseases. 2020;**79**:1340-1348

[519] Nakai T, Fukui S, Kidoguchi G, et al. Effect and safety profile of belimumab and tacrolimus combination therapy in thirty-three patients with systemic lupus erythematosus. Clinical Rheumatology. 2022;**41**:3735-3745

[520] Teng YKO, Bruce IN, Diamond B, et al. Phase III, multicentre, randomized, double-blind, placebo-controlled, 104-week study of subcutaneous belimumab administered in combination with rituximab in adults with systemic lupus erythematosus (SLE): Bliss-believe study protocol. BMJ Open. 2019;**9**:e025687

[521] Shipa M, Embleton-Thirsk A, Parvaz M, et al. Effectiveness of belimumab after rituximab in systemic lupus erythematosus: A randomized controlled trial. Annals of Internal Medicine. 2021;**174**:1647-1657

[522] Merrill JT, Wallace DJ, Petri M, et al. Safety profile and clinical activity of sifalimumab, a fully human anti-interferon α monoclonal antibody, in systemic lupus erythematosus: A phase I, multicentre, double-blind randomized study. Annals of the Rheumatic Diseases. 2011;**70**:1905-1913

[523] McBride JM, Jiang J, Abbas AR, et al. Safety and pharmacodynamics of rontalizumab in patients with systemic lupus erythematosus: Results of a phase I, placebo-controlled, double-blind, dose-escalation study. Arthritis and Rheumatism. 2012;**64**:3666-3676

[524] Kalunian KC, Merrill JT, Maciuca R, et al. A Phase II study of the efficacy and safety of rontalizumab (rhuMAb interferon-α) in patients with systemic lupus erythematosus (ROSE). Annals of the Rheumatic Diseases. 2016;**75**:196-202

[525] Doroudchi M-A, Thauland TJ, Patel BA, et al. Anifrolumab to treat a monogenic interferonopathy. The Journal of Allergy and Clinical Immunology in Practice. 2024;**12**:1374-1376.e1

[526] Rachubinski AL, Estrada BE, Norris D, et al. Janus kinase inhibition in Down syndrome: 2 cases of therapeutic benefit for alopecia areata. JAAD Case Reports. 2019;**5**:365-367

[527] Rodriguez S, Sahin A, Schrank BR, et al. Genome-encoded cytoplasmic double-stranded RNAs, found in C9ORF72 ALS-FTD brain, propagate neuronal loss. Science Translational Medicine. 2021;**13**. DOI: 10.1126/scitranslmed.aaz4699

[528] Vanderver A, Adang L, Gavazzi F, et al. Janus kinase inhibition in the Aicardi-Goutières syndrome. The New England Journal of Medicine. 2020;**383**:986-989

[529] Neven B, Al Adba B, Hully M, et al. JAK inhibition in the Aicardi-Goutières syndrome. The New England Journal of Medicine. 2020;**383**:2190-2191

[530] Li W, Wang W, Wang W, et al. Janus kinase inhibitors in the treatment of type I interferonopathies: A case series from a single center in china. Frontiers in Immunology. 2022;**13**:825367

[531] Frémond M-L, Hully M, Fournier B, et al. JAK inhibition in Aicardi-Goutières syndrome: A monocentric multidisciplinary real-world approach study. Journal of Clinical Immunology. 2023;**43**:1436-1447

[532] Jafarpour S, Suddock J, Hawes D, et al. Neuropathologic impacts of JAK inhibitor treatment in Aicardi-Goutières syndrome. Journal of Clinical Immunology. 2024;**44**:68

[533] Chougule A, Taur P, Gowri V, et al. SPENCD presenting with Evans phenotype and clinical response to JAK1/2 inhibitors-A report of 2 cases. Journal of Clinical Immunology. 2023;**43**:331-334

[534] Kothur K, Bandodkar S, Chu S, et al. An open-label trial of JAK 1/2 blockade in progressive IFIH1-associated neuroinflammation. Neurology. 2018;**90**:289-291

[535] Cattalini M, Galli J, Zunica F, et al. Case report: The JAK-inhibitor ruxolitinib use in Aicardi-Goutieres syndrome due to ADAR1 mutation. Frontiers in Pediatrics. 2021;**9**:725868

[536] Galli J, Cattalini M, Loi E, et al. Treatment response to Janus kinase inhibitor in a child affected by Aicardi-Goutières syndrome. Clinical Case Reports. 2023;**11**:e7724

[537] Rice GI, Meyzer C, Bouazza N, et al. Reverse-transcriptase inhibitors in the Aicardi–Goutières syndrome. The New England Journal of Medicine. 2018;**379**:2275-2277

[538] Sullivan AC, Zuniga G, Ramirez P, et al. A pilot study to investigate the safety and feasibility of antiretroviral therapy for Alzheimer's disease (ART-AD). medRxiv. 2024. DOI: 10.1101/2024.02.26.24303316

[539] Kulkarni JA, Witzigmann D, Thomson SB, et al. The current landscape of nucleic acid therapeutics. Nature Nanotechnology. 2021;**16**:630-643

[540] Finkel RS, Mercuri E, Darras BT, et al. Nusinersen versus Sham control in

infantile-onset spinal muscular atrophy. The New England Journal of Medicine. 2017;**377**:1723-1732

[541] Miller TM, Cudkowicz ME, Genge A, et al. Trial of antisense oligonucleotide tofersen for SOD1 ALS. The New England Journal of Medicine. 2022;**387**:1099-1110

[542] Viengkhou B, Hong C, Mazur C, et al. Interferon-α receptor antisense oligonucleotides reduce neuroinflammation and neuropathology in a mouse model of cerebral interferonopathy. The Journal of Clinical Investigation. 2024;**134**. DOI: 10.1172/JCI169562

[543] Terstappen GC, Meyer AH, Bell RD, et al. Strategies for delivering therapeutics across the blood–brain barrier. Nature Reviews. Drug Discovery. 2021;**20**:362-383

[544] Oller-Salvia B, Sánchez-Navarro M, Giralt E, et al. Blood–brain barrier shuttle peptides: An emerging paradigm for brain delivery. Chemical Society Reviews. 2016;**45**:4690-4707

[545] Niewoehner J, Bohrmann B, Collin L, et al. Increased brain penetration and potency of a therapeutic antibody using a monovalent molecular shuttle. Neuron. 2014;**81**:49-60

[546] Das T, Chen Z, Hendriks RW, et al. A20/tumor necrosis factor α-induced protein 3 in immune cells controls development of autoinflammation and autoimmunity: Lessons from mouse models. Frontiers in Immunology. 2018;**9**:104

[547] Deverman BE, Pravdo PL, Simpson BP, et al. Cre-dependent selection yields AAV variants for widespread gene transfer to the adult brain. Nature Biotechnology. 2016;**34**:204-209

[548] Mullard A. NfL makes regulatory debut as neurodegenerative disease biomarker. Nature Reviews. Drug Discovery. 2023;**22**:431-434

[549] Benatar M, Ostrow LW, Lewcock JW, et al. Biomarker qualification for neurofilament light chain in amyotrophic lateral sclerosis: Theory and practice. Annals of Neurology. 2024;**95**:211-216

[550] Hauser SL, Kappos L, Arnold DL, et al. Five years of ocrelizumab in relapsing multiple sclerosis: OPERA studies open-label extension. Neurology. 2020;**95**:e1854-e1867

[551] Younossi ZM, Stepanova M, Esteban R, et al. Superiority of interferon-free regimens for chronic Hepatitis C: The effect on health-related quality of life and work productivity. Medicine (Baltimore). 2017;**96**:e5914

[552] Borden EC. Interferons α and β in cancer: Therapeutic opportunities from new insights. Nature Reviews. Drug Discovery. 2019;**18**:219-234

[553] Kirkwood JM, Strawderman MH, Ernstoff MS, et al. Interferon Alfa-2b adjuvant therapy of high-risk resected cutaneous melanoma: The eastern cooperative oncology group trial EST 1684. Journal of Clinical Oncology. 2023;**41**:425-435

Chapter 3

Preclinical Validation of FTY720 and FTY720-Mitoxy in Mouse Models of Parkinsons Disease and Multiple System Atrophy (MSA): Evidence for Treating Lewy Body Disease Synucleinopathies Including MSA

Guadalupe Vidal-Martinez, Haiyan Lou and Ruth G. Perez

Abstract

We assessed FTY720 and our patented-mitochondria-localizing-FTY720-derivative, FTY720-Mitoxy, in mouse models of Parkinson's disease (PD) and MSA. FTY720 and FTY720-Mitoxy were given by gavage, injection, or osmotic pump. We used symptomatic transgenic alpha-Synuclein (aSyn) PD mice (A53T aSyn) and MSA mice (CNP-aSyn), as well as transgenic GM2 +/− PD mice. We also tested toxin PD and MSA models. We measured movement, constipation, gut motility, sweat ability, and bladder function. We counted blood lymphocytes 24 h after FTY720 or FTY720-Mitoxy. We measured Brain Derived Neurotrophic Factor (BDNF), Glial Cell Line Derived Neurotrophic Factor (GDNF), and Nerve Growth Factor (NGF) mRNA and protein. We assessed aSyn insolubility in gut, brain, and spinal cord by sequential protein extraction and immunoblot. We assessed fecal genomic DNA using 16S rRNA sequencing. In PD mice FTY720 normalized body and gut movement, urinary bladder function while increasing trophic factors and eliminating synucleinopathy. In MSA mice FTY720-Mitoxy normalized body and gut movement, sweat ability, mitochondrial function, improved microbiota while increasing trophic factors and eliminating synucleinopathy. FTY720 and FTY720-Mitoxy improve function and counteract synucleinopathy. As FTY720-Mitoxy is not immunosuppressive, it may be safer for treating PD and/or MSA.

Keywords: alpha-synuclein (aSyn), multiple system atrophy (MSA), Parkinson's disease (PD), transgenic (Tg) mice, A53T aSyn PD mouse model (A53T), aSyn MSA mouse model (CNP-aSyn), GM2 PD mouse model (GM2 +/−), toxin model of PD (6-OHDA), toxin model of MSA (3NP).

1. Introduction

PD and MSA are progressive neurodegenerative disorders with overlapping movement and autonomic symptoms that typically manifest over time during the aging process. Fortunately, there are mouse models that manifest symptoms of both diseases which allows for modeling them for drug testing. PD and MSA are both what are called "synucleinopathies" because they occur after the small chaperone-like protein, alpha-synuclein (aSyn), accumulates primarily inside neurons in PD and glial cells in MSA, leading to brain and body dysfunction [1, 2]. But one may wonder, why does the aSyn aggregation induce mainly neuronal problems in PD [3] and glial abnormalities followed by neuronal loss in MSA [4, 5]?

One clue about how this happens arises from data showing that PD motor impairment occurs only after a marked loss of substantia nigra dopaminergic neurons [6, 7], while surviving nigral neurons typically contain intracellular aSyn aggregates known as Lewy bodies (LBs) [8]. Only rare PD cases are associated with aSyn mutations and/or multiplications that are causative of the disease [9]. Recent evidence has shown that there are different conformationally and biologically distinct strains of pathological aSyn in PD and MSA [10]. Regardless of its strong association with PD and MSA, it is also very well documented that aSyn has important normal functions, some of which are especially vital for dopaminergic neurons where aSyn interacts with key proteins that modulate not only dopamine synthesis [11, 12] but also dopamine release [13, 14]. This modulation occurs, at least in part, because aSyn binds to and stimulates the activity of protein phosphatase 2A (PP2A), a major Ser/Thr phosphatase that regulates the phosphorylation state of the enzyme tyrosine hydroxylase (TH), the rate-limiting enzyme in dopamine synthesis, and also key proteins that modulate cell signaling [15, 16]. Significantly, in vivo silencing of aSyn expression in mature nigrostriatal neurons in vivo causes neuronal dysfunction and subsequent brain neuroinflammation to occur [17]. Additionally, when aSyn aggregates in human brains and tissues from animal models, dysregulation of PP2A activity occurs [18] which can lead to an excess of intracellular and extracellular dopamine, reactive oxygen species, and dopamine quinones, which are highly toxic to the nigral dopaminergic neurons [19–21]. Furthermore, another major enzyme, monoamine oxidase B, which helps degrade dopamine, is modulated by interaction with aSyn [22]. Together these data confirm that aSyn plays a key role in regulating brain pathways that control normal body movement.

In MSA, aSyn accumulates inside the myelinating glial cells of brain, the oligodendrocytes, which then forms two different types of lesions (1) glial cytoplasmic inclusions (GCI) and (2) glial nuclear inclusions (GNI) [23–25]. When this occurs, neuronal demyelination occurs along with a loss of trophic factors required to support neurons, ultimately impairing function [26–28]. MSA can manifest as two different forms, (1) a condition that primarily affects the basal ganglia, thus producing Parkinsonian symptoms (MSA-P) or (2) primarily as cerebellar dysfunction and ataxia (MSA-C) [27]. Because transgenic PD and MSA mouse models recapitulate many of the age-onset changes associated with PD and MSA [29–35] they have been used to assess potential therapies [36–43]. While many therapeutics for PD and MSA are in development [44, 45], the focus of this review is on our preclinical validation of FTY720 (along with data from other laboratories who studied FTY720), and our patented derivative, FTY720-Mitoxy, as possible therapies for PD and MSA.

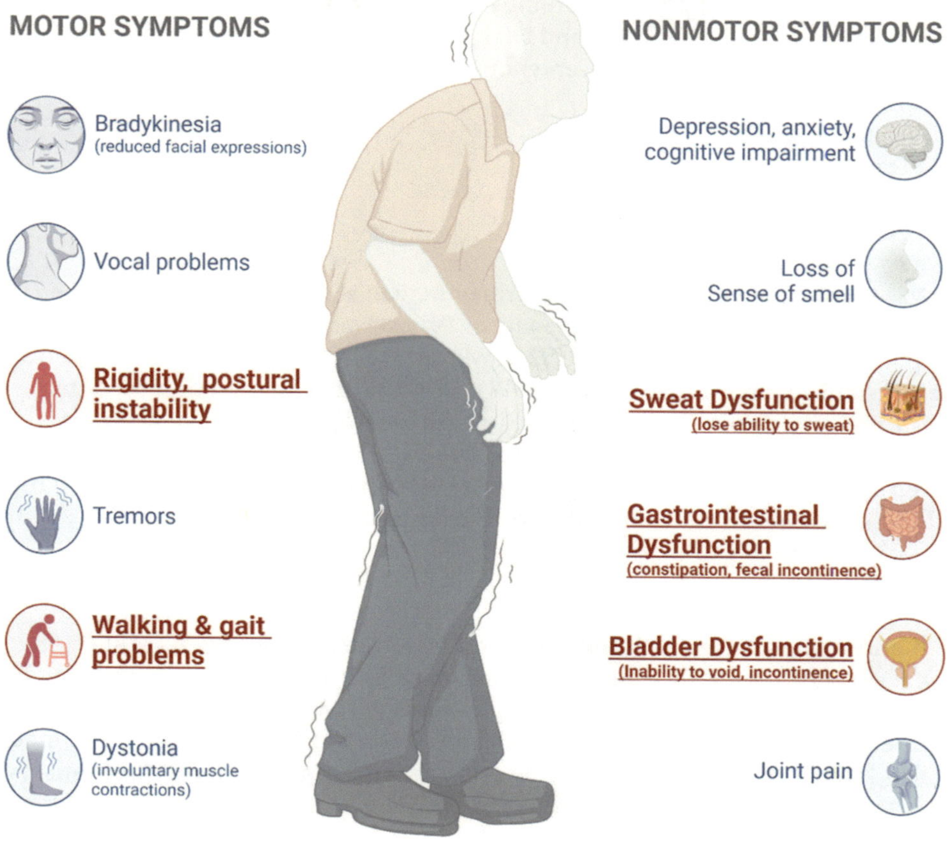

Figure 1.
PD and MSA both manifest after the onset of motor symptoms (listed on the left) and/or nonmotor symptoms (listed on the right), with symptoms in red and underlined, occurring in aging PD and MSA mouse models. Figure created with BioRender.com.

Because many symptoms of PD and MSA arise over time in humans and can be modeled in aging mice, drugs can be evaluated over time for their ability to slow, halt, or reverse PD or MSA symptoms. For the purposes of review in this chapter, we focus on the symptoms that are labeled in red font and underlined in **Figure 1**.

To test the efficacy of FTY720 and FTY720-Mitoxy as potential therapies for PD and MSA we, and others, evaluated several mouse models and tested multiple methods. *Though this chapter is a review of our published data, we included an abbreviated Materials and Methods section below (Section 2) to help more clearly summarize all of the models and methods employed over many years of study, in order to simplify data interpretation.*

2. Materials and methods

2.1 Mice as models of PD and MSA

Briefly, all of the mice studied in our laboratories were housed in barrier cages on ventilated racks in temperature and humidity-controlled rooms on 12-h light/dark cycles with food and water available ad libitum. Mice underwent behavioral testing in clean quiet test rooms after acclimation as previously described. Ethical treatment of mice followed AALAC, ARRIVE, and NIH guidelines on approved protocols at Texas Tech University Health Sciences Center or at Shandong University as also previously described.

2.2 PD mouse models

2.2.1 A53T aSyn Tg mice

Mice expressing the A53T mutant form of human aSyn were generated in the laboratory of Dr. Virginia Lee (University of Pennsylvania, Philadelphia, PA) [46]. We purchased the heterozygous (B6:C3-Tg-Prnp/SNCA*A53T/83Vle/J) breeders from the Jackson Laboratories (Bar Harbor, ME). Our cohort of Tg mice thus consisted of WT non-transgenic littermates as well as and heterozygous and homozygous offspring that overexpressed either one or two copies of mutant human A53T aSyn driven by a prion promoter [46]. Genotyping was performed as described [47]. Onset of PD-like symptoms were verified prior to drug treatment.

2.2.2 GM2 Tg mice

Mature gangliosides are ligands for myelin associated glycoprotein (MAG) [48] that act to enhance myelin stability [49] and contribute to normal brain function. It has been shown that immature GM3 gangliosides are elevated in PD brain [50], while mature GM1 ganglioside levels are significantly lower in PD patients and in PD mouse models [51, 52]. Transgenic B4galnt1 heterozygous mice, gift of Drs. Ledeen and Wu (Rutgers New Jersey Medical School), were used to generate our colony of wild type mice (WT, +/+) with two normal copies of the GM2 Synthase gene, and heterozygous mice with a single GM2 Synthase gene (GM2, +/−). Genotyping was performed as described [53, 54]. Thus, the GM2+/− heterozygous mice, with excess GM3 and reduced GM1 levels, closely model human PD. Onset of PD-like symptoms were verified prior to drug treatment.

2.2.3 6-OHDA toxin model

6-OHDA has been widely used to model PD in which striatal injections produce nigral dopamine neuron loss over 1–3 weeks' time, allowing for longitudinal assessment of the mice [55]. Briefly, C57BL/6 mice were pretreated with 0.5 mg/kg FTY720 or vehicle by intraperitoneal injection for 7 days prior to 6-OHDA. On the 7th day, 1 h after final FTY720 dosing, mice were placed in a stereotaxic apparatus under anesthesia and injected with 6 μg of 6-OHDA (prepared in 2 μL of normal saline with 0.02% ascorbic acid) or saline alone into two different sites of the right striatum. All mice were assessed at 7-, 14-, or 21-days post injection [56].

2.2.4 1-Methyl-4-phenyl-1,2,3,6-tetrahydropyridine (MPTP) model

Two different laboratories studied the impact of FTY720 in the MPTP toxin model of PD. Komnig et al. [57], used a subacute dose of MPTP, while Motyl et al. [58] used an acute MPTP treatment to induce PD like changes. Komnig found no benefit with FTY720 while Motyl and colleagues reported significant protection against MPTP toxicity using FTY720.

2.2.5 Rotenone model

Zhao et al. [59], used rotenone to induce PD-like symptoms in their mice, which caused systemic mitochondrial impairment, oxidative damage, microglial activation, selective nigrostriatal dopaminergic degeneration, L-DOPA-responsive motor deficits, aSyn aggregation and formation of Lewy body-like inclusions. FTY720 was reported to be highly protective in this model. Another laboratory tested FTY720-Chitosan against a rotenone model and also saw protection [60].

2.3 MSA mouse models

2.3.1 CNP-aSyn Tg mice

CNP-aSyn mice (B6:C3-Tg-CNP-SNCA-M2Vle) were obtained from a repository established by Dr. Virginia Lee at the Jackson Laboratories (Bar Harbor, ME). Heterozygous, non-littermate Tg mice were used to generate our CNP-aSyn mouse colony. Heterozygous or homozygous Tg mice express either one or two copies of WT human SNCA with expression driven by a CNP promoter in the myelinating cells of CNS (oligodendroglia) and peripheral nervous system (PNS, Schwann cells) [61, 62]. This CNP-aSyn model develops progressive motor and autonomic problems as well as neuronal and white matter damage in response to aSyn overexpression, similar to what occurs in subjects suffering with MSA-P and MSA-C [39, 63]. Onset of MSA-like symptoms was verified prior to drug treatment.

2.3.2 The 3NP toxin model of MSA

MSA models can also be generated using the mitochondrial toxin 3-nitropropionic acid (3NP) (Cat # N5634, Sigma-Aldrich, St. Louis, MO, USA), which inhibits mitochondrial succinate dehydrogenase (SDH) activity, also known as mitochondrial Complex II resulting in MSA like symptoms [64]. We prepared 3NP with sterile saline (pH 7.4) and sterile saline used along as the control. Aging CNP-aSyn mice (8.5 mo) were given subcutaneous injections of 3NP twice daily at escalating doses—10 mg/kg (day 9.5), 20 mg/kg (days 11 and 12), and 30 mg/kg (days 13 and 14) exactly as described [39, 65].

2.4 Drugs evaluated

All FTY720 and FTY720-Mitoxy (**Figure 2**) used in our studies, were evaluated for purity and stability prior to use [39, 66]. FTY720 is a synthetic sphingosine-1-phosphate receptor modulator approved to treat relapsing remitting multiple sclerosis (MS) [67]. MS patients benefit from FTY720 by both its anti-inflammatory and neuroprotective effects, which we have also demonstrated to occur in response to FTY720-Mitoxy, both in vitro and in vivo [68, 69].

Notably, both drugs increase the expression of brain derived neurotrophic factor (BDNF), while FTY720-Mitoxy also significantly increases the expression of nerve growth factor (NGF) and glial-cell-line derived neurotrophic factor (GDNF) in neuronal and oligodendroglial cells [39, 53, 68, 70, 71].

The major difference between the drugs is the fact that FTY720, which is phosphorylated in vivo by Sphingosine Kinase, causes immunosuppression. In stark contrast, FTY720-Mitoxy, which also rapidly crosses the blood brain barrier but is not phosphorylated [66] does not suppress the immune system [72].

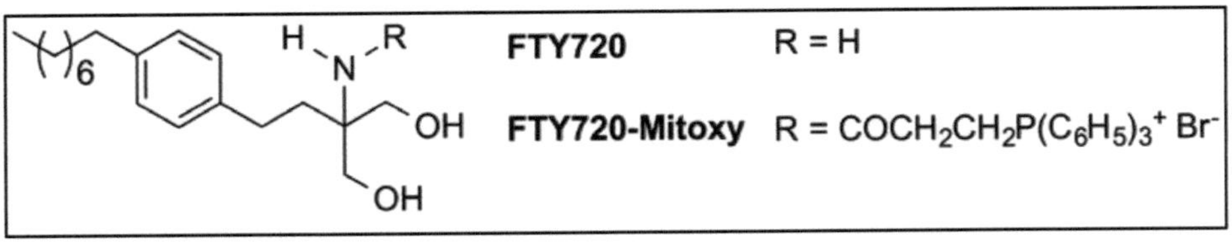

Figure 2.
FTY720 and FTY720-Mitoxy chemical structures. Figure is reprinted with permission of Elsevier Science and Technology Journals, Experimental Neurology [39] from the Copyright Clearance Center.

2.5 Behavioral tests to assess drug efficacy in mice

2.5.1 Movement tests

- *Rotarod* (Cat # LE8200, Harvard Apparatus, Holliston, MA), measures balance, coordination, and endurance. Timing as "latency to fall" from the apparatus was recorded in sec using established methods [46, 73]. Briefly, mice were familiarized with the rotarod during initial trainings of 2 sessions on 2 consecutive days. Each training session consisted of 2 runs lasting 2 min each, one at 4 revolutions per min (rpm) and the other at 8 rpm. Experimental data were collected in 3 runs/day on 2 different days for each mouse, with rotation increasing from 4 to 40 rpm over 5 min. A minimum 5 min rest period was allowed between runs for all mice [39, 71].

- *Open field* locomotor activity was monitored using the TruScan™ open field apparatus (Coulbourn Instruments, Whitehall, PA, USA). Mice were acclimated to the test room for 15 min prior to being placed individually in the center of the arena with total movement monitored for 15 min. Total movement was measured as successive coordinate movements made across the floor plane while mice were continuously active. Mice were tested in random order on two independent occasions with established methods [53, 74].

- *Apomorphine-induced rotations* were monitored over 3 weeks' time, from 1 week post 6-OHDA lesioning as before [11]. Apomorphine was subcutaneously injected into mice at a dose of 0.1 mg/kg (Sigma), with mice placed individually in plastic beakers (diameter: 13 cm), and videotaped from above for 30 min. Quantitative analyses of completed (360°) left and right rotations were made off-line by an investigator blinded to the experimental conditions.

- *Hindlimb reflex tests* were performed as follows. Each mouse was suspended by the tail for 5 sec during which the position of the hindlimbs was scored. Data were collected over 3 trials performed on 2 different days, with short breaks given between trials. Scores ranging from impaired to normal were as follows: 0 = one or both hindlimbs paralyzed, 1 = hindlimbs and paws close to the body with clasping toes, 2 = loss of flexion of hindlimbs, 3 = hindlimbs extended <90° angle, and 4 = hindlimbs extended >90° angle.

2.5.2 Gut function and gut health

- *Fecal pellets.* When food moves through the gut slowly, the colon absorbs more water, so consequently the feces become dryer and hardened. Thus, water content in feces was measured using methods described by Taylor et al., with total stool collected in the afternoon from individual mice placed in clean cages for 1 h. Feces were immediately transferred to 1.5-mL Eppendorf tubes that were labeled, capped, and weighed. Tubes were opened to allow fecal desiccation, and heated at 65°C overnight. Tubes were capped and weighed again, with water content calculated by computing the difference between wet and dry weights [47, 71].

- *Gastrointestinal transit time.* Whole gut transit time was assessed after oral gavage of a 0.2-mL volume of 6% (w/v) carmine red dye in 0.5% methylcellulose (Sigma-Aldrich). Post-gavage, all mice were observed up to 9 h for excretion of the first red stool, with the time recorded for each mouse. Mice that had not passed any red stool by 9 h scored >9 h [47, 75].

- *Colonic motility* was measured in old mice using the bead expulsion test. Briefly, a glass bead (3 mm; Sigma-Aldrich, Z143928-1EA) was gently pushed 2.0 cm into the colon using the smooth end of a plastic inoculating loop (Nunc, 253287). The total time from bead insertion to bead ejection was recorded for each mouse [47].

- *Microbiota* were analyzed by 16S rRNA sequencing at Texas Tech in Lubbock after extracting fecal genomic DNA in our laboratory at Texas Tech in El Paso. Briefly, human subjects collected their own fecal samples at home into a container filled with stool DNA stabilizer (PSP® Spin Stool DNA PlusKit, Stratec Molecular). After transfer to the laboratory, samples were stored at −80°C until processing. Mouse feces were collected into sterile tubes during 1 h periods in the morning, with feces preserved and stored exactly as above. Total fecal DNA was extracted using QIAamp fast DNA stool Mini kits (Cat # 51604, Qiagen Inc., Valencia, CA) followed by 16S rRNA analysis as described [76].

2.5.3 *Sweat function*

- *The starch iodine test* was used to assess sweating in mice with MSA-like changes. Sweat droplets were measured using established methods [77] with minor modifications. Specifically, mice were gently and firmly manually restrained by one experimenter throughout each test. Another experimenter cleaned the left hind paw with a water-moistened cotton tipped swab then painted that paw using a small artist brush dipped in a freshly prepared solution of 2% iodine (Cat # 207772, Sigma-Aldrich, St. Louis, MO, USA) in ethanol. After the paw dried, it was then painted with a starch solution prepared in castor oil (1 g/mL, Cat # S9765 in Cat # 259853, Sigma-Aldrich, St. Louis, MO, USA). The paw was then photographed through a 10X magnifier lens at 0.0, 2.5 and 5 min timepoints to record the presence of dark purple precipitates. Digital images were blind coded and the main paw areas (excluding digits) were analyzed using ImageQuant 5.2 (GE Healthcare, Waukesha, WI) to quantify droplets in arbitrary units [39].

2.5.4 *Bladder function*

- *Water intake* was confirmed for individually housed mice with water being delivered using a 50 mL conical tube sealed with a #7, single hole rubber stopper and a double-ball water sipper. Tubes were weighed before tests and again the

Symptom evaluated	Test employed
Postural instability	Hindlimb reflexes
Walking and gait problems	Rotarod, open field, apomorphine induced rotation
Sweat function	Starch iodine
Gastrointestinal (GI) function/GI health	Fecal pellets, GI transit time, bead expulsion, microbiota
Bladder function	Urinary patterns

Table 1.
Summary of symptoms evaluated and tests employed.

next morning to calculate water intake for all mice [53]. This was done to assure that mice were hydrated for urine pattern tests.

- *Urine patterns* were assessed as a measure of autonomic function. *Collection of urine.* Food and water were removed during tests. Five independent tests were conducted per mouse at each time point. Each mouse was individually placed in a clean cage for 1 h (10:00–11:00 am) with the cage bottom covered with a fitted white filter paper (Bio-Rad, Hercules, CA, USA, cat# 1650962). Filter papers were collected, labeled, and dried. *Analysis.* Urine spots were illuminated by UV light and categorized as small (<0.2 cm^2) or large (>0.2 cm^2). Counting was done by individuals blinded to genotypes. If overlapping urine spots were detected, those were excluded from counts (**Table 1**) [53, 71].

2.6 aSyn solubility to measure synucleinopathy

- *Sequential protein extraction* was performed using tissues from treated mice by well-established methods [18, 78]. This method does not isolate cellular or subcellular fractions but rather soluble from insoluble proteins using a series of buffers and ultracentrifugation with pellet re-extractions. The concentration of protein was confirmed by bicinchoninic acid assay (BCA, Thermo Pierce, Rockford, IL, USA). Laemmli buffer was added to samples, that were then heated to 95°C for 5 min before SDS-PAGE, with the exception of SDS/Urea samples, which were not boiled before gel loading. Proteins were transferred to nitrocellulose, with equivalent protein loading verified by Ponceau S stain.

- *Immunoblots*. Blots were blocked 1 h in 10% milk-PBS then incubated overnight at 4°C in aSyn antibody (sc-7011R, Santa Cruz Biotechnologies, Santa Cruz, CA, USA), 610786 (BD Biosciences, San Jose, CA, USA). Infrared signal was obtained using anti-mouse, anti-goat, or anti-rabbit secondary antibodies coupled to IgG IRDye680 or IgG IRDye800 (1:5000–1:10,000; Rockland Immunochemical, Boyertown, PA, USA) with blots imaged using Odyssey (LiCor Biosciences, Lincoln, NB, USA).

2.7 Trophic factor expression

- *Total mRNA* was extracted from brain or paw sweat glands using RNeasy Plus Mini Kit (Cat # 74134, Qiagen Inc., Valencia, CA) followed by retrotranscription with a RNA-to-cDNA Kit (Cat # 4387406, Thermo Fisher Scientific), as per manufacturer. *Total miRNA* from brain was extracted using miRNeasy Mini Kits

(Cat # 217004, Qiagen). *Mature miRNAs* were retrotranscribed with miScript II RT Kit (Cat # 218160, Qiagen). *RNA concentrations and purity* were confirmed by NanoDrop 2000 spectrophotometry (Thermo Fisher Scientific). Integrity of RNAs and assessment of genomic DNA contamination were done by evaluating 28S/18S rRNAs band ratios on RNA "bleach" gels as previously described [39].

- *BDNF, GDNF, and NGF Protein* were assessed on immunoblots loaded with equivalent amounts of total protein for each condition, as determined using the BCA assay as described in Section 2.5.

2.8 Mitochondrial assessment

- *Dounce homogenization* of 200 mg cerebellum/mouse was performed on ice to isolate brain mitochondria using a kit (Cat # 89801, Thermo Fisher Scientific). Protease inhibitors: 17 μg/mL aprotinin, 1 mM benzamidine, and 1 mM AEBSF were added to all solutions. The final pellet contained mitochondria suspended in 50 μL sterile PBS. Total protein concentrations of isolated mitochondria were determined by BCA as described in Section 2.5.

- *Succinate dehydrogenase (SDH) activity* was measured using 60 μg of purified mitochondria and a colorimetric assay (Cat # MAK1971KT, Sigma-Aldrich, St. Louis, MO USA), as previously described [39].

3. Results

3.1 Benefits of FTY720 and FTY720-Mitoxy in PD and MSA mouse models

Data from multiple publications are summarized below in tabular and graphic format confirm that FTY720, whose international patent recently expired and is now available in generic form, as well as our patented derivative FTY720-Mitoxy, show that both are extremely protective in PD and MSA mouse models. Both drugs reverse symptoms of abnormal body and gut movement as well as autonomic dysfunction including constipation, abnormal sweating, and abnormal urination. Both drugs also reduce or eliminate synucleinopathy as measured by sequential protein extraction evaluated by aSyn immunoblot (**Figure 3** and **Table 2**).

3.1.1 Trophic factors

Both drugs increase the expression of brain derived neurotrophic factor (BDNF), while FTY720-Mitoxy also significantly increases expression of nerve growth factor (NGF) and glial-cell-line derived neurotrophic factor (GDNF) in neurons and oligodendroglia cells [39, 53, 68, 70, 71].

3.1.2 Safety

A major difference between FTY720 and FTY720-Mitoxy is the fact that FTY720 becomes phosphorylated in vivo by Sphingosine Kinases, which leads to its immunosuppressive effects. Having FTY720 act in an immunosuppressive manner, while beneficial for MS patients with that autoimmune disorder, could be problematic for

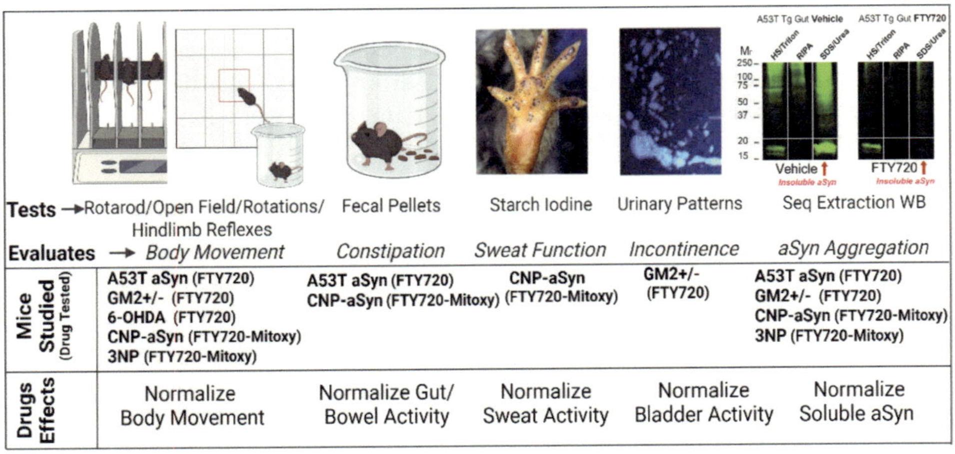

Figure 3.
Summary of FTY720 and FTY720-Mitoxy data that support taking the necessary next steps to test the safety and efficacy of FTY720 and FTY720-Mitoxy to slow PD or MSA. Top row: drawings and images illustrating tests and variables used to assess body movement, constipation, sweating, incontinence, and aSyn pathology in PD and MSA mouse models. Middle row: models of PD (A53T, GM2 +/−, 6-OHDA) and MSA (CNP-aSyn, 3NP), showing drugs tested in that model, in parentheses. Bottom row: drug effects on body movement, gut/bowel activity, sweat function, bladder function, and ability to sustain soluble aSyn and counteract synucleinopathy. Figure was created using BioRender.com.

Mice studied	Modeling	Variable measured	FTY720	FTY720-Mitoxy	Reference
A53T aSyn	PD	Movement (body/gut)	Protects	NT	[47]
GM2 +/−	PD	Movement (body)	Protects	NT	[53]
		Bladder function	Protects	NT	[53]
Rotenone	PD	Movement (body)	Protects	NT	[59]
MPTP	PD	Movement (body)	Protects	NT	[58]
6-OHDA	PD	Movement (body)	Protects	NT	[56, 59]
CNP aSyn	MSA	Movement (body/gut)	NT	Protects	[39]
3NP	MSA	Mitochondrial SDH	NT	Protects	[39]
Control mice	Normals	Immunosuppression	Positive	Negative	[72]
Rotenone/ Chitosan-FTY	PD	aSyn phosphorylation, PP2A modulation	Protects	NT	[60]

Table 2.
Data confirming FTY720 and FTY720-Mitoxy protection in vivo. PD or MSA onset was confirmed before initiating drugs (NT = not tested).

aging individuals suffering with PD or MSA as will be further described below. In stark contrast, FTY720-Mitoxy, which also rapidly crosses the blood brain barrier but is not phosphorylated [66] does not suppress the immune system [72], making it a potentially safer drug for treating patients with PD or MSA aSyn pathology.

3.1.3 Microbiota

We saw an increase in *Ruminococcus* in all mice after FTY720-Mitoxy, but an increase in *Bacteroides* only in FTY720-Mitoxy treated CNP-aSyn MSA mice (**Figure 4**).

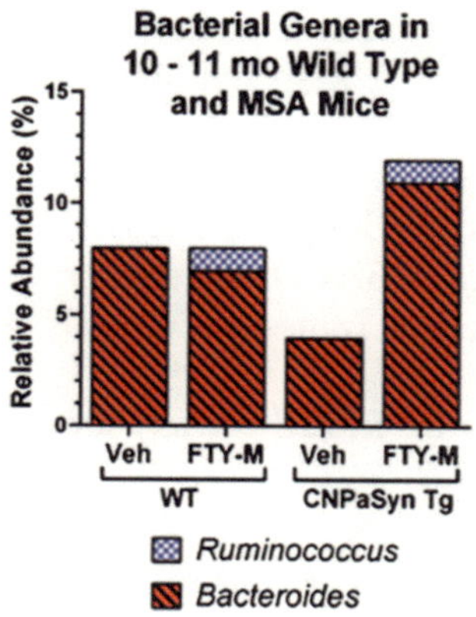

Figure 4.
Data from wild type (WT) control mice and CNP-aSyn MSA littermate mice collected 8–12 weeks post FTY720-Mitoxy treatment. This figure from Vidal-Martinez et al. [76], is re-printed with permission of iospress.nl.

Ruminococcus is considered beneficial. *Bacteroides* are considered "friendly commensals" when residing in the gut, where they act to functionally out-compete other bacteria and/or viruses to prevent infection [79]. Because all FTY720-Mitoxy treated CNP-aSyn MSA mice appeared healthy and had improved behavioral functions [39, 76], it is believed that *Bacteroides* in their gut were also beneficial.

3.1.4 Succinate dehydrogenase (SDH) activity

After FTY720-Mitoxy treatment of 3NP treated MSA mice, we isolated cerebellar mitochondria and measured their SDH activity relative to freshly prepared standards using established protocols. FTY720-Mitoxy significantly enhanced mitochondrial function in both WT and CNP-aSyn MSA 3NP mice. Specifically, 3NP treatment alone reduces SDH activity in WT and CNP-aSyn mitochondria. 3NP + FTY720-Mitoxy double treatment returns SDH activity to normal baseline values in WT and CNP-aSyn mitochondria as did FTY720-Mitoxy in WT mitochondria, but most significantly, FTY720-Mitoxy treatment improved SDH activity in the mitochondria isolated from transgenic CNP-aSyn MSA mice [39].

4. Discussion/conclusions

Herein, we demonstrate robust in vivo protection by FTY720 and FTY720-Mitoxy in several different mouse models of PD and/or MSA. Both drugs significantly slowed or even reversed disease progression while nearly totally counteracting aSyn pathology, also known as synucleinopathy. These are key requirements for drugs that are urgently needed for treating PD and MSA. Notably, FTY720 (fingolimod, Gilenya) could now be used off-label for PD or MSA should a doctor choose to prescribe it. It is worth noting that we used low dose FTY720 when treating our mice, and low dose FTY720 has been made available for treating children with multiple sclerosis. However, a major concern for using FTY720 for PD or MSA still remains because its immunosuppressive effects sometimes induce the opportunistic infection known as progressive multifocal leukoencephalopathy (PML) [73], which can be fatal.

This concern is what encouraged us to create novel FTY720-derivatives, FTY720-C2 and FTY720-Mitoxy, that are not phosphorylated and do not cause immune suppression [72]. And although FTY720-Mitoxy is not an oral drug, it very rapidly enters the brain when given by injection or when delivered over time and it also is highly stable, which allowed long-term delivery (over several weeks). Thus, we have demonstrated the preclinical proof of concept for FTY720-Mitoxy, which like insulin could be given by injection, transdermal patch, or pump to help improve a patient's quality of life [75].

Our preclinical findings with FTY720-Mitoxy show that it is highly beneficial in MSA models, which supports taking the necessary next steps in drug development to move this patented compound toward the clinic. While ours is currently the only laboratory to have published preclinical data regarding FTY720-Mitoxy, others now have the opportunity to test the drug in their own laboratories, as several vendors now offer FTY720-Mitoxy for sale.

Prior to embarking on Phase I safety or pharmacodynamics studies in healthy human subjects and/or affected subjects, FTY720-Mitoxy requires further characterization to verify its safety and dosing requirements. Importantly, because MSA is an Orphan disorder, with MSA patients often progressing rapidly, such steps to add FTY720-Mitoxy to the arsenal of potential therapies for MSA would be highly beneficial not only for MSA but perhaps also for more common synucleinopathies like PD, dementia with Lewy bodies, and even for Alzheimer's disease.

5. Patents

The corresponding author holds patents "Compositions and Methods for the Treatment of Parkinson's Disease" in the USA (#10,391,066) and Canada (#2,888,634) for the FTY720-derivatives, FTY720-C2 and FTY720-Mitoxy.

Acknowledgements

We appreciate support from the Steven Hoy family, Glanville/Reynolds/Perez Families, Anna Mae Doyle, Michael J. Fox Foundation, US National Institutes of Health, NINDS (R01-NS42094), Fogarty International Center (NCOD-5D43TW008333), TTUHSC Graduate Program, Multiple System Atrophy Coalition, Coldwell Foundation, El Paso Community Foundation, Paso Del Norte Foundation (to R.G.P.); Chinese Ministry of Education (BS2010YY036), National Natural Science Foundation (81274124, 81200982) and Shandong Province Science & Technology Program (2014GSF118038, 2016GSF201061) (to H.L.). Funders played no role in study design, data collection, analysis, data interpretation; manuscript writing; or decision about where to publish.

Author contributions

Dr. Perez did most of the writing, Table and Figure preparation. Dr. Vidal-Martinez performed most animal studies, wrote key portions on gut microbiota, and provided essential editorial feedback. Dr. Lou did key mouse experiments and provided editorial feedback. All authors approved the final version before submission.

Author details

Guadalupe Vidal-Martinez[1], Haiyan Lou[2] and Ruth G. Perez[3]*

1 Department of Psychiatry, Paul L. Foster School of Medicine, Texas Tech University Health Sciences Center, El Paso, TX, USA

2 Department of Pharmacology, Shandong University School of Medicine, Jinan, Shandong, China

3 R&R Perez LLC, Drug Development, El Paso, TX, USA

*Address all correspondence to: rperezllc@gmail.com

References

[1] Goedert M, Spillantini MG, Del Tredici K, Braak H. 100 years of Lewy pathology. Nature Reviews. Neurology. 2013;**9**:13-24. DOI: 10.1038/nrneurol.2012.242

[2] Jellinger KA, Lantos PL. Papp–Lantos inclusions and the pathogenesis of multiple system atrophy: An update. Acta Neuropathologica. 2010;**119**:657-667. DOI: 10.1007/s00401-010-0672-3

[3] Sulzer D. Clues to how alpha-synuclein damages neurons in Parkinson's disease. Movement Disorders: Official Journal of the Movement Disorder Society. 2010;**25**(Suppl. 1):S27-S31. DOI: 10.1002/mds.22639

[4] Miller DW, Johnson JM, Solano SM, Hollingsworth ZR, Standaert DG, Young AB. Absence of alpha-synuclein mRNA expression in normal and multiple system atrophy oligodendroglia. Journal of Neural Transmission. 2005;**112**:1613-1624. DOI: 10.1007/s00702-005-0378-1

[5] Kisos H, Pukass K, Ben-Hur T, Richter-Landsberg C, Sharon R. Increased neuronal alpha-synuclein pathology associates with its accumulation in oligodendrocytes in mice modeling alpha-synucleinopathies. PLoS ONE. 2012;**7**:e46817. DOI: 10.1371/journal.pone.0046817

[6] Burke RE, Dauer WT, Vonsattel JP. A critical evaluation of the Braak staging scheme for Parkinson's disease. Annals of Neurology. 2008;**64**:485-491. DOI: 10.1002/ana.21541

[7] Burke RE, O'Malley K. Axon degeneration in Parkinson's disease. Experimental Neurology. 2013;**246**:72-83. DOI: 10.1016/j.expneurol.2012.01.011

[8] Olanow CW, Tatton WG. Etiology and pathogenesis of Parkinson's disease. Annual Review of Neuroscience. 1999;**22**:123-144

[9] Nussbaum RL. The identification of alpha-synuclein as the first Parkinson disease gene. Journal of Parkinson's Disease. 2017;**7**:S45-S51. DOI: 10.3233/JPD-179003

[10] Peng C, Gathagan RJ, Covell DJ, Medellin C, Stieber A, Robinson JL, et al. Cellular milieu imparts distinct pathological alpha-synuclein strains in alpha-synucleinopathies. Nature. 2018;**557**:558-563. DOI: 10.1038/s41586-018-0104-4

[11] Perez RG, Waymire JC, Lin E, Liu JJ, Guo F, Zigmond MJ. A role for alpha-synuclein in the regulation of dopamine biosynthesis. The Journal of Neuroscience: The Official Journal of the Society for Neuroscience. 2002;**22**:3090-3099

[12] Tehranian R, Montoya SE, Van Laar AD, Hastings TG, Perez RG. Alpha-synuclein inhibits aromatic amino acid decarboxylase activity in dopaminergic cells. Journal of Neurochemistry. 2006;**99**:1188-1196. DOI: 10.1111/j.1471-4159.2006.04146.x

[13] Larsen KE, Schmitz Y, Troyer MD, Mosharov E, Dietrich P, Quazi AZ, et al. Alpha-synuclein overexpression in PC12 and chromaffin cells impairs catecholamine release by interfering with a late step in exocytosis. The Journal of Neuroscience: The Official Journal of the Society for Neuroscience. 2006;**26**:11915-11922

[14] Mosharov EV, Staal RG, Bove J, Prou D, Hananiya A, Markov D, et al.

Alpha-synuclein overexpression increases cytosolic catecholamine concentration. The Journal of Neuroscience: The Official Journal of the Society for Neuroscience. 2006;**26**:9304-9311. DOI: 10.1523/JNEUROSCI.0519-06.2006

[15] Peng X, Tehranian R, Dietrich P, Stefanis L, Perez RG. Alpha-synuclein activation of protein phosphatase 2A reduces tyrosine hydroxylase phosphorylation in dopaminergic cells. Journal of Cell Science. 2005;**118**:3523-3530. DOI: 10.1242/jcs.02481

[16] Benskey MJ, Perez RG, Manfredsson FP. The contribution of alpha synuclein to neuronal survival and function—Implications for Parkinson's disease. Journal of Neurochemistry. 2016;**137**:331-359. DOI: 10.1111/jnc.13570

[17] Benskey MJ, Sellnow RC, Sandoval IM, Sortwell CE, Lipton JW, Manfredsson FP. Silencing alpha synuclein in mature nigral neurons results in rapid neuroinflammation and subsequent toxicity. Frontiers in Molecular Neuroscience. 2018;**11**:1-21. DOI: 10.3389/fnmol.2018.00036

[18] Wu J, Lou H, Alerte TN, Stachowski EK, Chen J, Singleton AB, et al. Lewy-like aggregation of alpha-synuclein reduces protein phosphatase 2A activity in vitro and in vivo. Neuroscience. 2012;**207**:288-297. DOI: 10.1016/j.neuroscience.2012.01.028

[19] Perez RG, Hastings TG. Could a loss of alpha-synuclein function put dopaminergic neurons at risk? Journal of Neurochemistry. 2004;**89**:1318-1324. DOI: 10.1111/j.1471-4159.2004.02423.x

[20] Berman SB, Zigmond MJ, Hastings TG. Modification of dopamine transporter function: Effect of reactive oxygen species and dopamine. Journal of Neurochemistry. 1996;**67**:593-600

[21] Chen L, Ding Y, Cagniard B, Van Laar AD, Mortimer A, Chi W, et al. Unregulated cytosolic dopamine causes neurodegeneration associated with oxidative stress in mice. The Journal of Neuroscience: The Official Journal of the Society for Neuroscience. 2008;**28**:425-433. DOI: 10.1523/JNEUROSCI.3602-07.2008

[22] Kang SS, Ahn EH, Zhang Z, Liu X, Manfredsson FP, Sandoval IM, et al. Alpha-synuclein stimulation of monoamine oxidase-B and legumain protease mediates the pathology of Parkinson's disease. The EMBO Journal. 2018;**37**:1-19. DOI: 10.15252/embj.201798878

[23] Tu PH, Galvin JE, Baba M, Giasson B, Tomita T, Leight S, et al. Glial cytoplasmic inclusions in white matter oligodendrocytes of multiple system atrophy brains contain insoluble alpha-synuclein. Annals of Neurology. 1998;**44**:415-422. DOI: 10.1002/ana.410440324

[24] Wakabayashi K, Yoshimoto M, Tsuji S, Takahashi H. Alpha-synuclein immunoreactivity in glial cytoplasmic inclusions in multiple system atrophy. Neuroscience Letters. 1998;**249**:180-182

[25] Dickson DW, Lin W, Liu WK, Yen SH. Multiple system atrophy: A sporadic synucleinopathy. Brain Pathology. 1999;**9**:721-732

[26] Jellinger KA. Multiple system atrophy: An oligodendroglioneural synucleinopathy. Journal of Alzheimer's Disease. 2018;**62**(3):1141-1179. DOI: 10.3233/JAD-170397

[27] Ubhi K, Low P, Masliah E. Multiple system atrophy: A clinical and

neuropathological perspective. Trends in Neurosciences. 2011;**34**:581-590. DOI: 10.1016/j.tins.2011.08.003

[28] Campese N, Fanciulli A, Stefanova N, Haybaeck J, Kiechl S, Wenning GK. Neuropathology of multiple system atrophy: Kurt Jellinger's legacy. Journal of Neural Transmission. 2021;**128**:1481-1494. DOI: 10.1007/s00702-021-02383-3

[29] Chesselet MF, Fleming S, Mortazavi F, Meurers B. Strengths and limitations of genetic mouse models of Parkinson's disease. Parkinsonism & Related Disorders. 2008;**14**(Suppl. 2): S84-S87. DOI: 10.1016/j.parkreldis.2008.04.004

[30] Kahle PJ. Alpha-synucleinopathy models and human neuropathology: Similarities and differences. Acta Neuropathologica. 2008;**115**:87-95

[31] Terzioglu M, Galter D. Parkinson's disease: Genetic versus toxin-induced rodent models. The FEBS Journal. 2008;**275**:1384-1391. DOI: 10.1111/j.1742-4658.2008.06302.x

[32] Fillon G, Kahle PJ. Alpha-synuclein transgenic mice: Relevance to multiple system atrophy. Movement Disorders: Official Journal of the Movement Disorder Society. 2005;**20**(Suppl. 12): S64-S66. DOI: 10.1002/mds.20542

[33] Fellner L, Wenning GK, Stefanova N. Models of multiple system atrophy. In: Current Topics in Behavioral Neurosciences. Mannheim, Germany: Springer; 2013. DOI: 10.1007/7854_2013_269

[34] Refolo V, Bez F, Polissidis A, Kuzdas-Wood D, Sturm E, Kamaratou M, et al. Progressive striatonigral degeneration in a transgenic mouse model of multiple system atrophy: Translational implications for interventional therapies. Acta Neuropathologica Communications. 2018;**6**:2. DOI: 10.1186/s40478-017-0504-y

[35] Marmion DJ, Peelaerts W, Kordower JH. A historical review of multiple system atrophy with a critical appraisal of cellular and animal models. Journal of Neural Transmission. 2021;**128**:1507-1527. DOI: 10.1007/s00702-021-02419-8

[36] Stefanova N, Poewe W, Wenning GK. Rasagiline is neuroprotective in a transgenic model of multiple system atrophy. Experimental Neurology. 2008;**210**:421-427. DOI: 10.1016/j.expneurol.2007.11.022

[37] Ubhi K, Rockenstein E, Mante M, Patrick C, Adame A, Thukral M, et al. Rifampicin reduces alpha-synuclein in a transgenic mouse model of multiple system atrophy. Neuroreport. 2008;**19**:1271-1276. DOI: 10.1097/WNR.0b013e32830b3661

[38] Heras-Garvin A, Weckbecker D, Ryazanov S, Leonov A, Griesinger C, Giese A, et al. Anle138b modulates alpha-synuclein oligomerization and prevents motor decline and neurodegeneration in a mouse model of multiple system atrophy. Movement Disorders: Official Journal of the Movement Disorder Society. 2019;**34**:255-263. DOI: 10.1002/mds.27562

[39] Vidal-Martinez G, Segura-Ulate I, Yang B, Diaz-Pacheco V, Barragan JA, De-Leon Esquivel J, et al. FTY720-Mitoxy reduces synucleinopathy and neuroinflammation, restores behavior and mitochondria function, and increases GDNF expression in multiple system atrophy mouse models. Experimental Neurology. 2020;**325**:113120. DOI: 10.1016/j.expneurol.2019.113120

[40] Heras-Garvin A, Refolo V, Schmidt C, Malfertheiner K, Wenning GK, Bradbury M, et al. ATH434 reduces α-synuclein-related neurodegeneration in a murine model of multiple system atrophy. Movement Disorders: Official Journal of the Movement Disorder Society. 2021;**36**:2605-2614. DOI: 10.1002/mds.28714

[41] Ledeen RW, Wu G. Gangliosides, alpha-synuclein, and Parkinson's disease. Progress in Molecular Biology and Translational Science. 2018;**156**:435-454. DOI: 10.1016/bs.pmbts.2017.12.009

[42] Bengoa-Vergniory N, Faggiani E, Ramos-Gonzalez P, Kirkiz E, Connor-Robson N, Brown LV, et al. CLR01 protects dopaminergic neurons in vitro and in mouse models of Parkinson's disease. Nature Communications. 2020;**11**:4885. DOI: 10.1038/s41467-020-18689-x

[43] Diwakarla S, McQuade RM, Constable R, Artaiz O, Lei E, Barnham KJ, et al. ATH434 reverses colorectal dysfunction in the A53T mouse model of Parkinson's disease. Journal of Parkinson's Disease. 2021;**11**:1821-1832. DOI: 10.3233/JPD-212731

[44] Romano R, Bucci C. Antisense therapy: A potential breakthrough in the treatment of neurodegenerative diseases. Neural Regeneration Research. 2024;**19**:1027-1035. DOI: 10.4103/1673-5374.385285

[45] Singh K, Bhushan B, Chanchal DK, Sharma SK, Rani K, Yadav MK, et al. Emerging therapeutic potential of cannabidiol (CBD) in neurological disorders: A comprehensive review. Behavioural Neurology. 2023;**2023**:8825358. DOI: 10.1155/2023/8825358

[46] Giasson BI, Duda JE, Quinn SM, Zhang B, Trojanowski JQ, Lee VM. Neuronal alpha-synucleinopathy with severe movement disorder in mice expressing A53T human alpha-synuclein. Neuron. 2002;**34**:521-533

[47] Vidal-Martinez G, Vargas-Medrano J, Gil-Tommee C, Medina D, Garza NT, Yang B, et al. FTY720/Fingolimod reduces synucleinopathy and improves gut motility in A53T mice: Contributions of pro-brain-derived neurotrophic factor (pro-BDNF) and mature BDNF. The Journal of Biological Chemistry. 2016;**291**:20811-20821. DOI: 10.1074/jbc.M116.744029

[48] Yang LJ, Zeller CB, Shaper NL, Kiso M, Hasegawa A, Shapiro RE, et al. Gangliosides are neuronal ligands for myelin-associated glycoprotein. Proceedings of the National Academy of Sciences of the United States of America. 1996;**93**:814-818

[49] Vyas AA, Schnaar RL. Brain gangliosides: Functional ligands for myelin stability and the control of nerve regeneration. Biochimie. 2001;**83**:677-682

[50] Chan RB, Perotte AJ, Zhou B, Liong C, Shorr EJ, Marder KS, et al. Elevated GM3 plasma concentration in idiopathic Parkinson's disease: A lipidomic analysis. PLoS ONE. 2017;**12**:e0172348. DOI: 10.1371/journal.pone.0172348

[51] Wu G, Lu ZH, Kulkarni N, Ledeen RW. Deficiency of ganglioside GM1 correlates with Parkinson's disease in mice and humans. Journal of Neuroscience Research. 2012;**90**:1997-2008. DOI: 10.1002/jnr.23090

[52] Hadaczek P, Wu G, Sharma N, Ciesielska A, Bankiewicz K, Davidow AL, et al. GDNF signaling implemented by GM1 ganglioside; failure in Parkinson's disease and GM1-deficient murine model. Experimental Neurology.

2015;**263**:177-189. DOI: 10.1016/j.expneurol.2014.10.010

[53] Gil-Tommee C, Vidal-Martinez G, Reyes CA, Vargas-Medrano J, Herrera GV, Martin SM, et al. Parkinsonian GM2 synthase knockout mice lacking mature gangliosides develop urinary dysfunction and neurogenic bladder. Experimental Neurology. 2019;**311**:265-273. DOI: 10.1016/j.expneurol.2018.10.014

[54] Wu G, Xie X, Lu ZH, Ledeen RW. Cerebellar neurons lacking complex gangliosides degenerate in the presence of depolarizing levels of potassium. Proceedings of the National Academy of Sciences of the United States of America. 2001;**98**:307-312. DOI: 10.1073/pnas.011523698

[55] Jagmag SA, Tripathi N, Shukla SD, Maiti S, Khurana S. Evaluation of models of Parkinson's disease. Frontiers in Neuroscience. 2015;**9**:503. DOI: 10.3389/fnins.2015.00503

[56] Ren M, Han M, Wei X, Guo Y, Shi H, Zhang X, et al. FTY720 attenuates 6-OHDA-associated dopaminergic degeneration in cellular and mouse Parkinsonian models. Neurochemical Research. 2017;**42**:686-696. DOI: 10.1007/s11064-016-2125-4

[57] Komnig D, Dagli TC, Habib P, Zeyen T, Schulz JB, Falkenburger BH. Fingolimod (FTY720) is not protective in the subacute MPTP mouse model of Parkinson's disease and does not lead to a sustainable increase of brain-derived neurotrophic factor. Journal of Neurochemistry. 2018;**147**:678-691. DOI: 10.1111/jnc.14575

[58] Motyl J, Przykaza Ł, Boguszewski PM, Kosson P, Strosznajder JB. Pramipexole and Fingolimod exert neuroprotection in a mouse model of Parkinson's disease by activation of sphingosine kinase 1 and Akt kinase. Neuropharmacology. 2018;**135**:139-150. DOI: 10.1016/j.neuropharm.2018.02.023

[59] Zhao P, Yang X, Yang L, Li M, Wood K, Liu Q, et al. Neuroprotective effects of fingolimod in mouse models of Parkinson's disease. FASEB Journal: Official Publication of the Federation of American Societies for Experimental Biology. 2017;**31**:172-179. DOI: 10.1096/fj.201600751R

[60] Sardoiwala MN, Boddu M, Biswal L, Karmakar S, Choudhury SR. FTY720 nanoformulation induces O-GlcNacylation of synuclein to alleviate synucleinopathy. ACS Chemical Neuroscience. 2024;**15**:71-77. DOI: 10.1021/acschemneuro.3c00545

[61] Giasson BI, Forman MS, Higuchi M, Golbe LI, Graves CL, Kotzbauer PT, et al. Initiation and synergistic fibrillization of tau and alpha-synuclein. Science. 2003;**300**:636-640

[62] Yazawa I, Giasson BI, Sasaki R, Zhang B, Joyce S, Uryu K, et al. Mouse model of multiple system atrophy alpha-synuclein expression in oligodendrocytes causes glial and neuronal degeneration. Neuron. 2005;**45**:847-859

[63] Minnerop M, Luders E, Specht K, Ruhlmann J, Schimke N, Thompson PM, et al. Callosal tissue loss in multiple system atrophy—A one-year follow-up study. Movement Disorders: Official Journal of the Movement Disorder Society. 2010;**25**:2613-2620. DOI: 10.1002/mds.23318

[64] Scallet AC, Nony PL, Rountree RL, Binienda ZK. Biomarkers of 3-nitropropionic acid (3-NPA)-induced mitochondrial dysfunction as indicators of neuroprotection. Annals of the New York Academy of Sciences. 2001;**939**:381-392. DOI: 10.1111/j.1749-6632.2001.tb03647.x

[65] Ubhi K, Lee PH, Adame A, Inglis C, Mante M, Rockenstein E, et al. Mitochondrial inhibitor 3-nitroproprionic acid enhances oxidative modification of alpha-synuclein in a transgenic mouse model of multiple system atrophy. Journal of Neuroscience Research. 2009;**87**:2728-2739. DOI: 10.1002/jnr.22089

[66] Enoru JO, Yang B, Krishnamachari S, Villanueva E, DeMaio W, Watanyar A, et al. Preclinical metabolism, pharmacokinetics and in vivo analysis of new blood-brain-barrier penetrant fingolimod analogues: FTY720-C2 and FTY720-Mitoxy. PLoS ONE. 2016;**11**:e0162162. DOI: 10.1371/journal.pone.0162162

[67] Brinkmann V, Billich A, Baumruker T, Heining P, Schmouder R, Francis G, et al. Fingolimod (FTY720): Discovery and development of an oral drug to treat multiple sclerosis. Nature Reviews. Drug Discovery. 2010;**9**:883-897. DOI: 10.1038/nrd3248

[68] Vargas-Medrano J, Segura-Ulate I, Yang B, Chinnasamy R, Arterburn JB, Perez RG. FTY720-Mitoxy reduces toxicity associated with alpha-synuclein and oxidative stress by increasing trophic factor expression and myelin protein in OLN-93 oligodendroglia cell cultures. Neuropharmacology. 2019;**158**:1-8. DOI: 10.1016/j.neuropharm.2019.107701

[69] Vargas-Medrano J, Yang B, Garza NT, Segura-Ulate I, Perez RG. Up-regulation of protective neuronal MicroRNAs by FTY720 and novel FTY720-derivatives. Neuroscience Letters. 2019;**690**:178-180. DOI: 10.1016/j.neulet.2018.10.040

[70] Vargas-Medrano J, Segura-Ulate I, Vidal-Martinez G, Yang B, Perez RG. FTY720-derivatives increase neurotrophic factor expression and protect oligodendroglia against hydrogen-peroxide-mediated oxidative stress. In: Proceedings of the Society for Neuroscience. Washington, DC: Society for Neuroscience; 2018

[71] Vidal-Martinez G, Najera K, Miranda JD, Gil-Tommee C, Yang B, Vargas-Medrano J, et al. FTY720 improves behavior, increases brain derived neurotrophic factor levels and reduces alpha-synuclein pathology in parkinsonian GM2+/− mice. Neuroscience. 2019;**411**:1-10. DOI: 10.1016/j.neuroscience.2019.05.029

[72] Segura-Ulate I, Belcher TK, Vidal-Martinez G, Vargas-Medrano J, Perez RG. FTY720-derivatives do not induce FTY720-like lymphopenia. Journal of Pharmacological Sciences. 2017;**133**:187-189

[73] Graham DR, Sidhu A. Mice expressing the A53T mutant form of human alpha-synuclein exhibit hyperactivity and reduced anxiety-like behavior. Journal of Neuroscience Research. 2010;**88**:1777-1783. DOI: 10.1002/jnr.22331

[74] Farrell KF, Krishnamachari S, Villanueva E, Lou H, Alerte TN, Peet E, et al. Non-motor parkinsonian pathology in aging A53T alpha-synuclein mice is associated with progressive synucleinopathy and altered enzymatic function. Journal of Neurochemistry. 2014;**128**:536-546. DOI: 10.1111/jnc.12481

[75] Kuo YM, Li Z, Jiao Y, Gaborit N, Pani AK, Orrison BM, et al. Extensive enteric nervous system abnormalities in mice transgenic for artificial chromosomes containing Parkinson disease-associated alpha-synuclein gene mutations precede central nervous system changes. Human Molecular Genetics. 2010;**19**:1633-1650. DOI: 10.1093/hmg/ddq038

[76] Vidal-Martinez G, Chin B, Camarillo C, Herrera GV, Yang B, Sarosiek I, et al. A pilot microbiota study in Parkinson's disease patients versus control subjects, and effects of FTY720 and FTY720-Mitoxy therapies in Parkinsonian and multiple system atrophy mouse models. Journal of Parkinson's Disease. IOS Press; 2020;**10**:185-192. DOI: 10.3233/JPD-191693

[77] Liu Y, Sebastian B, Liu B, Zhang Y, Fissel JA, Pan B, et al. Sensory and autonomic function and structure in footpads of a diabetic mouse model. Scientific Reports. 2017;**7**:41401. DOI: 10.1038/srep41401

[78] Waxman EA, Giasson BI. Specificity and regulation of casein kinase-mediated phosphorylation of alpha-synuclein. Journal of Neuropathology and Experimental Neurology. 2008;**67**:402-416

[79] Zafar H, Saier MH Jr. Gut bacteroides species in health and disease. Gut Microbes. 2021;**13**:1-20. DOI: 10.1080/19490976.2020.1848158

Chapter 4

Neuroprotective Properties of Peptides

Oytun Erbas, İlknur Altuntaş, Pemra Nesil, Hadi Sasani and Mehtap Odabaşı

Abstract

The development of a treatment strategy for neurodegenerative disorders is a serious issue for the healthcare world and a crucial subject of discussion. In the past two decades, a lot of focus has been placed on identifying the pathophysiological processes involved in neuronal death linked to neurodegenerative disorders and developing a variety of treatment options for neuroprotection. Numerous research teams have studied the use of peptides as neuroprotective treatments for different types of neurodegenerative disorders for a long time. The review aims to provide details about the roles of erythropoietin (EPO), glucagon-like peptide-1 (GLP-1), granulocyte colony-stimulating factor (G-CSF), and oxytocin (OXT) in neurodegenerative disorders as well as what cellular and molecular mechanisms they trigger to elicit the neuroprotective action, with a focus on neurodegenerative disorders.

Keywords: erythropoietin, glucagon-like peptide-1, granulocyte colony-stimulating factor, oxytocin, peptides, neurodegenerative disorders, neuropeptides, neuroprotection

1. Introduction

It is becoming more well-accepted that secondary biochemical alterations that result in tissue loss, which are secondary to acute neurodegenerative disorders, play a significant role in the development of chronic neurological impairment. Neurodegenerative disorders such as motor neuron disease, Alzheimer's disease (AD), Parkinson's disease (PD), ataxia, spinal muscular atrophy, autism, amyotrophic lateral sclerosis, Huntington's disease, epilepsy, ischemic brain diseases, and central nervous system (CNS) diseases, such as stroke have also been linked to molecular pathways that contribute to cell damage and cell loss. Due to a lack of clinical efficacy or unpleasant side effects, several neuroprotective therapies intended to reduce neuronal death have been ineffective. This prompted researchers to investigate alternative therapeutic applications, such as peptides as neuroprotective agents [1–5]. Notably, several peptides have been applied in clinical settings, including erythropoietin (EPO), glucagon-like peptide-1 (GLP-1), granulocyte colony-stimulating factor (G-CSF), and oxytocin (OXT) [6–12]. **Figure 1** shows the synergistic neuroprotective effects of G-CSF, GLP-1, and EPO.

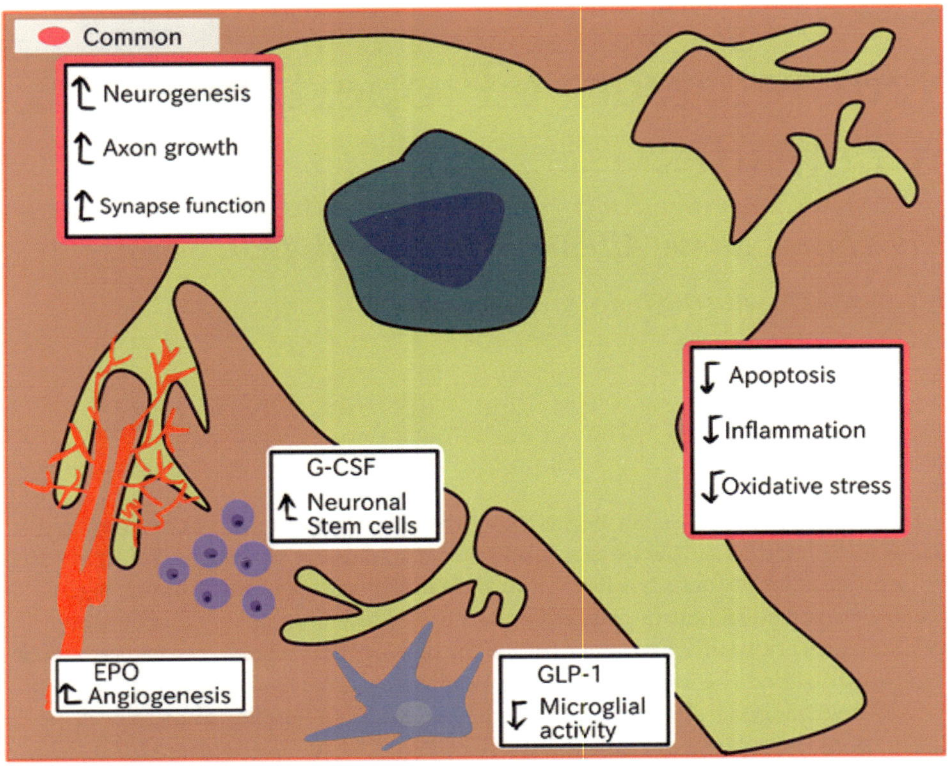

Figure 1.
The synergistic neuroprotective effects of G-CSF, GLP-1, and EPO promote neurogenesis, axon growth, and synaptic functioning while decreasing cell apoptosis, inflammation, and oxidative stress. Individually, G-CSF stimulates neural stem cells, EPO enhances angiogenesis, and GLP-1 decreases microglial activity.

2. Neuroprotective properties of erythropoietin

Human erythropoietin (EPO) is a 34 kilodalton (kDa) glycoprotein hormone formed up of four-helix loops. The gene for it is found on chromosome 7q11.22 and produces a 193-amino acid polypeptide chain [13]. The approaches of glycosylation and sialylation are also required for EPO to operate normally as they increase EPO's molecule's longevity and prolong its stay in circulation. The liver is the main site of EPO synthesis in individuals during fetal and neonatal life, but renal EPO messenger ribonucleic acid levels rise exponentially following 30 weeks of gestation, demonstrating the shift from the liver to the kidneys as the EPO production zone [14]. Also generated by cells from numerous organs, with the heart, spleen, lung, testis, ovaries, retina, and brain, where it exerts non-erythropoietic roles [15]. The discovery that the brain is one of these EPO-producing locations has captured the most interest. It is worth noting that prior line analyzing research has found that the pericytes in the brain and kidney both are transformed from the neural crest, which might also explain why they serve the same role in separate locations. The hippocampus, cortex, and midbrain were all reported to yield and express EPO inside the CNS. EPO has also been shown to have a crucial role in fostering and boosting neurogenesis, which is important for the growth of the brain and blood system [16], restricts cell damage, and prevents oxidation reactions. The peptide may have a favorable impact on the reduction of neuronal disorder due to its protective effects and ability to reduce reactive oxygen species (ROS) [6].

Erythropoietin receptor (EPOR) has a 225-amino acid subunit, a 23-amino-acid outer membrane segment, and a 235-amino-acid intracellular subunit. EPO activates secondary chemical signals like the signal transducer and activator of transcription 5 (STAT5), phosphatidylinositol 3-kinase (PI3K), and mitogen-activated protein kinase (MAPK) through the hematopoietic system's attachment of EPO to its target, which proceeds in homodimerization [17]. EPO is a bioactive molecule that is formed in the brain and has an essential function in neural growth and synapse formation control. EPOR has been detected in vitro grown rat oligodendrocytes and astrocytes, and recombinant human EPO (rhEPO) treatment increases their development and reproduction, hinting that the EPO/EPOR linkage is vital in angiogenesis after trauma. The four specific EPOR versions that are present in various tissues are described [18].

1. The brain has the canonical isoform, which is primarily expressed in the hematopoietic system. EPO activates this subunit, which modulates EPO's activity in inflammation and hypoxia in neurons [19].

2. Neuronal cell safeguard is an expression of EPOR's second form. In this scenario, the EPOR monomer connects the beta common receptor (βcR; CD131), a characteristic target portion of interleukin (IL)-3, IL-5, and granulocyte-macrophage colony-stimulating factor (GM-CSF). The most prominent theory is that dimerization causes the development of a particular tissue-building receptor. The classical homodimer upregulating tends to be activated by the stimulation of this sensor in an identical method [20].

3. The substantia nigra's dopaminergic neurons have a tertiary version of the receptors, which is shorter than the full-length form and causes an alteration in the known to possess subdomain. The absence of STAT phosphorylation in the EPOR abridged isoform raises the possibility of another, as of before unidentified, mode of action [7].

4. Finally, it has been confirmed that the rat brain has a periplasmic soluble form of the receptor. Besides the subsequent mediators being activated, this isoform engages with EPO. Therefore, EPO's contact with other EPOR forms is limited due to its decreased accessibility. When there is ischemia, this isoform's translation is significantly suppressed, which starts a process that fights comprehensive EPOR [19].

EPO's main purpose is to manage the growth of hematopoietic cells, so it is essential to identify if targeting neural cells may have a strong effect. The modulatory effects of EPO on neuroplasticity may affect neural precursor cells of other sources as well. These actions may include rapid maturation and enhanced progenitor growth, which has been seen in hypoxic mesencephalic progenitor cells [21]. Additionally, brain stem cells generated from the spinal cord exhibited EPO-driven neurogenesis. Brain-derived neurotrophic factors can be induced by EPO to potentially stimulate neurogenesis. EPO promotes regeneration while also assisting in the suppression of apoptosis. Apoptosis is diminished by the engagement of the cascade EPOR molecules Janus kinase 2 and PI3K and the control of the regulatory protein Bad (the Bcl-2 associated agonist of cell death) [22].

EPO is synthesized in the kidneys and released into circulation in response to hypoxia. By focusing on EPO as a cascade protein controlled by hypoxia, the hypoxia-inducible factor-1 alpha (HIF-1α) was in effect discovered [19]. Conversely, it currently appears that HIF-2α, also known as endothelial PAS domain protein 1, is much more essential than HIF-1 in driving the overexpression of EPO under deprivation [23]. The finding is that EPO and EPOR are generated in the brain's hippocampus and telencephalon, the two areas particularly vulnerable to hypoxia. Hence, it is theoretical to assume that EPO has a biological process in the brain that serves as a defense against hypoxia and perhaps ischemia [18]. In several additional neurodegenerative disorders, ROS also plays a role in causing cell damage and neuronal loss. In a rat model of vascular dementia reported by Erbas et al., EPO anti-oxidative capabilities particularly decrease beta-amyloid-induced apoptosis and boost tyrosine hydroxylase (TH) positive neural cells [24]. A crucial additional point in the stability of HIF and, thus, the synthesis of EPO is the creation of ROS generation in both hypoxia and hyperoxia. Although enhanced prolyl hydroxylation and thus reduced HIF function are heavily related to ROS blocking, it is unclear how extra or insufficient oxygen affects cell damage in the brain [25].

EPO has become a versatile tissue-protective mediator, in part because of its anti-inflammatory characteristics [26]. In fact, rhEPO penetrates the blood–brain barrier (BBB) whenever given to rats with localized ischemic injury, reducing the extent of the lesion by 50 to 75% [27]. In a laboratory autoimmune encephalitis form of multiple sclerosis, rhEPO inhibited the production and secretion of proinflammatory cytokines and growth factors, as well as the migration of cytokines through into the site of inflammation [23].

The second most prevalent neurodegenerative disorder is PD. Bradykinesia, stiffness, and tremor are only a few examples of motor and nonmotor features. Alpha-synuclein clusters, which are essential parts of Lewy bodies, and the growth of dopaminergic neurons in the atrophied substantia nigra pars compacta are two crucial pathogenic indicators [28]. According to a particular report of autophagy signals along with AMP-activated protein kinase and Unc-51-like autophagy activating kinase 1, EPO therapy stimulates the autophagy mechanism in rotenone-treated SH-SY5Y neurons (a neuroblastoma cell line called SK-N-SH that has triple-subcloned) [29]. EPO has various neuroprotective effects on astrocytes, microglia, and synapses and is implicated in the control of neuroinflammation. In fact, EPO prevents the death of vascular endothelium and the arousal of astrocytes, which maintains the BBB [30]. According to studies, EPO reduces levels of tumor necrosis factor-alpha (TNF-α) and increases levels of TH in rats that have had parkinsonism brought on by rotenone or 6-hydroxydopamine. This suggests that EPO may function through modulating neuro-inflammation in order to achieve its goals [24]. In a lipopolysaccharide-induced autistic rat model, EPO was also effective in enhancing cognition and neurochemistry [31].

The most prevalent kind of dementia, AD, is clinically defined by a memory deficit that worsens with time and a deterioration in cognitive abilities. Extracellular neuritic plaques induced by amyloid-beta (Aβ) formation and internal neuro-fibrillary bundles caused by hyperphosphorylation of the tau protein are the disease's defining features. The earliest signs that EPO could help with cognitive skills came from studies on non-neurological diseases when individuals receiving EPO during hemodialysis showed an increase in their mental abilities. Traditional pharmaceutical therapy for AD comprises acetylcholinesterase inhibitors, N-methyl-D-aspartate antagonists, and their potential combinations since no cure has been discovered [32]. EPO's health benefits have first been investigated at the molecular scale, employing both robust cell cultures and primary hippocampus neurons [16]. The chemical appears to be effective by blocking the apoptotic mechanism and protecting against Aβ toxicity [33].

Additionally, it is probable to notice a decline in the inflammatory activity and an elevation in antioxidant responses. EPO seemed to minimize cell damage, inflammation, and tau hyperphosphorylation while enhancing neurogenesis [25]. On abnormalities in neuroplasticity, the chemical appears to have a repair impact [33]. This, in addition to the fact that EPOR is present in the hippocampus, raises the prospect that EPO may have clinical benefits in this situation [31].

Acute ischemic stroke is caused by a temporary or irreversible decrease in cerebral blood flow that is typically related to the blockage of a cerebral artery, an embolization, or localized thrombosis. A protective effect against ischemia injury is provided by the stimulation of HIFs, which stimulates downstream factors including EPO and vascular endothelial growth factor [23]. In hypoxic *in vitro* models, EPO expression levels in both rat astrocytes and neurons. EPO begins to act on frontal neuron progenitor cells, implying its role in neurogenesis. Bioactivity rises after EPO administration in primary hippocampal and cortical neurons exposed to cerebral ischemia, indicating its role in apoptosis and cell healing. By recovering hippocampal CA1 neurons from deadly ischemic damage, rhEPO treatment reduced ischemia-induced memory deficit. Other researchers reported that the indigenous EPO/EPOR system protects hypoxic astrocytes and oligodendrocyte progenitor cells, indicating that suppressing endogenous EPO in astrocytes results in diminished preservation of oligodendrocyte precursor cells and cell apoptosis [34].

High EPO dosages are beneficial in term neonates with hypoxic–ischemic encephalopathy (HIE) when the damage has not yet been established [35]. Animal studies have revealed that EPO can be given at high dosages around 6 hours after the beginning of brain damage to have a meaningful neuroprotective role. EPO potentially impacts the processes of cerebral flow restitution, angiogenesis, and neuroregeneration in this environment, reducing ischemia damage. Research data also show that EPO can be used as an adjuvant therapy with hypothermia or as a supplement for hypothermia in HIE [2].

3. Neuroprotective properties of glucagon-like peptide-1

The glucagon-like peptide-1 (GLP-1), a 30-amino acid peptide hormone, is synthesized in the intestinal endocrine L-cells by differential processing of the proglucagon gene. It is a member of the incretin subfamily. The "incretin effect" is when incretins cause the pancreas to release more insulin when blood sugar levels are high. Even before it leaves the gut, the hormone GLP-1 is quickly digested and rendered inactive by the enzyme dipeptidyl peptidase IV. This raises the probability that GLP-1 receptor (GLP-1R)-expressing sensory neurons in the liver and intestine communicate GLP-1 effects [36, 37]. There are the highest concentrations of GLP-1R in the pancreas, the gut, and the CNS, although they are also found in small amounts in the heart, the vasculature, the kidneys, and the lungs [38].

The GLP-1 is a complex hormone with a wide range of metabolic effects, including the glucose-dependent stimulation of insulin secretion, a reduction in stomach emptying and food intake, an increase in natriuresis and diuresis, and a modification of rodent B-cell proliferation. GLP-1 primarily acts as an incretin hormone by stimulating insulin secretion and inhibiting glucagon release, which together help to reduce postprandial glucose excursions. It has consequences for learning and memory, reward behavior, and palatability and has cardio-neuroprotective effects, reducing inflammation and apoptosis. In addition to many GLP-1-based pharmacotherapies being tested in clinical settings for the treatment of obesity, GLP-1R agonists are successfully used in the clinic to treat type 2 diabetes mellitus (T2DM) and its related complications such as diabetic nephropathy [37, 39, 40].

Different from the intestinal system, GLP-1 is also produced in the brain, notably in the nucleus tractus solitarius (NTS) in the brainstem in particular. The paraventricular nucleus and arcuate nucleus are two regions of the hypothalamus that have GLP-1-expressing neurons. The management of appetite is aided by GLP-1 release, which also promotes a feeling of satiety [8, 41].

GLP-1 receptors are found in the substantia nigra, amygdala, hippocampus, hypothalamus, and NTS, as well as in cortical regions such as the lateral prefrontal cortex. These receptors may be stimulated to promote neurogenesis and synaptogenesis and to guard against oxidative stress, neuroinflammation, and apoptosis [41–44]. It is important to note that while blood-borne GLP-1 and GLP-1R agonists rapidly penetrate the BBB, incretins and their receptors are expressed in the CNS [3, 9].

In both humans and animals, GLP-1 modulates autonomic function and the stress response by activating the hypothalamic–pituitary–adrenal axis. It has antiapoptotic, neuroprotective, and neuromodulatory properties. GLP-1 agonism may have neuroprotective effects by lowering microglial activation, which in turn lowers the release of M1 macrophages (e.g. TNF-α and IL-1β). GLP-1 affects synaptic transmission and plasticity in the rat hippocampus, at least in part through glutamate absorption. Additionally, it has been shown that astrocytes express the GLP-1R, which is linked to the suppression of neural inflammation. In cell cultures, activation of the GLP-1R was associated with neurite outgrowth and neurotrophic impacts, such as hippocampus neurogenesis. Additionally, the receptor's upregulation in the hippocampus was connected to improvements in learning and memory [44]. On the other hand, GLP-1R expression in the hypothalamus was reported to be reduced in people with T2DM [45].

Preproglucan and consequently GLP-1 are mostly produced by proprotein convertase 1/3 expressing neurons in the caudal region of the dorsal vagal complex's (DVC) medial NTS and, to a lesser extent, the area postrema. Afferent vagal inputs, such as gastric distention, the activation of peripheral GLP-1Rs, or the release of the satiety-related hormones leptin and cholecystokinin, enhance the activity of preproglucagon-expressing neurons in the NTS. The NTS neurons create proglucagon and/or GLP-1-positive projections that are directed into the olfactory bulb, several hypothalamic nuclei, the bed nucleus of the stria terminalis, the lateral and medial septal nuclei, the amygdaloid complex, the septohippocampal area, the nucleus accumbens, and, less frequently, the medullary reticular formation, dorsal motor nucleus of the vagus, and the cortex. The GLP-1R is broadly distributed in the CNS, in contrast to the NTS, where GLP-1 production and distribution are limited [4].

In the treatment of stroke and neurodegenerative disorders such as AD, PD, amyotrophic lateral sclerosis, autism, schizophrenia, and other diseases such as diabetic retinopathy, ocular hypertension, and glaucoma, GLP-1 and GLP-1R have demonstrated remarkable neuroprotective effectiveness [3, 46–50].

GLP-1 analogs (including liraglutide, lixisenatide, semaglutide, exendin-4, and NLY01) exhibit strong anti-inflammatory effects. GLP-1R/gastric inhibitory polypeptide receptor (GIPR) dual agonists inhibited microgliosis, astrogliosis, and the expression of toll-like receptor-4 in a manner comparable to GLP-1 mimetics, however, they had a greater impact. Analogs of the GLP-1R (such as oxyntomodulin and exenatide) promote synaptogenesis, preserve synapses, increase hippocampus synaptic plasticity, and improve learning and memory [4, 49].

Alzheimer's disease and PD, both kinds of neurodegenerative disorders, have been linked to impaired insulin signaling [51]. The main clinical sign of AD is progressive ongoing dementia, which can be distinguished from other forms of dementia by intellectual symptoms such as memory loss and behavioral issues as well as cognitive symptoms such as reduced cognition. Similarities between AD and T2DM, which is thought to be a high-risk factor. Neurofibrillary tangles, which are shaped by hyperphosphorylated tau protein and can build up into oligomers and/or Aβ plaques, are one of the neuro-pathological characteristics of AD. Aβ buildup in AD has the potential to damage synapses and cause neuroinflammation by triggering astroglia and microglia cells [4, 52, 53].

Additionally, *in vivo* research using PD models has shown that unusually elevated levels of TNF-α and interferon-gamma (IFN-γ) secretion support the TNF-α/Janus kinase/signal transducer and activator of transcription and IFN-γ/MAPK/extracellular signal-regulated kinase-mediated activation of nuclear factor kappa-B in microglia and astroglia, respectively. Therefore, chronic neuroinflammation in AD and PD results in the permeabilization of the BBB by TNF-α and IL-1β; immune cell infiltration into the CNS; mitochondrial and axonal abnormalities; synaptic damage; and insulin resistance in the brain, as well as microglial, astrocyte, and neuronal malfunction and death [4].

GLP-1 directly promotes neurite development and synaptogenesis, in addition to shielding synapses from amyloid and oxidative damage. Additionally, GLP-1R activation has demonstrated synapto-protective qualities by promoting cytoskeletal actin/tubulin polymerization to induce neurite multiplication, branching, outgrowth in cell cultures (PC12, SH-SY5Y), and adult sensory neurons. It has been demonstrated in the rat model that lixisenatide, a GLP-1R agonist, also inhibits synaptic damage brought on by Aβ buildup, supporting spatial memory by influencing the PI3K pathway [4, 54].

Exenatide (exendin-4, a synthetic peptide containing 39 amino acids) was shown in studies to protect against ischemia-induced neuronal death by upregulating GLP-1R expression, primarily in gamma-aminobutyric acid–releasing (GABAergic) interneurons or astrocytes in the gerbils' hippocampal CA1 region. After a stroke in mice, it reduced neurological impairments. When administered 4 weeks before and 2–4 weeks after generating stroke in diabetic rats, a clinical dose of exendin-4 also decreased cell damage, stopped microglial infiltration, and enhanced stroke-induced neuroblast production and proliferation of neural stem cells [3]. GLP-1 and GLP-1R agonists provide protection for many systems as well as CNS, by promoting neurogenesis and synaptogenesis and preventing oxidative stress, neuroinflammation, and apoptosis.

4. Neuroprotective properties of granulocyte colony-stimulating factor

Granulocyte colony-stimulating factor (G-CSF), now referred to as colony-stimulating factor 3 (CSF-3), is a 25-kDa glycoprotein that is encoded by the Csf3 gene on the human chromosome 17 [55]. It is a growth factor that promotes the proliferation, differentiation, and survival of hematopoietic progenitor cells. G-CSF is essential for the migration of hematopoietic stem cells as well as the proliferation and differentiation of granulocyte progenitors. It promotes the differentiation of hematopoietic progenitor cells into neutrophils and modulates neutrophil migration, as well as having trophic effects on several cell types, including neurons [56–58].

G-CSF typically influences myeloid cell development from progenitor cells to mature neutrophil granulocytes during hematopoiesis [59–61]. It functions via a homodimeric granulocyte colony-stimulating factor receptor (GCSF-R) and is expressed on myeloid cells ranging from myeloblasts to mature neutrophils. GCSF-R is found at a low density on the cell surface (700–1500 per cell) and has a strong affinity for G-CSF. Low occupancy at the receptors is adequate to achieve the maximum biological response. G-CSFR is composed of a single extracellular domain, a transmembrane domain, and an intracellular domain [62, 63]. The extracellular domain contains immunoglobulin (Ig)-like domains, a cytokine receptor homologous (CRH) domain, and three fibronectin (FN)-III-like repeats. The Ig-like domains and the CRH domain are important in G-CSF binding, whereas the FN-III-like repeats are involved in receptor dimer stability [64]. Numerous cells, including bone marrow, fibroblasts, macrophages, endothelial cells, glial cells, and neurons of various brain regions, all contain G-CSFRs [65–67]. G-CSF regulates hematopoietic cell proliferation, differentiation, and survival primarily via activating the Janus kinase/STAT, Ras/MAPK, and AKT/PI3K pathways [58].

G-CSF has been demonstrated to increase neutrophil chemotaxis and phagocytosis, as well as increase bactericidal and fungicidal activities, antibody-induced cell toxicity, and complement receptor expression (CD11b, CG18b, CD35) [67]. G-CSF administration stimulated monocytes to produce IL-10 and mobilizes T helper type 2 cells, promoting dendritic cells, which may contribute to the reduction of T cell reactivity [68]; G-CSF also increases the survival of neutrophils and their progenitors, including stem cells. Clinical studies have shown that the duration of severe neutropenia following chemotherapy is shortened and neutrophil counts recover more quickly when G-CSF is administered to cancer patients who have had both allogeneic and autologous bone marrow transplantation [69].

Recent research has demonstrated the neuroprotective impact of G-CSF treatment, which is due to its high antioxidant, anti-inflammatory, and antiapoptotic properties [10, 11]. In a number of ischemic rodent models, G-CSF has been demonstrated to provide long-term neuroprotection by encouraging somatic growth and improving sensorimotor and neurocognitive skills [70, 71]. The neuro-regenerative and neuroprotective properties of G-CSF have also been demonstrated in preclinical studies in a number of neurodevelopmental disorders, including autism, spinal cord injury, cerebral ischemia, PD, and AD [5, 10, 72–74]. To investigate the possibility of using G-CSF for AD treatment, two different Aβ protein aggregate-induced AD mice models were used. Interestingly, they found that G-CSF-induced bone marrow stem cell release enhanced neurogenesis around Aβ plaques in mouse brains and greatly restored the neurological function of AD mice [75]. Recombinant human G-CSF (filgrastim) was authorized for use by the Food and Drug Administration in 1991 to treat cancer patients receiving myelotoxic chemotherapy [76]. According to a wealth of research, the G-CSF molecule and its recombinant form, filgrastim, have the potential to treat cerebral ischemia, stroke, and neurodegenerative disorders such as Huntington's disease, amyotrophic lateral sclerosis, AD, and PD [58, 77]. The therapeutic efficacy and safety of G-CSF are supported by all available clinical and preclinical research data, establishing its value as a treatment for neurodegenerative disorders.

5. Neuroprotective properties of oxytocin

The CNS's glial, microglial, and neuronal interactions are incredibly dynamic and responsive to various stimuli. As chemical messengers that communicate both within the brain and between the brain and the body, hormones are essential for the body's homeostasis. OXT is a nonapeptide generated in the hypothalamic paraventricular (PVN), supraoptic (SON), and accessory nuclei (AN) [78, 79]. Via G-protein-coupled receptors, OXT affects the central and peripheral nervous systems. Various peripheral tissues, including the pancreas, blood vessels, ovary, thymus, skin, placenta, testis, heart, adipocytes, and kidney, also generate it [80]. OXT is crucial for aggression, sexual and maternal behavior, neuromodulation, social memory, and bonding. It helps in the evacuation of milk from the mammary gland during breastfeeding and is a powerful stimulator of uterine contractions [81]. The structure of vasopressin, a similar nonapeptide with only two amino acid differences from OXT, is extremely similar to that of OXT. Oxytocin receptor (OXTR), which together with the related V1a, V1b, and V2 vasopressin receptor subtypes form a subfamily of the large G protein-coupled receptor superfamily, is the sole receptor for OXT that is currently known [82].

Studies have shown that lower levels of central endogenous OXTergic activity are related to social behavior profiles that are compromised [83, 84]. Several psychiatric disorders such as social anxiety, major depressive disorder, autism spectrum disorder, addiction, depression, and schizophrenia have been connected to disturbed brain OXTergic signaling [78, 85]. Numerous animal experiments published in the literature demonstrate OXT's neuroprotective properties. The immune system regulation, social neuroprotection, antiapoptotic, anti-inflammatory, and antioxidative actions of the OXT hormone are among its neuroprotective properties. It also controls the immunological and autonomic nervous systems in addition to the brain and reproductive system [86]. There are several medicines that have side effects including autotoxicity, neurotoxicity, and nephrotoxicity. Since oxidative stress and inflammation are important in the pathogenesis of neurological disorders, and the antioxidant/anti-inflammatory properties of OXT are widely recognized, there has been numerous research on OXT's positive effects in neurotoxicity prevention [85, 87]. Microglia, the brain, and the spinal cord's resident macrophages are the innate immune system's main line of defense. Microglia and astrocyte intercommunication controls the inflammatory response in the brain. TNF-α, IL-1, IL-6, and IL-12 are a few proinflammatory cytokines that are produced and secreted in relation to M1 microglia polarization, which in general react to defend tissue and increase the elimination of infections. Overactivation or dysregulation of the M1 microglia phenotype, on the other hand, may increase neuronal damage caused by pathogenic stimuli and toxins, resulting in more extensive damage to neighboring neurons. Recent studies showed that OTX is important in the regulation of microglial reactivity in the growing brain [88, 89]. The relationship between neuroinflammation, microglial activation, and neuronal death has also been explored in several neurodegenerative disorders, including autism, frontotemporal dementia (FTD), ALS, PD, AD, and Huntington's disease. Recent research has revealed that autistic brains have activated microglia. OXT treatment has been shown to diminish activated microglia in the hippocampus and amygdala and enhance the behaviors of autistic mice, lowering anxiety, depression, and repetitive behavior, as well as improving social contact [90]. According to a study, depending on the type of memory test and the psychobiological importance of the stimuli, the effects of intranasally administered OXT in humans revealed that the hormone selectively affected memory performance [91]. In their research, Erbaş et al. investigated the neuroprotective effects of OXT on rotenone-induced PD in rats. According to their research, oxytocin may protect dopaminergic neurons from rotenone-induced injury while also restoring them [92]. Postmortem brain tissue from patients with Huntington's disease with varying

Peptides	Role in neuroprotection	Function
EPO	Neurogenesis↑ Neurotrophic effects↑	Promotes and enhances neurogenesis by activating brain-derived neurotrophic factors and acting on neural progenitor cells
	Oxidative stress↓ Mitochondrial dysfunction↓	Restricts cell damage and reduces neurological dysfunction via its protective effects and ability to minimize reactive oxygen species
	Neural growth↑ Synaptic plasticity↑	Activates secondary chemical signals (STAT5, PI3K, and MAPK) and functions in neural growth and synapse formation control
	Functional recovery↑	Promotes rapid maturation and enhanced progenitor growth in hypoxic mesencephalic progenitor cells
	Regeneration↑	Promotes regeneration assisting in the suppression of apoptosis
	Maintains the blood–brain barrier↑	Prevents the death of vascular endothelium and the arousal of astrocytes
	Neuroinflammation↓	Reduces levels of tumor necrosis factor-alpha, declines the inflammatory activity, and elevates antioxidant responses
	Inhibition of apoptosis↑	Blocks the apoptotic mechanism and protects against amyloid beta toxicity, minimizes cell damage, and tau hyperphosphorylation in Alzheimer's disease
	Cognition↑	Reduces ischemia-induced memory deficit, protects hypoxic astrocytes and oligodendrocyte progenitor cells in acute ischemic stroke
	Neurodegeneration↓	Impacts the processes of cerebral flow restitution, angiogenesis, and neuroregeneration reducing the effects of ischemia in hypoxic–ischemic encephalopathy
GLP-1	Apoptosis↓	Promotes neuroprotective, neuromodulatory, and antiapoptotic activities.
	Inflammation↓	Lowers microglial activation and the release of M1 macrophages
	Cognition↑	Promotes synaptogenesis, preserves synapses, increases hippocampal synaptic plasticity, and improves learning and memory
	Synaptogenesis↑	Promotes neurite development and synaptogenesis shielding synapses from amyloid and oxidative damage.
	Neuroprotection↑	Reduces neurological impairments
G-CSF	Cell survival↑ Apoptosis↓	Regulates hematopoietic cell proliferation, differentiation, and survival via activating the Janus kinase/STAT, Ras/MAPK, and AKT/PI3K pathways
	Neuroinflammation↓ Regeneration↑	Increases neutrophil chemotaxis and phagocytosis
	Neurotrophic effects↑	Stimulates monocytes to produce IL-10, mobilizes T helper type 2 cells, and promotes dendritic cells
	Neurogenesis↑	Releases enhanced neurogenesis around Aβ plaques and restores the neurological function of Alzheimer's disease

Peptides	Role in neuroprotection	Function
OXT	Neuroprotection↑	Mediates social neuroprotection, antiapoptotic, and antioxidative actions
	Neural growth↑ Neurogenesis↑	Controls the immunological and autonomic nervous systems
	Brain development↑	Regulates the microglial reactivity in the growing brain to diminish activated microglia in the hippocampus and amygdala
	Cognition↑	Lowers anxiety, depression, and repetitive behavior and improves social contact
	Neurodegeneration↓ Neuroinflammation↓	Protects dopaminergic neurons from rotenone-induced injury and restores

EPO: erythropoietin, GLP-1: glucagon-like peptide-1, G-CSF: granulocyte colony-stimulating factor, OXT: oxytocin.
↑: enhance.
↓: decrease.

Table 1.
An overview of the roles and effects of peptides in neuroprotection.

Vonsattel grades (grades 2–4) that had been immunohistochemically processed showed a selective 45% loss of OXT neurons and smaller cell sizes in the remaining OXT neurons [93]. Individuals with the mutant HTT gene had a significant 38% reduction in OXT cerebrospinal fluid levels, according to a recent study [94]. Patients with motor manifest and premanifest Huntington's disease have been found to have a positive correlation between OXT plasma levels and depression in a clinical study [95]. Additionally, a selective OXT loss in HD, ALS, and FTD has been linked to hypothalamic pathology [96]. OXT's anti-inflammatory and neuroprotective effects suggest that it may represent a possible therapeutic approach for the treatment of neurodegenerative and neurodevelopmental disorders.

Table 1 summarizes the functions and neuroprotective properties of peptides (EPO, GLP-1, G-CSF, and OXT).

6. Conclusion

Although neurodegenerative disorders are pathological conditions linked to aging, neurodegeneration frequently goes undetected for a long time and neuronal death happens gradually over the course of a lifetime before the first clinical signs can be observed. Increasing preclinical and clinical evidence demonstrating the efficacy of EPO, GLP-1, G-CSF, and OXT in treating various brain diseases shows that these molecules are versatile and have strong immunomodulatory, anti-inflammatory, anti-apoptotic, and neuroprotective properties. Given their beneficial effects on the brain, immunological system, reproductive system, and autonomic nervous system, these peptides hold promise as potential future treatments for neurodegenerative disorders.

Acknowledgements

A bibliometric research was performed on research and review articles published in the Scopus and PubMed databases using the keywords "erythropoietin," "glucagon-like peptide-1," "granulocyte colony-stimulating factor," and "oxytocin" and their neuroprotective effects on neurodegenerative disorders such as "Alzheimer's disease," "Parkinson's disease," "ataxia," "spinal muscular atrophy," "autism," "amyotrophic lateral sclerosis," "Huntington's disease," "epilepsy," "ischemic brain diseases," and "stroke". Current research and literature have been reviewed.

Declaration of conflicting interests

The authors declared no conflicts of interest with respect to the authorship and/or publication of this article.

Author details

Oytun Erbas[1,2]*, İlknur Altuntaş[1,2], Pemra Nesil[1,2], Hadi Sasani[3]
and Mehtap Odabaşı[4]

1 ERBAS Institute of Experimental Medicine, USA

2 ERBAS Institute of Experimental Medicine, Türkiye

3 Faculty of Medicine, Department of Radiology, Tekirdağ Namık Kemal University, Tekirdağ, Türkiye

4 Republic of Türkiye Ministry of Agriculture And Forestry, İstanbul Food Control Laboratory Directorate, İstanbul, Turkey

*Address all correspondence to: oytunerbas@yahoo.com

References

[1] Faden AI, Knoblach SM, Movsesyan VA, Cernak I. Novel small peptides with neuroprotective and nootropic properties. Journal of Alzheimer's Disease. 2004;**6**(Suppl. 6): S93-S97. DOI: 10.3233/jad-2004-6s603

[2] Perrone S, Lembo C, Gironi F, Petrolini C, Catalucci T, Corbo G, et al. Erythropoietin as a neuroprotective drug for newborn infants: Ten years after the first use. Antioxidants (Basel). 2022;**11**(4):652. DOI: 10.3390/antiox11040652

[3] Yang X, Qiang Q, Li N, Feng P, Wei W, Hölscher C. Neuroprotective mechanisms of glucagon-like peptide-1-based therapies in ischemic stroke: An update based on preclinical research. Frontiers in Neurology. 2022;**13**:844697. DOI: 10.3389/fneur.2022.844697

[4] Reich N, Hölscher C. The neuroprotective effects of glucagon-like peptide 1 in Alzheimer's and Parkinson's disease: An in-depth review. Frontiers in Neuroscience. 2022;**16**:970925. DOI: 10.3389/fnins.2022.970925

[5] Saklani P, Khan H, Gupta S, Kaur A, Singh TG. Neuropeptides: Potential neuroprotective agents in ischemic injury. Life Sciences. 2022;**288**:120186. DOI: 10.1016/j.lfs.2021.120186 Epub 2021 Nov 28

[6] Bartnicki P, Kowalczyk M, Rysz J. The influence of the pleiotropic action of erythropoietin and its derivatives on nephroprotection. Medical Science Monitor. 2013;**19**:599-605. DOI: 10.12659/MSM.889023

[7] Marcuzzi F, Zucchelli S, Bertuzzi M, Santoro C, Tell G, Carninci P, et al. Isoforms of the Erythropoietin receptor in dopaminergic neurons of the Substantia Nigra. Journal of Neurochemistry. 2016;**139**(4):596-609. DOI: 10.1111/jnc.13757 Epub 2016 Sep 30

[8] Holt MK, Llewellyn-Smith IJ, Reimann F, Gribble FM, Trapp S. Serotonergic modulation of the activity of GLP-1 producing neurons in the nucleus of the solitary tract in mouse. Molecular Metabolism. 2017;**6**(8):909-921. DOI: 10.1016/j.molmet.2017.06.002

[9] Kastin AJ, Akerstrom V, Pan W. Interactions of glucagon-like peptide-1 (GLP-1) with the blood-brain barrier. Journal of Molecular Neuroscience. 2002;**18**(1-2):7-14. DOI: 10.1385/JMN:18:1-2:07

[10] Durankuş F, Albayrak Y, Erdoğan F, Albayrak N, Erdoğan MA, Erbaş O. Granulocyte colony-stimulating factor has a sex-dependent positive effect in the maternal immune activation-induced autism model. International Journal of Developmental Neuroscience. Dec 2022;**82**(8):716-726. DOI: 10.1002/jdn.10221 [Epub 2022 Aug 12]

[11] Modi J, Menzie-Suderam J, Xu H, Trujillo P, Medley K, Marshall ML, et al. Mode of action of granulocyte-colony stimulating factor (G-CSF) as a novel therapy for stroke in a mouse model. Journal of Biomedical Science. 2020;**27**(1):19. DOI: 10.1186/s12929-019-0597-7

[12] Akman T, Akman L, Erbas O, Terek MC, Taskiran D, Ozsaran A. The preventive effect of oxytocin to Cisplatin-induced neurotoxicity: An experimental rat model. BioMed Research International. 2015;**2015**:167235. DOI: 10.1155/2015/167235 Epub 2015 Jan 22

[13] Law ML, Cai GY, Lin FK, Wei Q, Huang SZ, Hartz JH, et al. Chromosomal assignment of the human erythropoietin gene and its DNA polymorphism. Proceedings of the National Academy of Sciences of the United States of America. 1986;**83**(18):6920-6924. DOI: 10.1073/pnas.83.18.6920

[14] Lombardero M, Kovacs K, Scheithauer BW. Erythropoietin: A hormone with multiple functions. Pathobiology. 2011;**78**(1):41-53. DOI: 10.1159/000322975 Epub 2011 Apr 5

[15] Weidemann A, Johnson RS. Nonrenal regulation of EPO synthesis. Kidney International. 2009;**75**(7): 682-688. DOI: 10.1038/ki.2008.687 Epub 2009 Jan 21

[16] Shingo T, Sorokan ST, Shimazaki T, Weiss S. Erythropoietin regulates the in vitro and in vivo production of neuronal progenitors by mammalian forebrain neural stem cells. The Journal of Neuroscience. 2001;**21**(24):9733-9743. DOI: 10.1523/JNEUROSCI.21-24-09733.2001

[17] Darnell JE Jr, Kerr IM, Stark GR. Jak-STAT pathways and transcriptional activation in response to IFNs and other extracellular signaling proteins. Science. 1994;**264**(5164):1415-1421. DOI: 10.1126/science.8197455

[18] Ostrowski D, Heinrich R. Alternative erythropoietin receptors in the nervous system. Journal of Clinical Medicine. 2018;**7**(2):24. DOI: 10.3390/jcm7020024

[19] Watts D, Gaete D, Rodriguez D, Hoogewijs D, Rauner M, Sormendi S, et al. Hypoxia pathway proteins are master regulators of erythropoiesis. International Journal of Molecular Sciences. 2020;**21**(21):8131. DOI: 10.3390/ijms21218131

[20] Brines M, Grasso G, Fiordaliso F, Sfacteria A, Ghezzi P, Fratelli M, et al. Erythropoietin mediates tissue protection through an erythropoietin and common beta-subunit heteroreceptor. Proceedings of the National Academy of Sciences of the United States of America. 2004;**101**(41):14907-14912. DOI: 10.1073/pnas.0406491101 Epub 2004 Sep 29

[21] Chong ZZ, Shang YC, Mu Y, Cui S, Yao Q, Maiese K. Targeting erythropoietin for chronic neurodegenerative diseases. Expert Opinion on Therapeutic Targets. 2013;**17**(6):707-720. DOI: 10.1517/14728222.2013.780599 Epub 2013 Mar 20

[22] Ma Y, Zhou Z, Yang GY, Ding J, Wang X. The effect of erythropoietin and its derivatives on ischemic stroke therapy: A comprehensive review. Frontiers in Pharmacology. 2022;**13**:743926. DOI: 10.3389/fphar.2022.743926

[23] Haase VH. Regulation of erythropoiesis by hypoxia-inducible factors. Blood Reviews. 2013;**27**(1):41-53. DOI: 10.1016/j.blre.2012.12.003 Epub 2013 Jan 3

[24] Erbaş O, Çınar BP, Solmaz V, Çavuşoğlu T, Ateş U. The neuroprotective effect of erythropoietin on experimental Parkinson model in rats. Neuropeptides. 2015;**49**:1-5. DOI: 10.1016/j.npep.2014.10.003 Epub 2014 Oct 30

[25] Li G, Ma R, Huang C, Tang Q, Fu Q, Liu H, et al. Protective effect of erythropoietin on beta-amyloid-induced PC12 cell death through antioxidant mechanisms. Neuroscience Letters. 2008;**442**(2):143-147. DOI: 10.1016/j.neulet.2008.07.007 Epub 2008 Jul 10

[26] Wang W, Kagaya Y, Asaumi Y, Fukui S, Takeda M, Shimokawa H. Protective effects of recombinant human erythropoietin against pressure

overload-induced left ventricular remodeling and premature death in mice. The Tohoku Journal of Experimental Medicine. 2011;**225**(2):131-143. DOI: 10.1620/tjem.225.131

[27] Jacquens A, Needham EJ, Zanier ER, Degos V, Gressens P, Menon D. Neuro-inflammation modulation and post-traumatic brain injury lesions: From bench to bed-side. International Journal of Molecular Sciences. 2022;**23**(19):11193. DOI: 10.3390/ijms231911193

[28] Faustini G, Longhena F, Varanita T, Bubacco L, Pizzi M, Missale C, et al. Synapsin III deficiency hampers α-synuclein aggregation, striatal synaptic damage and nigral cell loss in an AAV-based mouse model of Parkinson's disease. Acta Neuropathologica. 2018;**136**(4):621-639. DOI: 10.1007/s00401-018-1892-1 Epub 2018 Jul 25

[29] Jang W, Kim HJ, Li H, Jo KD, Lee MK, Song SH, et al. 1,25-Dyhydroxyvitamin D_3 attenuates rotenone-induced neurotoxicity in SH-SY5Y cells through induction of autophagy. Biochemical and Biophysical Research Communications. 2014;**451**(1):142-147. DOI: 10.1016/j.bbrc.2014.07.081 Epub 2014 Jul 29

[30] Bond WS, Rex TS. Evidence that erythropoietin modulates neuroinflammation through differential action on neurons, astrocytes, and microglia. Frontiers in Immunology. 2014;**5**:523. DOI: 10.3389/fimmu.2014.00523

[31] Solmaz V, Erdoğan MA, Alnak A, Meral A, Erbaş O. Erythropoietin shows gender dependent positive effects on social deficits, learning/memory impairments, neuronal loss and neuroinflammation in the lipopolysaccharide induced rat model of autism. Neuropeptides. 2020;**83**:102073. DOI: 10.1016/j.npep.2020.102073 Epub 2020 Jul 17

[32] Raulin AC, Doss SV, Trottier ZA, Ikezu TC, Bu G, Liu CC. ApoE in Alzheimer's disease: Pathophysiology and therapeutic strategies. Molecular Neurodegeneration. 2022;**17**(1):72. DOI: 10.1186/s13024-022-00574-4

[33] Cevik B, Solmaz V, Yigitturk G, Cavusoğlu T, Peker G, Erbas O. Neuroprotective effects of erythropoietin on Alzheimer's dementia model in rats. Advances in Clinical and Experimental Medicine. 2017;**26**(1):23-29. DOI: 10.17219/acem/61044

[34] Davis CM, Lyon-Scott K, Varlamov EV, Zhang WH, Alkayed NJ. Role of endothelial STAT3 in cerebrovascular function and protection from ischemic brain injury. International Journal of Molecular Sciences. 2022;**23**(20):12167. DOI: 10.3390/ijms232012167

[35] Fauchère JC, Dame C, Vonthein R, Koller B, Arri S, Wolf M, et al. An approach to using recombinant erythropoietin for neuroprotection in very preterm infants. Pediatrics. 2008;**122**(2):375-382. DOI: 10.1542/peds.2007-2591

[36] Drucker DJ, Nauck MA. The incretin system: Glucagon-like peptide-1 receptor agonists and dipeptidyl peptidase-4 inhibitors in type 2 diabetes. Lancet. 2006;**368**(9548):1696-1705. DOI: 10.1016/S0140-6736(06)69705-5

[37] Holst JJ. The physiology of glucagon-like peptide 1. Physiological Reviews. 2007;**87**(4):1409-1439. DOI: 10.1152/physrev.00034.2006

[38] Campbell JE, Drucker DJ. Pharmacology, physiology, and mechanisms of incretin hormone action. Cell Metabolism. 2013;**17**(6):819-837. DOI: 10.1016/j.cmet.2013.04.008 Epub 2013 May 16

[39] Çavusoglu T, Erbas O, Karadeniz T, Akdemir O, Acikgoz E, Karadeniz M, et al. Comparison of nephron-protective effects of enalapril and GLP analogues (exenatide) in diabetic nephropathy. Experimental and Clinical Endocrinology & Diabetes. 2014;**122**(6):327-333. DOI: 10.1055/s-0034-1372584 Epub 2014 Jun 18

[40] Müller TD, Finan B, Bloom SR, D'Alessio D, Drucker DJ, Flatt PR, et al. Glucagon-like peptide 1 (GLP-1). Molecular Metabolism. 2019;**30**:72-130. DOI: 10.1016/j.molmet.2019.09.010 Epub 2019 Sep 30

[41] Heppner KM, Kirigiti M, Secher A, Paulsen SJ, Buckingham R, Pyke C, et al. Expression and distribution of glucagon-like peptide-1 receptor mRNA, protein and binding in the male nonhuman primate (Macaca mulatta) brain. Endocrinology. 2015;**156**(1):255-267. DOI: 10.1210/en.2014-1675

[42] Athauda D, Foltynie T. The glucagon-like peptide 1 (GLP) receptor as a therapeutic target in Parkinson's disease: Mechanisms of action. Drug Discovery Today. 2016;**21**(5):802-818. DOI: 10.1016/j.drudis.2016.01.013 Epub 2016 Feb 3

[43] Jensen CB, Pyke C, Rasch MG, Dahl AB, Knudsen LB, Secher A. Characterization of the glucagonlike peptide-1 receptor in male mouse brain using a novel antibody and in situ hybridization. Endocrinology. 2018;**159**(2):665-675. DOI: 10.1210/en.2017-00812

[44] Mansur RB, Fries GR, Trevizol AP, Subramaniapillai M, Lovshin J, Lin K, et al. The effect of body mass index on glucagon-like peptide receptor gene expression in the post mortem brain from individuals with mood and psychotic disorders. European Neuropsychopharmacology. 2019;**29**(1):137-146. DOI: 10.1016/j.euroneuro.2018.10.007 Epub 2018 Nov 6

[45] Ten Kulve JS, van Bloemendaal L, Balesar R, IJzerman RG, Swaab DF, Diamant M, et al. Decreased hypothalamic glucagon-like peptide-1 receptor expression in type 2 diabetes patients. The Journal of Clinical Endocrinology and Metabolism. 2016;**101**(5):2122-2129. DOI: 10.1210/jc.2015-3291 Epub 2015 Dec 16

[46] Erbaş O, Akseki HS, Solmaz V, Aktuğ H, Taşkıran D. Fatty liver-induced changes in stereotypic behavior in rats and effects of glucagon-like peptide-1 analog on stereotypy. The Kaohsiung Journal of Medical Sciences. 2014;**30**(9):447-452. DOI: 10.1016/j.kjms.2014.05.007 Epub 2014 Jun 25

[47] Mouhammad ZA, Vohra R, Horwitz A, Thein AS, Rovelt J, Cvenkel B, et al. Glucagon-like peptide 1 receptor agonists - potential game changers in the treatment of glaucoma? Frontiers in Neuroscience. 2022;**16**:824054. DOI: 10.3389/fnins.2022.824054

[48] Ramos H, Bogdanov P, Sampedro J, Huerta J, Simó R, Hernández C. Beneficial effects of glucagon-like peptide-1 (GLP-1) in diabetes-induced retinal abnormalities: Involvement of oxidative stress. Antioxidants (Basel). 2020;**9**(9):846. DOI: 10.3390/antiox9090846

[49] Solmaz V, Tekatas A, Erdoğan MA, Erbaş O. Exenatide, a GLP-1 analog, has healing effects on LPS-induced autism model: Inflammation, oxidative stress, gliosis, cerebral GABA, and serotonin interactions. International Journal of Developmental Neuroscience. 2020;**80**(7):601-612. DOI: 10.1002/jdn.10056 Epub 2020 Aug 11

[50] Sterling JK, Adetunji MO, Guttha S, Bargoud AR, Uyhazi KE, Ross AG, et al. GLP-1 receptor agonist NLY01 reduces retinal inflammation and neuron death secondary to ocular hypertension. Cell Reports. 2020;**33**(5):108271. DOI: 10.1016/j.celrep.2020.108271

[51] Andersen A, Lund A, Knop FK, Vilsbøll T. Glucagon-like peptide 1 in health and disease. Nature Reviews. Endocrinology. 2018;**14**(7):390-403. DOI: 10.1038/s41574-018-0016-2

[52] Hendrix RD, Ou Y, Davis JE, Odle AK, Groves TR, Allen AR, et al. Alzheimer amyloid-β- peptide disrupts membrane localization of glucose transporter 1 in astrocytes: Implications for glucose levels in brain and blood. Neurobiology of Aging. 2021;**97**:73-88. DOI: 10.1016/j.neurobiolaging.2020.10.001 Epub 2020 Oct 10

[53] Ikeda Y, Nagase N, Tsuji A, Kitagishi Y, Matsuda S. Neuroprotection by dipeptidyl-peptidase-4 inhibitors and glucagon-like peptide-1 analogs via the modulation of AKT-signaling pathway in Alzheimer's disease. World Journal of Biological Chemistry. 2021;**12**(6):104-113. DOI: 10.4331/wjbc.v12.i6.104

[54] Cai HY, Yang JT, Wang ZJ, Zhang J, Yang W, Wu MN, et al. Lixisenatide reduces amyloid plaques, neurofibrillary tangles and neuroinflammation in an APP/PS1/tau mouse model of Alzheimer's disease. Biochemical and Biophysical Research Communications. 2018;**495**(1):1034-1040. DOI: 10.1016/j.bbrc.2017.11.114 Epub 2017 Nov 22

[55] Panopoulos AD, Watowich SS. Granulocyte colony-stimulating factor: Molecular mechanisms of action during steady state and 'emergency' hematopoiesis. Cytokine. 2008; **42**(3):277-288. DOI: 10.1016/j.cyto.2008.03.002 Epub 2008 Apr 8

[56] Tekgunduz SA, Aycicek A, Bayram C, Uysalol EP, Akici F, Ozdemir GN. The effect of granulocyte colony-stimulating factors on survival parameters in pediatric patients with acute lymphoblastic leukemia: A retrospective study. Transfusion and Apheresis Science. 2022;**61**(1):103366. DOI: 10.1016/j.transci.2022.103366 Epub 2022 Jan 25

[57] Theyab A, Algahtani M, Alsharif KF, Hawsawi YM, Alghamdi A, Alghamdi A, et al. New insight into the mechanism of granulocyte colony-stimulating factor (G-CSF) that induces the mobilization of neutrophils. Hematology. 2021;**26**(1):628-636. DOI: 10.1080/16078454.2021.1965725

[58] Rahi V, Jamwal S, Kumar P. Neuroprotection through G-CSF: Recent advances and future viewpoints. Pharmacological Reports. 2021;**73**(2): 372-385. DOI: 10.1007/s43440-020-00201-3 Epub 2021 Jan 2

[59] Yadav S, Priya A, Borade DR, Agrawal-Rajput R. Macrophage subsets and their role: Co-relation with colony-stimulating factor-1 receptor and clinical relevance. Immunologic Research. 21 Oct 2022:1-23. DOI: 10.1007/s12026-022-09330-8 Epub ahead of print

[60] Metcalf D. The colony-stimulating factors and cancer. Cancer Immunology Research. 2013;**1**(6):351-356. DOI: 10.1158/2326-6066.CIR-13-0151

[61] Ding J, Wang J, Cai X, Yin T, Zhang Y, Yang C, et al. Granulocyte colony-stimulating factor in reproductive-related disease: Function, regulation and therapeutic effect. Biomedicine & Pharmacotherapy. 2022;**150**:112903. DOI: 10.1016/j.biopha.2022.112903 Epub 2022 Apr 14

[62] Park SD, Saunders AS, Reidy MA, Bender DE, Clifton S, Morris KT. A

review of granulocyte colony-stimulating factor receptor signaling and regulation with implications for cancer. Frontiers in Oncology. 2022;**12**:932608. DOI: 10.3389/fonc.2022.932608

[63] Rapoport AP, Abboud CN, DiPersio JF. Granulocyte-macrophage colony-stimulating factor (GM-CSF) and granulocyte colony-stimulating factor (G-CSF): Receptor biology, signal transduction, and neutrophil activation. Blood Reviews. 1992;**6**(1):43-57. DOI: 10.1016/0268-960x(92)90007-d

[64] de Koning JP, Dong F, Smith L, Schelen AM, Barge RM, van der Plas DC, et al. The membrane-distal cytoplasmic region of human granulocyte colony-stimulating factor receptor is required for STAT3 but not STAT1 homodimer formation. Blood. 1996;**87**(4):1335-1342

[65] Taşkıran E, Erdoğan MA, Yiğittürk G, Erbaş O. Therapeutic effects of liraglutide, oxytocin and granulocyte colony stimulating factor in doxorubicin-induced cardiomyopathy model: An experimental animal study. Cardiovascular Toxicology. 2019;**19**(6):510-517. DOI: 10.1007/s12012-019-09524-x

[66] Solaroglu I, Cahill J, Jadhav V, Zhang JH. A novel neuroprotectant granulocyte-colony stimulating factor. Stroke. 2006;**37**(4):1123-1128. DOI: 10.1161/01.STR.0000208205.26253.96 Epub 2006 Mar 2

[67] Dale DC, Liles WC, Summer WR, Nelson S. Review: Granulocyte colony-stimulating factor–role and relationships in infectious diseases. The Journal of Infectious Diseases. 1995;**172**(4):1061-1075. DOI: 10.1093/infdis/172.4.1061

[68] Rutella S, Zavala F, Danese S, Kared H, Leone G. Granulocyte colony-stimulating factor: A novel mediator of T cell tolerance. Journal of Immunology. 2005;**175**(11):7085-7091. DOI: 10.4049/jimmunol.175.11.7085

[69] Ozer H, Armitage JO, Bennett CL, Crawford J, Demetri GD, Pizzo PA, et al. American society of clinical oncology. 2000 update of recommendations for the use of hematopoietic colony-stimulating factors: Evidence-based, clinical practice guidelines. American society of clinical oncology growth factors expert panel. Journal of Clinical Oncology. 2000;**18**(20):3558-3585. DOI: 10.1200/JCO.2000.18.20.3558

[70] da Ros PB, Monteiro BL, Aires R, Silva CME, MCC G, Vasquez EC, et al. Low doses of G-CSF prevent cerebral infarction and maintain muscle strength in an experimental model of global ischemic stroke. Current Pharmaceutical Biotechnology. 2018;**19**(6):514-519. DOI: 10.2174/1389201019666180718094334

[71] Sugiyama Y, Yagita Y, Oyama N, Terasaki Y, Omura-Matsuoka E, Sasaki T, et al. Granulocyte colony-stimulating factor enhances arteriogenesis and ameliorates cerebral damage in a mouse model of ischemic stroke. Stroke. 2011;**42**(3):770-775. DOI: 10.1161/STROKEAHA.110.597799 Epub 2011 Jan 21

[72] Kim NK, Choi BH, Huang X, Snyder BJ, Bukhari S, Kong TH, et al. Granulocyte-macrophage colony-stimulating factor promotes survival of dopaminergic neurons in the 1-methyl-4-phenyl-1,2,3,6-tetrahydropyridine-induced murine Parkinson's disease model. The European Journal of Neuroscience. 2009;**29**(5):891-900. DOI: 10.1111/j.1460-9568.2009.06653.x Epub 2009 Feb 24

[73] Sanchez-Ramos J, Song S, Sava V, Catlow B, Lin X, Mori T, et al. Granulocyte

colony stimulating factor decreases brain amyloid burden and reverses cognitive impairment in Alzheimer's mice. Neuroscience. 2009;**163**(1):55-72. DOI: 10.1016/j.neuroscience.2009.05.071 Epub 2009 Jun 14

[74] Koda M, Nishio Y, Kamada T, Someya Y, Okawa A, Mori C, et al. Granulocyte colony-stimulating factor (G-CSF) mobilizes bone marrow-derived cells to the injured spinal cord and promotes functional recovery after compression-induced spinal cord injury in mice. Brain Research. 2007;**1149**:223-231. DOI: 10.1016/j.brainres.2007.02.058 Epub 2007 Mar 1

[75] Tsai KJ, Tsai YC, Shen CK. G-CSF rescues the memory impairment of animal models of Alzheimer's disease. The Journal of Experimental Medicine. 2007;**204**(6):1273-1280. DOI: 10.1084/jem.20062481 Epub 2007 May 21

[76] American Society of Clinical Oncology. Recommendations for the use of hematopoietic colony-stimulating factors: Evidence-based, clinical practice guidelines. Journal of Clinical Oncology. 1994;**12**(11):2471-2508. DOI: 10.1200/JCO.1994.12.11.2471

[77] Azmy MS, Menze ET, El-Naga RN, Tadros MG. Neuroprotective effects of filgrastim in rotenone-induced parkinson's disease in rats: Insights into its anti-inflammatory, neurotrophic, and antiapoptotic effects. Molecular Neurobiology. 2018;**55**(8):6572-6588. DOI: 10.1007/s12035-017-0855-1 Epub 2018 Jan 11

[78] Erdoğan MA, Taşkıran E, Yiğittürk G, Erbaş O, Taşkıran D. The investigation of therapeutic potential of oxytocin and liraglutide on vincristine-induced neuropathy in rats. Journal of Biochemical and Molecular Toxicology. 2020;**34**(1):e22415. DOI: 10.1002/jbt.22415 Epub 2019 Nov 4

[79] Panaro MA, Benameur T, Porro C. Hypothalamic neuropeptide brain protection: Focus on oxytocin. Journal of Clinical Medicine. 2020;**9**(5):1534. DOI: 10.3390/jcm9051534

[80] Lee HJ, Macbeth AH, Pagani JH, Young WS 3rd. Oxytocin: The great facilitator of life. Progress in Neurobiology. 2009;**88**(2):127-151. DOI: 10.1016/j.pneurobio.2009.04.001 Epub 2009 Apr 10

[81] Kiss A, Mikkelsen JD. Oxytocin–Anatomy and functional assignments: A minireview. Endocrine Regulations. 2005;**39**(3):97-105

[82] Muratspahić E, Monjon E, Duerrauer L, Rogers SM, Cullen DA, Vanden Broeck J, et al. Oxytocin/vasopressin-like neuropeptide signaling in insects. Vitamins and Hormones. 2020;**113**:29-53. DOI: 10.1016/bs.vh.2019.08.011 Epub 2019 Oct 18

[83] Winslow JT, Insel TR. The social deficits of the oxytocin knockout mouse. Neuropeptides. 2002;**36**(2-3):221-229. DOI: 10.1054/npep.2002.0909

[84] Dhungel S, Rai D, Terada M, Orikasa C, Nishimori K, Sakuma Y, et al. Oxytocin is indispensable for conspecific-odor preference and controls the initiation of female, but not male, sexual behavior in mice. Neuroscience Research. 2019;**148**:34-41. DOI: 10.1016/j.neures.2018.11.008 Epub 2018 Nov 28

[85] Gümüs B, Kuyucu E, Erbas O, Kazimoglu C, Oltulu F, Bora OA. Effect of oxytocin administration on nerve recovery in the rat sciatic nerve damage model. Journal of Orthopaedic Surgery and Research. 2015;**10**:161. DOI: 10.1186/s13018-015-0301-x

[86] Carter CS, Kenkel WM, MacLean EL, Wilson SR, Perkeybile AM,

Yee JR, et al. Is oxytocin "Nature's Medicine"? Pharmacological Reviews. 2020;**72**(4):829-861. DOI: 10.1124/pr.120.019398

[87] Zhu J, Li Y, Liang J, Li J, Huang K, Li J, et al. The neuroprotective effect of oxytocin on vincristine-induced neurotoxicity in mice. Toxicology Letters. 2021;**340**:67-76. DOI: 10.1016/j.toxlet.2021.01.008 Epub 2021 Jan 8

[88] Liddelow SA, Guttenplan KA, Clarke LE, Bennett FC, Bohlen CJ, Schirmer L, et al. Neurotoxic reactive astrocytes are induced by activated microglia. Nature. 2017;**541**(7638):481-487. DOI: 10.1038/nature21029 Epub 2017 Jan 18

[89] Takano T. Role of microglia in autism: Recent advances. Developmental Neuroscience. 2015;**37**(3):195-202. DOI: 10.1159/000398791 Epub 2015 May 21

[90] Wang Y, Zhao S, Liu X, Zheng Y, Li L, Meng S. Oxytocin improves animal behaviors and ameliorates oxidative stress and inflammation in autistic mice. Biomedicine & Pharmacotherapy. 2018;**107**:262-269. DOI: 10.1016/j.biopha.2018.07.148 Epub 2018 Aug 8

[91] Heinrichs M, Meinlschmidt G, Wippich W, Ehlert U, Hellhammer DH. Selective amnesic effects of oxytocin on human memory. Physiology & Behavior. 2004;**83**(1):31-38. DOI: 10.1016/j.physbeh.2004.07.020

[92] Erbaş O, Oltulu F, Taşkiran D. Amelioration of rotenone-induced dopaminergic cell death in the striatum by oxytocin treatment. Peptides. 2012;**38**(2):312-317. DOI: 10.1016/j.peptides.2012.05.026 Epub 2012 Sep 14

[93] Vonsattel JP, Myers RH, Stevens TJ, Ferrante RJ, Bird ED, Richardson EP Jr. Neuropathological classification of Huntington's disease. Journal of Neuropathology and Experimental Neurology. 1985;**44**(6):559-577. DOI: 10.1097/00005072-198511000-00003

[94] Hellem MNN, Cheong RY, Tonetto S, Vinther-Jensen T, Hendel RK, Larsen IU, et al. Decreased CSF oxytocin relates to measures of social cognitive impairment in Huntington's disease patients. Parkinsonism & Related Disorders. 2022;**99**:23-29. DOI: 10.1016/j.parkreldis.2022.05.003 Epub 2022 May 13

[95] Fisher ER, Rocha NP, Morales-Scheihing DA, Venna VR, Furr-Stimming EE, Teixeira AL, et al. The relationship between plasma oxytocin and executive functioning in huntington's disease: A pilot study. Journal of Huntington's Disease. 2021;**10**(3):349-354. DOI: 10.3233/JHD-210467

[96] Bergh S, Cheong RY, Petersén Å, Gabery S. Oxytocin in Huntington's disease and the spectrum of amyotrophic lateral sclerosis-frontotemporal dementia. Frontiers in Molecular Neuroscience. 2022;**15**:984317. DOI: 10.3389/fnmol.2022.984317

Chapter 5

Genetic Treatments for Rare Neurodegenerative Disorders

Christina A. Kousparou

Abstract

Rare neurodegenerative disorders encompass a diverse group of conditions characterized by the progressive degeneration of the nervous system. Usually, a combination of genetic, biochemical, and clinical features characterizes these disorders. An overview, classification, and investigation of the genetic mutations and variants linked to rare neurodegenerative diseases are included in this chapter on genetic therapy for these diseases. The article discusses novel approaches to treating genetic illnesses, including gene therapy, CRISPR-based interventions, and RNA-based therapeutics. It includes case studies and particular instances of effective genetic treatments as well as ongoing clinical trials. In addition, difficulties and moral issues are discussed, covering issues like delivery strategies, side effects, and moral questions about the use of gene editing in the treatment of various illnesses. Lastly, future outlooks and conjectures regarding possible developments, avenues for further study, and the prospects for genetic therapies in the treatment of uncommon neurodegenerative illnesses are discussed.

Keywords: rare, neurodegenerative, genetic, gene therapy, CRISPR, RNA, ethics, gene delivery, adeno-associated virus

1. Introduction

Rare neurodegenerative diseases represent a critical area of study in biomedical research due to their profound impact on individuals' lives and the broader healthcare landscape. Despite their rarity, these conditions collectively affect a significant number of people worldwide, often leading to debilitating symptoms and premature death.

Understanding the underlying causes of these illnesses offers prospective options for therapeutic action in addition to fundamental understanding of neurobiology. Furthermore, research on rare neurodegenerative illnesses can reveal common pathways with more prevalent neurological disorders, which can guide the development of treatments across a spectrum of conditions. Furthermore, new genetic abnormalities linked to various illnesses have been found thanks to developments in genomic technologies, which have made it easier to classify diseases accurately, diagnose patients early, and develop individualized treatment plans.

Figure 1 shows a simplified flowchart to outline a generic overview and the general process for diagnosing and managing rare neurodegenerative disorders.

Classification of these disorders can be based on a number of criteria, including disease onset and progression. Early-onset diseases are those that manifest symptoms at a young age, frequently before adulthood. Tay-Sachs disease, Niemann-Pick disease, and juvenile Huntington's disease [1] are a few examples. The genetic foundation, pathophysiology, and clinical manifestations of Tay-Sachs disease, Niemann-Pick disease, and juvenile Huntington's disease are summarized in **Figure 2**. The figure

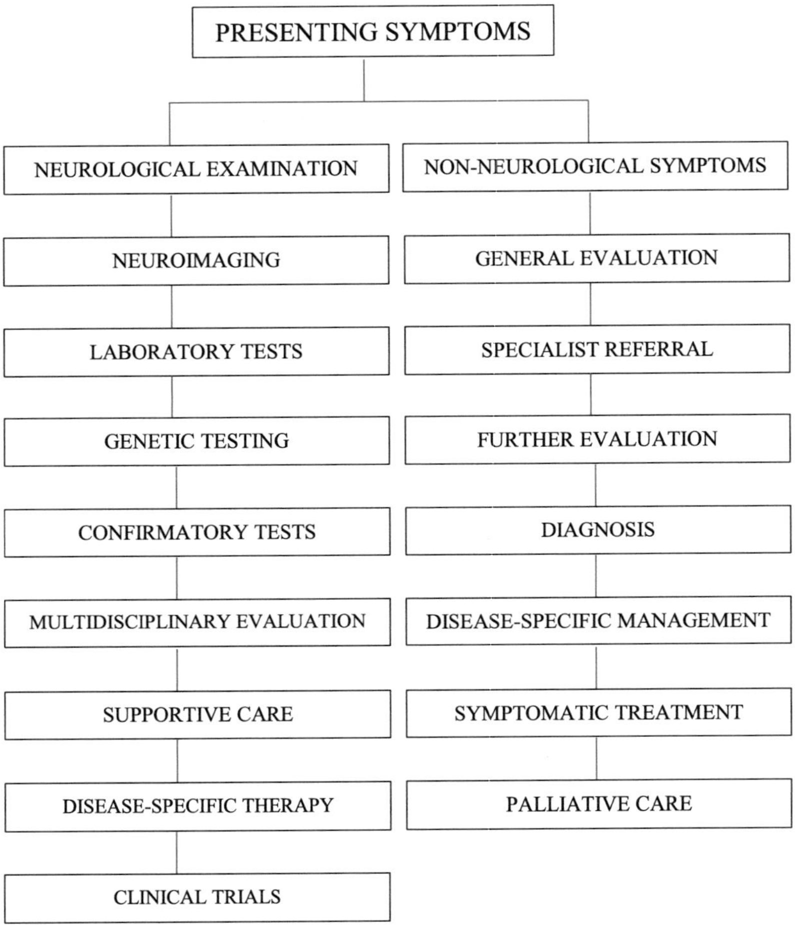

Figure 1.
The process begins with the identification of presenting symptoms suggestive of a neurological disorder. These may include motor or cognitive impairment, sensory changes, or autonomic dysfunction. A comprehensive neurological examination is conducted to assess motor function, sensation, reflexes, coordination, and cognitive status. Imaging studies such as MRI or CT scans may be performed to visualize structural abnormalities in the brain or spinal cord. Blood tests, cerebrospinal fluid analysis, or other laboratory investigations may be conducted to assess metabolic, infectious, or autoimmune factors that could contribute to neurological symptoms. In cases where a genetic cause is suspected, genetic testing may be performed to identify specific mutations associated with neurodegenerative disorders. Additional tests or procedures may be necessary to confirm the diagnosis, such as muscle biopsy, nerve conduction studies, or specialized imaging techniques. A multidisciplinary team, including neurologists, geneticists, neuropsychologists, and other specialists, may be involved in the evaluation and management of rare neurodegenerative disorders. Patients may receive supportive care to address symptoms and improve quality of life, including physical therapy, occupational therapy, speech therapy, and psychological support. If available, disease-specific treatments or therapies targeting the underlying cause of the disorder may be initiated. Patients may be eligible to participate in clinical trials investigating novel therapies or interventions for rare neurodegenerative disorders. The process concludes with ongoing monitoring, management of symptoms, and support for patients and their families.

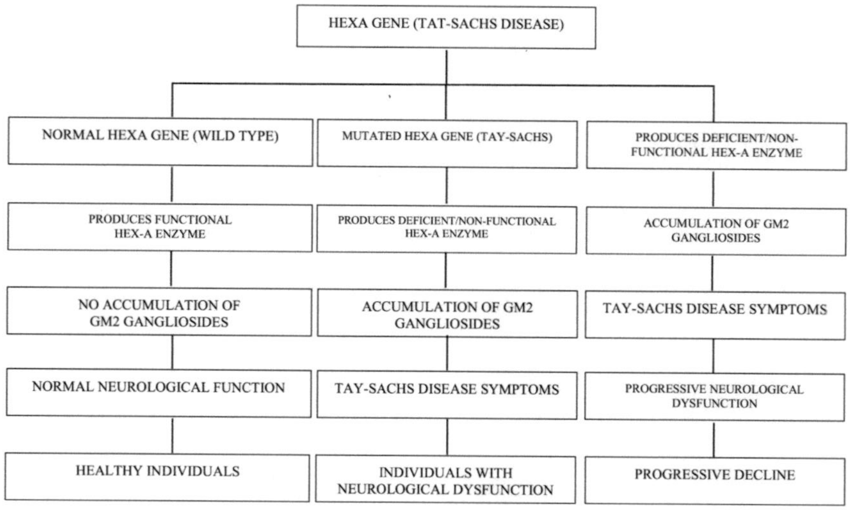
HEXA GENE (TAT-SACHS DISEASE)
NORMAL HEXA GENE (WILD TYPE)
MUTATED HEXA GENE (TAY-SACHS)
PRODUCES DEFICIENT/NON-FUNCTIONAL HEX-A ENZYME
PRODUCES FUNCTIONAL HEX-A ENZYME
PRODUCES DEFICIENT/NON-FUNCTIONAL HEX-A ENZYME
ACCUMULATION OF GM2 GANGLIOSIDES
NO ACCUMULATION OF GM2 GANGLIOSIDES
ACCUMULATION OF GM2 GANGLIOSIDES
TAY-SACHS DISEASE SYMPTOMS
NORMAL NEUROLOGICAL FUNCTION
TAY-SACHS DISEASE SYMPTOMS
PROGRESSIVE NEUROLOGICAL DYSFUNCTION
HEALTHY INDIVIDUALS
INDIVIDUALS WITH NEUROLOGICAL DYSFUNCTION
PROGRESSIVE DECLINE

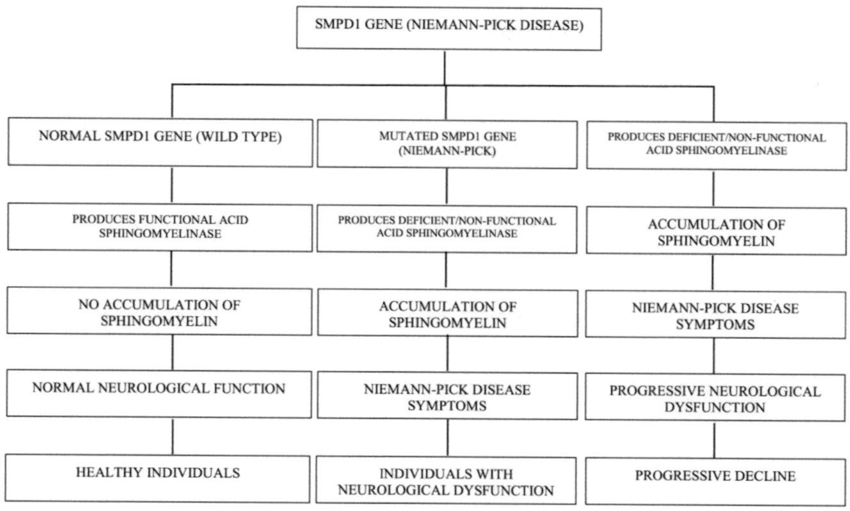
SMPD1 GENE (NIEMANN-PICK DISEASE)
NORMAL SMPD1 GENE (WILD TYPE)
MUTATED SMPD1 GENE (NIEMANN-PICK)
PRODUCES DEFICIENT/NON-FUNCTIONAL ACID SPHINGOMYELINASE
PRODUCES FUNCTIONAL ACID SPHINGOMYELINASE
PRODUCES DEFICIENT/NON-FUNCTIONAL ACID SPHINGOMYELINASE
ACCUMULATION OF SPHINGOMYELIN
NO ACCUMULATION OF SPHINGOMYELIN
ACCUMULATION OF SPHINGOMYELIN
NIEMANN-PICK DISEASE SYMPTOMS
NORMAL NEUROLOGICAL FUNCTION
NIEMANN-PICK DISEASE SYMPTOMS
PROGRESSIVE NEUROLOGICAL DYSFUNCTION
HEALTHY INDIVIDUALS
INDIVIDUALS WITH NEUROLOGICAL DYSFUNCTION
PROGRESSIVE DECLINE

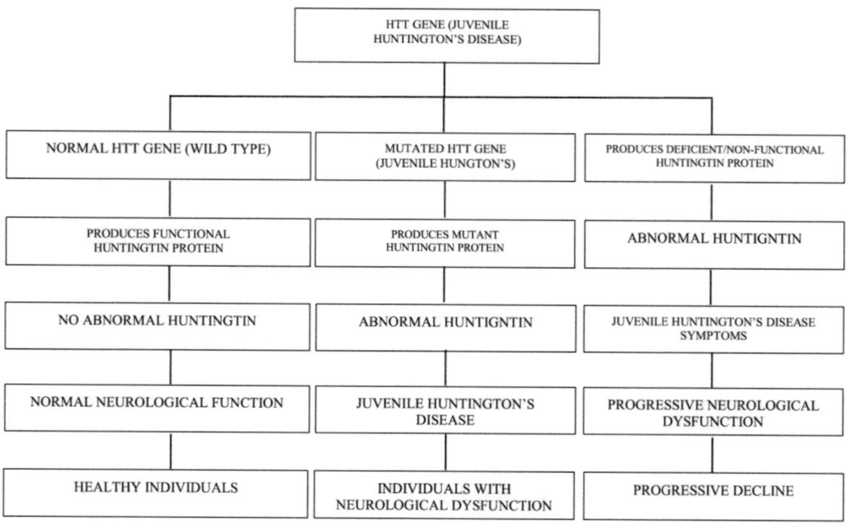
HTT GENE (JUVENILE HUNTINGTON'S DISEASE)
NORMAL HTT GENE (WILD TYPE)
MUTATED HTT GENE (JUVENILE HUNGTON'S)
PRODUCES DEFICIENT/NON-FUNCTIONAL HUNTINGTIN PROTEIN
PRODUCES FUNCTIONAL HUNTINGTIN PROTEIN
PRODUCES MUTANT HUNTINGTIN PROTEIN
ABNORMAL HUNTIGNTIN
NO ABNORMAL HUNTINGTIN
ABNORMAL HUNTIGNTIN
JUVENILE HUNTINGTON'S DISEASE SYMPTOMS
NORMAL NEUROLOGICAL FUNCTION
JUVENILE HUNTINGTON'S DISEASE
PROGRESSIVE NEUROLOGICAL DYSFUNCTION
HEALTHY INDIVIDUALS
INDIVIDUALS WITH NEUROLOGICAL DYSFUNCTION
PROGRESSIVE DECLINE

Figure 2.
Three genetic disorders: Tay-Sachs disease, Niemann-Pick disease, and Juvenile Huntington's disease, along with the associated mutations and their effects on neurological function. HEXA gene (Tay-Sachs disease): results from mutations in the HEXA gene, leading to deficient or non-functional Hex-A enzyme. Accumulation of GM2 gangliosides in neurons causes progressive neurological dysfunction. Individuals with Tay-Sachs disease experience developmental regression, muscle weakness, seizures, and early death. SMPD1 gene (Niemann-Pick disease): caused by mutations in the SMPD1 gene, resulting in deficient or non-functional acid sphingomyelinase (ASM) enzyme. Accumulation of sphingomyelin in cells leads to progressive neurological dysfunction. Niemann-Pick disease is characterized by hepatosplenomegaly, progressive neurological decline, and early death. HTT gene (Juvenile Huntington's disease): disease arises from mutations in the HTT gene, causing an abnormal expansion of CAG repeats and production of mutant huntingtin protein. Accumulation of mutant huntingtin protein in neurons leads to progressive neurological dysfunction. The disease manifests with movement disorders, cognitive decline, and behavioral changes, typically starting in childhood or adolescence.

also provides the genes linked to each disease, the consequences of mutations on enzyme or protein function, and the symptoms that result from each disorder. Each gene is depicted with its normal function, mutation, and the effect of the mutation on nervous system performance.

Contrary to disorders that typically occur later in life, such as some forms of atypical Parkinsonism or certain types of hereditary ataxias, which are classified as late-onset. An alternative way of approaching these disorders is through their clinical manifestations. Conditions affecting motor functions, including Parkinson's disease, Huntington's disease, and certain forms of ataxia, are termed movement disorders; these are diseases primarily characterized by cognitive decline and dementia, like frontotemporal dementia, certain forms of familial Alzheimer's disease, and prion diseases are presenting cognitive impairment. And finally, there are those who manifest mixed phenotypic profiles, such as amyotrophic lateral sclerosis (ALS), which present with a combination of motor impairment and cognitive decline.

The genetic basis of the disease varies, and the number of genes involved. Polygenic or multifactorial disorders, like sporadic forms of Alzheimer's disease, which are influenced by multiple genetic and environmental factors, are more complex to understand than monogenic conditions (conditions caused by a single genetic mutation), such as Huntington's disease or familial forms of ALS. Nevertheless, there are differences in the involvement of cellular components. For instance, disorders like Tay-Sachs disease and Niemann-Pick disease, which arise from the build-up of substances within lysosomes, differ from protein aggregation disorders, which are marked by the aggregation of proteins in the brain, such as prion diseases, Parkinson's disease, and Alzheimer's disease.

Other examples of diseases featuring abnormal aggregation of the protein tau, including conditions like frontotemporal dementia and certain forms of atypical parkinsonism (tauopathies), are classified differently from synucleinopathies, which are marked by the accumulation of alpha-synuclein, like Parkinson's disease and multiple system atrophy.

This classification is wide and subject to change when new genetic and molecular pathways underlying various illnesses are discovered through continued research. A range of distinct diseases with their own clinical manifestations, underlying genetic causes, and modes of disease progression may fall under each classification.

2. Genetic mutations and rare neurological diseases: understanding the underlying conditions

Understanding the genetic alterations associated with rare neurological disorders is essential for creating targeted treatments and precision medicine methodologies.

New gene variants and molecular pathways are being found by means of advanced genetic sequencing technology, which opens up new avenues for the development of therapeutic medicines targeted at reducing or repairing the underlying genetic defects responsible for these debilitating neurological illnesses.

All are characterized by the progressive degeneration of the nervous system due to mutations and variations in specific genes which play a pivotal role in the system's pathogenesis. These underpinnings are crucial for accurate diagnosis, prognosis, and the development of targeted treatments.

Trinucleotide repeat expansions are a prominent class of uncommon neurological illnesses in which the amplification of particular DNA sequences results in aberrant protein synthesis and cellular malfunction. A classic example is Huntington's disease (HD), which is defined by an expanded CAG repeat in the chromosome 4 HTT gene. The age at which symptoms appear and the severity of the disease are correlated with the length of this repeat sequence. Similar to this, a CGG repeat expansion in the FMR1 gene causes fragile X syndrome, which manifests as a variety of neurological and behavioral problems along with intellectual incapacity.

Spinal Muscular Atrophy (SMA) is primarily caused by mutations in the Survival Motor Neuron 1 (SMN1) gene, which is located on chromosome 5q13.2 [2]. The SMN1 gene encodes the survival motor neuron (SMN) protein, which is essential for the maintenance and function of motor neurons in the spinal cord. Without adequate levels of SMN protein, motor neurons degenerate, leading to muscle weakness and atrophy characteristic of SMA. The most common mutation associated with SMA is a deletion of exon 7 in the SMN1 gene. Exon 7 deletion results in a truncated or non-functional SMN protein. Individuals with SMA typically have two copies of the SMN1 gene, one inherited from each parent. However, in SMA patients, both copies of the SMN1 gene are usually affected by mutations, leading to a deficiency in functional SMN protein.

In addition to SMN1 gene mutations, there is a closely related gene called SMN2, which is nearly identical to SMN1 but differs in a critical region that affects alternative splicing. The SMN2 gene produces a smaller amount of full-length SMN protein compared to SMN1 due to alternative splicing events that often exclude exon 7. However, some portion of SMN2 transcripts retain exon 7, resulting in the production of functional SMN protein. The severity of SMA is influenced by the number of copies of the SMN2 gene and the level of functional SMN protein produced. Generally, individuals with more copies of the SMN2 gene tend to have milder forms of SMA due to higher levels of functional SMN protein. However, other genetic and environmental factors can also modulate disease severity.

Another group comprises lysosomal storage disorders, such as Tay-Sachs Disease and Niemann-Pick Disease, resulting from mutations in genes involved in lysosomal function [3–5]. Tay-Sachs Disease is caused by mutations in the HEXA gene, leading to the accumulation of GM2 gangliosides in nerve cells and subsequent neurodegeneration [6]. Niemann-Pick Disease involves mutations in NPC1 or NPC2 genes, causing impaired lipid metabolism and the buildup of lipids in cells, particularly in the brain [7].

Neurodegenerative conditions like Alzheimer's Disease (AD) and Parkinson's Disease (PD) are associated with protein misfolding and aggregation. AD involves mutations in genes like APP, PSEN1, and PSEN2, resulting in the aberrant processing of amyloid precursor protein and the accumulation of beta-amyloid plaques in the brain. PD, while often sporadic, can be linked to mutations in genes like SNCA (alpha-synuclein), LRRK2, and Parkin, leading to the formation of Lewy bodies and dopaminergic neuron degeneration.

Polyglutamine disorders, exemplified by various Spinocerebellar Ataxias (SCAs), are characterized by CAG repeat expansions in different genes (e.g., ATXN1, ATXN2, ATXN3), resulting in ataxia, movement impairment, and other neurological symptoms. These disorders exhibit genetic anticipation, wherein successive generations tend to have earlier disease onset and increased severity due to repeat expansion.

Amyotrophic Lateral Sclerosis (ALS) is a motor neuron disease with both sporadic and familial forms. Familial ALS can result from mutations in genes like C9orf72, SOD1, FUS, and TARDBP, impacting motor neuron function and survival. These mutations disrupt cellular processes, including RNA metabolism, protein quality control, and cytoskeletal dynamics, leading to motor neuron degeneration and subsequent muscle weakness and paralysis.

Prion diseases, such as Creutzfeldt-Jakob Disease (CJD), involve the misfolding of the prion protein (PRNP gene), leading to the accumulation of abnormal prion proteins in the brain. This results in rapid neurological deterioration, cognitive decline, and movement abnormalities.

3. Emerging therapeutic approaches

Emerging and novel therapy modalities for rare neurological illnesses are varied and always changing. They show the increasing sophistication and diversity of solutions being created to deal with difficult situations. Research in these areas needs to continue receiving substantial funding in order to improve patient outcomes and quality of life.

Gene therapy involves delivering functional copies of a gene to compensate for mutations causing the disorder. In rare neurological disorders, this approach aims to correct genetic defects responsible for the condition. Techniques such as viral vectors, including adeno-associated viruses (AAV), are often used to deliver therapeutic genes to target cells. Recent advancements in gene editing technologies like CRISPR-Cas9 hold promise for precise gene correction.

Onasemnogene abeparvovec (Zolgensma) is an innovative gene therapy approved by the FDA for the treatment of pediatric patients less than 2 years of age diagnosed with SMA [8–15]. It works by delivering a functional copy of the SMN1 gene to replace the defective gene responsible for SMA, addressing the root cause of the disease. This therapy is administered via a one-time intravenous infusion. Clinical trials and real-world experiences have shown promising results with Zolgensma. Many infants treated with this gene therapy have demonstrated significant improvements in motor function, increased muscle strength, and milestone achievements that would not have been possible without treatment. Some children who received Zolgensma have achieved the ability to sit, stand, or even walk independently, depending on the severity and type of SMA.

However, a number of variables, such as the age at which treatment is started, the severity of the illness, and other individual characteristics, may affect how each person reacts to Zolgensma. It is important to remember that, despite Zolgensma's impressive efficacy, it might not always fully reverse the symptoms of SMA or restore motor function, particularly in situations where irreversible motor neuron loss has already taken place.

As patients are followed up after treatment, researchers are still examining the long-term effects and durability of Zolgensma to assess the therapy's long-term safety, efficacy, and influence on the course of the disease. CRISPR-based interventions have shown significant potential in addressing rare neurodegenerative diseases by offering precise genome editing capabilities. While this technology is still in its early stages for clinical use in treating these conditions, research and preclinical studies have demonstrated promising results in targeting genetic mutations associated with these disorders.

In precision editing of mutations, CRISPR/Cas9 technology enables precise modification of the DNA sequence, allowing for targeted correction of disease-causing mutations responsible for various rare neurodegenerative disorders [16]. Researchers are exploring ways to utilize CRISPR to edit out or correct genetic mutations linked to conditions such as Huntington's disease, certain forms of familial ALS, and other monogenic neurodegenerative diseases. One potential approach involves correcting or modifying the genetic mutations responsible for these diseases in affected cells or tissues. For instance, in Huntington's disease, researchers aim to reduce or eliminate the production of the mutant huntingtin protein using CRISPR-based strategies. Another approach involves modifying the expression of genes associated with disease progression to potentially slow down or halt neurodegeneration.

However, efficiently getting CRISPR components into the brain and into particular types of neurons is a big hurdle. For CRISPR-based therapeutics to be safe and effective, precise editing without unwanted genomic modifications is essential (prevention of off-target effects). Furthermore, regulation and careful consideration must be given to the ethical concerns of germline editing, potential unexpected consequences, and long-term impacts of genetic modifications.

Clinical trials assessing the use of CRISPR/Cas9 technology in treating certain neurodegenerative diseases, are being planned or are in early stages to assess safety and therapeutic potential [17–22]. Specifically, Leber congenital amaurosis 10 (LCA10) is a rare genetic disorder causing early-onset blindness. EDIT-101, developed by Editas Medicine, is a CRISPR-based gene editing therapy designed to treat LCA10 by targeting mutations in the CEP290 gene. Editas Medicine has initiated clinical trials for EDIT-101. In Huntington's disease, CRISPR-based gene editing approaches are being investigated to selectively silence or correct the mutant HTT gene. However, clinical trials specifically using CRISPR-Cas9 for Huntington's disease are still in the very early stages. In ALS, CRISPR-Cas9 technology has been used in preclinical research to target genes associated with ALS, such as C9orf72 or SOD1, for potential therapeutic intervention. Clinical trials involving CRISPR-Cas9 for ALS are not yet underway, but the technology holds promise for future treatments.

Short, synthetic nucleic acid molecules that target RNA are used in antisense oligonucleotide treatment (ASO), which modifies gene expression [23]. This method is especially helpful for conditions like spinal muscular atrophy (SMA) and different types of muscular dystrophy that are brought on by abnormal RNA processing or splicing. Small compounds can interact with particular targets, such as enzymes or receptors, to regulate biological processes. Finding new targets or repurposing current medications for different applications are common steps in the development of small-molecule treatments for uncommon neurological illnesses. These treatments can focus on a number of pathways, including neurotransmitter signaling, protein aggregation, and neuroinflammation, that are implicated in the pathophysiology of disease.

Stem cell-based therapies hold promise for rare disorders by replacing damaged or lost cells, promoting tissue repair, or modulating the immune response. These approaches involve transplanting stem cells, either from exogenous sources or through the reprogramming of patient-derived cells, into the affected tissues. Stem cell therapy is being explored for conditions like Parkinson's disease, Huntington's disease, and certain types of leukodystrophies. Enzyme Replacement Therapy (ERT) is a treatment approach used for rare neurological disorders caused by enzyme deficiencies, such as lysosomal storage disorders (e.g., Gaucher disease, Pompe disease). It involves administering recombinant enzymes to replace the deficient enzyme and restore normal metabolic function [24]. ERT can improve symptoms and slow disease progression in affected individuals. RNA Interference (RNAi) is a mechanism for silencing specific genes by targeting complementary RNA sequences. RNAi-based therapies utilize small interfering RNAs (siRNAs) or short hairpin RNAs (shRNAs) to degrade target mRNAs, thereby reducing the expression of disease-causing genes. This approach is being investigated for various rare neurological disorders, including amyotrophic lateral sclerosis (ALS) and Huntington's disease. And lastly, immunotherapy strategies aim to modulate the immune system's response to treat neuroinflammatory and autoimmune disorders. Approaches include monoclonal antibodies targeting specific immune cells or cytokines, as well as immune checkpoint inhibitors to enhance immune responses against pathogens or tumor cells. Immunomodulatory therapies are being explored for conditions like multiple sclerosis, neuromyelitis optica, and certain autoimmune encephalitides.

4. Challenges and considerations

There are several hurdles such as delivery methods, off-target effects, and ethical considerations related to gene editing in the context of treating rare neurological diseases.

Regarding delivery modalities, a significant challenge is delivering gene editing tools across the BBB to target specific cells within the central nervous system (CNS). Various strategies are being explored, including viral vectors, nanoparticles, exosomes, and cell-penetrating peptides, to facilitate efficient delivery into the CNS. Achieving cell specificity and ensuring that gene editing tools reach the desired cell types without affecting non-targeted cells is also extremely critical. Selective targeting methodologies, such as engineered viruses or nanoparticles with cell-specific ligands, are under investigation to enhance precision. Furthermore, developing techniques that allow direct *in vivo* delivery of gene editing tools to specific regions of the brain or spinal cord while minimizing systemic side effects is proving difficult [25].

Unintended genetic modifications causing off-target effects must be avoided, in turn to avoid unintended non-specific alterations in the genome. Enhancing the precision and accuracy of gene editing technologies, such as CRISPR/Cas systems, to minimize off-target effects must be of primary focus. A comprehensive assessment of potential long-term consequences, including genomic stability, unintended mutations, and potential tumorigenesis, is essential before the widespread clinical application of these technologies. Scientists are investigating involving modified Cas enzymes and guide RNAs to enhance the specificity of gene editing tools, reducing off-target effects while maintaining on-target efficiency.

Ethically, germline editing raises concerns regarding the permanent alteration of the genome and potential heritability of edited genes, impacting future generations. Stringent ethical guidelines and regulatory frameworks are essential to address the ethical implications of germline editing in the context of rare (and other) diseases. Ensuring informed consent and respecting patient autonomy, particularly in vulnerable populations or pediatric cases, is crucial when considering experimental gene editing therapies. But it does not stop there: ethical considerations extend to ensuring equitable *access* to gene editing therapies disparities in availability, affordability, and distribution of these treatments across different populations.

Addressing these hurdles requires collaborative efforts among researchers, clinicians, regulatory bodies, and ethicists for developing innovative, safe, and effective gene editing approaches diseases. Rigorous preclinical studies continued advancements in delivery technologies, thorough assessment of safety profiles, and transparent ethical frameworks are essential in navigating these challenges and ensuring responsible development and implementation of gene editing therapies for neurodegenerative disorders.

5. Conclusion

Rare neurodegenerative diseases encompass a heterogeneous group of disorders characterized by progressive degeneration of the nervous system, resulting in debilitating neurological symptoms. Despite their rarity individually, and collectively, these disorders pose significant challenges to patients, families, and healthcare systems worldwide. Over the past few decades, substantial progress has been made in understanding the underlying pathophysiology, genetic mechanisms, and potential therapeutic strategies for these conditions. In this conclusive scientific section, we will explore recent advancements, challenges, and future directions in the field of rare neurodegenerative diseases.

Recent advancements in rare neurodegenerative diseases have been propelled by breakthroughs in genetics, molecular biology, and neuroscience. The advent of next-generation sequencing technologies has revolutionized the identification of disease-causing genetic variants, enabling the discovery of novel genes associated with rare neurodegenerative disorders. Furthermore, advancements in animal models and induced pluripotent stem cell (iPSC) technology have facilitated the elucidation of disease mechanisms and the development of preclinical models for drug discovery and testing. One of the most significant advancements in recent years has been the emergence of gene therapy as a promising treatment approach for rare neurodegenerative diseases. Gene therapy holds great potential for correcting underlying genetic defects, slowing disease progression, or even providing a cure for some disorders. Clinical trials utilizing gene therapy vectors, such as adeno-associated viruses (AAVs) [26–29], have shown promising results in diseases like spinal muscular atrophy (SMA), Batten disease, and familial amyloid polyneuropathy (FAP), among others. In addition to gene therapy, other therapeutic modalities, such as small molecule drugs, antisense oligonucleotides (ASOs), and monoclonal antibodies, are also being investigated for their potential to target specific pathways implicated in rare neurodegenerative diseases. These advancements highlight the growing momentum in the field and the increasing hope for effective treatments for patients with these devastating disorders.

Despite significant progress, rare neurodegenerative diseases continue to present formidable challenges to researchers, clinicians, and patients alike. One of the most pressing challenges is the heterogeneity of these disorders, both in terms of clinical presentation and underlying genetic etiology. The rarity of individual diseases poses difficulties in conducting large-scale clinical trials and accruing sufficient patient cohorts for meaningful research studies. Another major challenge is the lack of disease-modifying treatments for many rare neurodegenerative diseases. While symptomatic therapies may help alleviate some symptoms and improve quality of life, they do not address the underlying cause of the disease or halt its progression. Developing effective disease-modifying therapies requires a deeper understanding of the molecular pathways involved in neurodegeneration and the identification of druggable targets. Furthermore, the translation of promising preclinical findings into clinically viable treatments faces numerous hurdles, including regulatory approvals, manufacturing challenges, and cost considerations. The high cost of developing and delivering novel therapies poses significant barriers to access for patients, particularly those in resource-limited settings or without adequate healthcare coverage.

Looking ahead, several promising avenues hold potential for addressing the challenges posed by rare neurodegenerative diseases and advancing the field toward effective treatments and cures. Collaborative efforts among researchers, clinicians, patient advocacy groups, and industry partners are essential for accelerating the pace of discovery and translation. Precision medicine approaches, leveraging advances in genomics, proteomics, and imaging technologies, offer the promise of personalized therapies tailored to individual patients' genetic and molecular profiles. Biomarker discovery and validation are critical for identifying disease progression markers, monitoring treatment response, and stratifying patients for clinical trials. Moreover, the continued development of innovative therapeutic modalities, such as RNA-based therapies, gene editing technologies (e.g., CRISPR-Cas9), and gene silencing approaches, holds tremendous potential for addressing the underlying genetic defects in rare neurodegenerative diseases [30]. Strategies for optimizing drug delivery to the central nervous system (CNS) and overcoming the blood-brain barrier are also being actively pursued to enhance therapeutic efficacy. In addition to therapeutic interventions, efforts to improve patient care and support services are essential for addressing the holistic needs of individuals and families affected by rare neurodegenerative diseases. Multidisciplinary care teams, including neurologists, genetic counselors, physical and occupational therapists, and social workers, play a crucial role in providing comprehensive care and support across the continuum of the disease.

In conclusion, rare neurodegenerative diseases represent a complex and challenging group of disorders with significant unmet medical needs. While recent advancements have provided hope for effective treatments, numerous challenges persist, including disease heterogeneity, lack of disease-modifying therapies, and barriers to translation. However, with continued investment in research, collaboration, and innovation, there is optimism for the future of rare neurodegenerative disease research and the development of transformative therapies that will improve the lives of patients and families affected by these devastating conditions.

Conflict of interest

The author was Head of Medical Affairs of Novartis Pharmaceuticals Islands. The company is the manufacturer of Zolgensma used in the treatment of SMA.

DOI: http://dx.doi.org/10.5772/intechopen.1005439

Author details

Christina A. Kousparou
European University Cyprus, Nicosia, Cyprus

*Address all correspondence to: c.kousparou@euc.ac.cy

References

[1] Peluso S, de Rosa A, De Michele G. Juvenile Huntington's disease: A mini-review. Geriatrics. 2023;**8**(1):24. DOI: 10.3390/geriatrics8010024

[2] Klein CJ, Mauermann ML, Dyck PJB. Spinal muscular atrophies. Neurologic Clinics. 2022;**40**(2):443-458. DOI: 10.1016/j.ncl.2021.11.011

[3] Wraith JE. Lysosomal disorders. Seminars in Neonatology. 2002;**7**(1): 75-83. DOI: 10.1053/siny.2001.0112

[4] Mehta A, Winchester B. Lysosomal storage disorders: A practical guide. The Indian Journal of Medical Research. 2018;**148**(5):601-610. DOI: 10.4103/ijmr.IJMR_198_18

[5] Walkley SU, Vanier MT. Secondary lipid accumulation in lysosomal disease. Biochimica et Biophysica Acta. 2009;**1793**(4):726-736. DOI: 10.1016/j.bbamcr.2008.12.002

[6] Tziomalos K. Tay-Sachs disease: An overview. The International Journal of Neuroscience. 2020;**130**(7):677-680. DOI: 10.1080/00207454.2019.1686237

[7] Vanier MT. Niemann-Pick diseases. Handbook of Clinical Neurology. 2013;**113**:1717-1721. DOI: 10.1016/B978-0-444-59565-2.00048-6

[8] Farrar MA, Teoh HL, Carey KA, et al. The outcome of spinal muscular atrophy (SMA) types 2 and 3. Journal of Neurology, Neurosurgery, and Psychiatry. 2016;**87**(2):209-215. DOI: 10.1136/jnnp-2015-310734

[9] Mercuri E, Finkel RS, Muntoni F, et al. Diagnosis and management of spinal muscular atrophy: Part 1—Recommendations for diagnosis, rehabilitation, orthopedic and nutritional care. Neuromuscular Disorders. 2018;**28**(2):103-115. DOI: 10.1016/j.nmd.2017.11.005

[10] D'Amico A, Mercuri E, Tiziano FD, Bertini E. Spinal muscular atrophy. Orphanet Journal of Rare Diseases. 2011;**6**:71. DOI: 10.1186/1750-1172-6-71

[11] Lefebvre S, Burglen L, Reboullet S, et al. Identification and characterization of a spinal muscular atrophy-determining gene. Cell. 1995;**80**(1):155-165. DOI: 10.1016/0092-8674(95)90460-3

[12] Kolb SJ, Kissel JT. Spinal muscular atrophy: A timely review. Archives of Neurology. 2011;**68**(8):979-984. DOI: 10.1001/archneurol.2011.161

[13] Shorrock HK, Gillingwater TH, Groen EJN. Overview of current drugs and molecules in development for spinal muscular atrophy therapy. Drugs. 2018;**78**(3):293-305. DOI: 10.1007/s40265-018-0861-y

[14] Prior TW. Spinal muscular atrophy diagnostics. Journal of Child Neurology. 2007;**22**(8):952-956. DOI: 10.1177/0883073807305666

[15] Jochmann E, Steinbach R, Jochmann T, et al. Update on spinal muscular atrophy genetics. Journal of Child Neurology. 2018;**33**(12):842-848. DOI: 10.1177/0883073818798516

[16] Kim EJ, Kang KH, Ju S, et al. CRISPR-Cas9: A promising tool for gene editing on induced pluripotent stem cells. The Korean Journal of Internal Medicine. 2017;**32**(1):42-61. DOI: 10.3904/kjim.2016.197

[17] Bakondi B, Lv W, Lu B, Jones MK, Tsai Y, Kim KJ. AAV-mediated CRISPR/Cas gene editing of retinal cells in

vivo. Investigative Ophthalmology & Visual Science. 2016;**57**(12):5581-5582. DOI: 10.1167/iovs.16-20512

[18] Park CY, Kim DH, Son JS, Sung JJ, Lee J, Bae S. Targeted genome engineering via zinc finger nucleases, transcription activator-like effector nucleases, and clustered regularly interspaced short palindromic repeat/Cas9 in neurological diseases. Seminars in Neurology. 2018;**38**(1):97-103. DOI: 10.1055/s-0037-1607433

[19] Qu B, Du Y, Chen Y, Zhang X, Wang J. CRISPR/Cas9 editing of APP C-terminus attenuates β-cleavage and promotes α-cleavage. Nature Communications. 2017;**8**:13863. DOI: 10.1038/ncomms13863

[20] Xu X, Tay Y, Sim B, et al. Reversal of phenotypic abnormalities by CRISPR/Cas9-mediated gene correction in Huntington disease patient-derived induced pluripotent stem cells. Stem Cell Reports. 2017;**8**(3):619-633. DOI: 10.1016/j.stemcr.2017.01.021

[21] Bakondi B, Lv W, Lu B, et al. In vivo CRISPR/Cas9 gene editing corrects retinal dystrophy in the S334ter-3 rat model of autosomal dominant retinitis pigmentosa. Molecular Therapy. 2016;**24**(3):556-563. DOI: 10.1038/mt.2015.220

[22] Liu KI, Ramli MN, Woo CW, Wang Y, Zhao T, Zhang X. A chemical-inducible CRISPR-Cas9 system for rapid control of genome editing. Nature Chemical Biology. 2016;**12**(11):980-987. DOI: 10.1038/nchembio.2205

[23] Bennett CF, Krainer AR, Cleveland DW. Antisense oligonucleotide therapies for neurodegenerative diseases. Annual Review of Neuroscience. 2019;**42**:385-406. DOI: 10.1146/annurev-neuro-070918-050409

[24] Wiatr K, Szlachcic WJ, Trzeciak M, Figlerowicz M, Figiel M. Huntington disease as a neurodevelopmental disorder and early signs of the disease in stem cells. Molecular Neurobiology. 2018;**55**(4):3351-3371. DOI: 10.1007/s12035-017-0500-2

[25] Gessler DJ, Gao G. Gene therapy for the treatment of neurological disorders: Metabolic disorders, neurodegenerative diseases, and brain cancer. Neurotherapeutics. 2019;**16**(1):156-177. DOI: 10.1007/s13311-018-00688-3

[26] Kotterman MA, Schaffer DV. Engineering adeno-associated viruses for clinical gene therapy. Nature Reviews. Genetics. 2014;**15**(7):445-451. DOI: 10.1038/nrg3742

[27] Wu Z, Asokan A, Samulski RJ. Adeno-associated virus serotypes: Vector toolkit for human gene therapy. Molecular Therapy. 2006;**14**(3):316-327. DOI: 10.1016/j.ymthe.2006.05.009

[28] Hocquemiller M, Giersch L, Audrain M, Parker S, Cartier N. Adeno-associated virus-based gene therapy for CNS diseases. Human Gene Therapy. 2016;**27**(7):478-496. DOI: 10.1089/hum.2016.091

[29] Mingozzi F, High KA. Immune responses to AAV vectors: Overcoming barriers to successful gene therapy. Blood. 2013;**122**(1):23-36. DOI: 10.1182/blood-2013-01-306647

[30] Kumar SRP, Markusic DM, Biswas M, High KA, Herzog RW. Clinical development of gene therapy: Results and lessons from recent successes. Molecular Therapy—Methods & Clinical Development. 2016;**3**:16034. DOI: 10.1038/mtm.2016.34

Chapter 6

Current Drugs Strategies for Treatment of Rare Neurodegenerative Diseases

Ali Gamal Al-kaf and Ali Abdullah Al-yahawi

Abstract

Nervous system problems affect around 600 million people worldwide. Among these, neurodegenerative illnesses are often distinguished by a late adult start, a progressive clinical course, and a localized loss of neurons in the central nervous system. These include, among others, multiple sclerosis, Parkinson's disease, amyotrophic lateral sclerosis (ALS, also known as Lou Gehrig's disease), Huntington's disease, Prion diseases, encephalitis, epilepsy, genetic brain disorders, hydrocephalus, stroke, and Alzheimer's and other less common dementias. The brain stem, cerebellum, thalamus, hypothalamus, basal ganglia, cerebral cortex, and intracranial white matter are among the areas that neurodegeneration typically affects. Mendelian inheritance is well-established, despite the fact that most neurodegenerative illnesses are sporadic. The neuropathological findings and clinical symptoms in hereditary neurodegenerative disorders are intriguing. Regretfully, there are few neurodegenerative diseases for which no effective treatments are available. The rare hereditary types of neurodegenerative diseases, such as ataxias, multiple system atrophy, spastic paraplegias, Parkinson's disease, dementias, motor neuron diseases, and uncommon metabolic disorders, are highlighted in this chapter along with their clinical and genetic characteristics.

Keywords: genetic diagnosis, neuromuscular, metabolic disorders, dementia, ataxia, movement disorders

1. Introduction

Rare neurodegenerative diseases are a group of disorders characterized by the progressive degeneration of the structure and function of the nervous system. These conditions are considered rare because they affect a small number of individuals in comparison to more common neurodegenerative diseases like Alzheimer's or Parkinson's. Many of these diseases are genetic in nature, resulting from mutations in specific genes. Here are some examples and basics about neurodegenerative diseases.

Neurodegenerative diseases are a subset of degenerative diseases that primarily affect the structure and function of the nervous system, leading to the progressive degeneration of neurons. These conditions often result in cognitive decline, motor dysfunction, and, in many cases, a reduced quality of life. Here are some examples and basics about neurodegenerative diseases [1, 2]:

1. Common neurodegenerative diseases

   - Alzheimer's disease (AD): It affects memory, thinking, and behavior. It is the most common cause of dementia.

   - Parkinson's disease (PD): It involves the malfunction and death of certain nerve cells in the brain, leading to movement-related symptoms.

   - Huntington's disease (HD): It is a genetic disorder that causes the progressive breakdown of nerve cells in the brain, leading to motor and cognitive impairments.

   - Amyotrophic lateral sclerosis (ALS): It affects nerve cells in the brain and spinal cord, leading to the loss of voluntary muscle control [1, 2].

2. Common features

   - Progressive degeneration: Neurodegenerative diseases are characterized by the gradual and irreversible loss of neurons and their function.

   - Accumulation of abnormal proteins: Many neurodegenerative diseases are associated with the buildup of abnormal protein that aggregates in the brain, such as beta-amyloid plaques in AD or Lewy bodies PD.

   - Inflammation: Neuroinflammation is often present, contributing to the progression of the disease [1, 2].

3. Symptoms

   - Symptoms vary depending on the specific disease but may include memory loss, cognitive decline, tremors, muscle stiffness, difficulty with movement and coordination, and changes in mood or behavior.

   - As the diseases progress, individuals may experience worsening symptoms and a decline in overall functioning [1, 2].

4. Causes

   - While the exact causes of neurodegenerative diseases are often complex and not fully understood, genetic factors, environmental influences, and the accumulation of abnormal proteins are commonly implicated.

   - Some neurodegenerative diseases have a genetic component, with mutations in specific genes increasing the risk of developing the condition [1, 2].

DOI: http://dx.doi.org/10.5772/intechopen.1005438

5. Diagnosis

    - Diagnosis involves a thorough medical history, neurological examinations, cognitive assessments, and often imaging studies (MRI, CT scans) to detect structural changes in the brain.

    - In some cases, genetic testing may be employed to identify specific mutations associated with familial forms of the diseases [1, 2].

6. Treatment

    - Most neurodegenerative diseases have no cure, however, treatment focuses on managing symptoms and improving the individual's quality of life.

    - Medications, physical therapy, occupational therapy, and supportive care are common approaches [1, 2].

7. Research and advances

    - Ongoing research aims to understand the underlying mechanisms of neurodegenerative diseases, identify potential biomarkers, and develop novel therapeutic strategies.

    - Clinical trials explore new medications, gene therapies, and interventions aimed at slowing or halting disease progression.

It is important to note that the field of neurodegenerative diseases is rapidly evolving, and ongoing research is critical for advancing our understanding and developing effective treatments.

Rare neurodegenerative diseases, also known as rare neurologic disorders, are a diverse group of conditions that affect the nervous system and are characterized by progressive degeneration. These diseases are considered rare because they affect a small number of individuals within the population. While each rare neurodegenerative disease is unique, there are some common features and considerations [1, 2]:

1. Limited prevalence

    - Rare neurodegenerative diseases are defined by their low prevalence, often affecting a small number of people within a population.

    - The rarity of these conditions can pose challenges for diagnosis, research, and the development of treatments due to limited awareness and resources [1, 2].

2. Heterogeneity

    - There is a significant heterogeneity among rare neurodegenerative diseases. Each disorder has distinct clinical features, genetic underpinnings, and disease progression.

    - Some examples of rare neurodegenerative diseases include Niemann-Pick disease, Batten disease, Ataxia-telangiectasia, and various forms of leukodystrophies [1, 2].

3. Genetic basis

    - Many rare neurodegenerative diseases have a genetic component, resulting from mutations in specific genes.
    - In some cases, these conditions follow an autosomal recessive, autosomal dominant, or X-linked inheritance pattern [3].

4. Early onset

    - Some rare neurodegenerative diseases manifest early in life, often during childhood or adolescence.
    - Early-onset forms may present unique challenges in terms of diagnosis, management, and the impact on the affected individuals and their families [3].

5. Multisystem involvement

    - Several rare neurodegenerative diseases involve multiple organ systems, not just the nervous system. This can lead to a wide range of symptoms and complications.
    - Examples include disorders affecting the nervous system, muscles, metabolism, and other organs [3].

6. Diagnostic challenges

    - Diagnosing rare neurodegenerative diseases can be challenging due to their low prevalence, the diversity of symptoms, and limited awareness among healthcare professionals.
    - Genetic testing and advanced imaging techniques may be crucial for accurate diagnosis [3].

7. Limited treatment options

    - Due to the rarity and often poorly understood nature of these diseases, treatment options are limited, and there may be no cure.
    - Management typically focuses on alleviating symptoms, providing supportive care, and improving the individual's quality of life [3].

8. Research and collaboration

    - Ongoing research efforts aim to understand the genetic basis, underlying mechanisms, and potential therapeutic targets for rare neurodegenerative diseases.
    - Collaboration between researchers, clinicians, and patient advocacy groups is essential for advancing knowledge and developing treatments.

Given the rarity and complexity of these diseases, specialized clinics and research centers often play a crucial role in the diagnosis, management, and research efforts related to rare neurodegenerative diseases.

These diseases pose significant challenges for both patients and their families due to their rarity, limited treatment options, and often rapid progression. Research efforts are ongoing to better understand the underlying mechanisms and develop potential therapies for these conditions [3, 4].

2. Pathogenesis of Alzheimer's disease (AD)

The pathogenesis of AD is complex and involves multiple factors, including genetic, environmental, and molecular contributors. While the exact mechanisms are not fully understood, several key features are associated with the development and progression of AD [5]:

1. Amyloid beta (Aβ) accumulation

    - One of the hallmarks of AD is the accumulation of abnormal protein aggregates called beta-amyloid plaques in the brain.

    - Aβ is a protein fragment derived from the larger amyloid precursor protein (APP). In AD, there is an imbalance in the production and clearance of Aβ, leading to its accumulation in the brain [6].

2. Tau protein pathology

    - Tau is a protein that plays a crucial role in maintaining the structural integrity of neurons by stabilizing microtubules.

    - In AD, abnormal modifications of tau lead to the formation of neurofibrillary tangles inside neurons. These tangles disrupt the normal functioning of neurons and contribute to their degeneration [7].

3. Neuroinflammation

    - Chronic inflammation in the brain is associated with the progression of AD. Immune cells, such as microglia, become activated and contribute to the inflammatory response.

    - Inflammation may exacerbate the accumulation of Aβ and tau pathology and contribute to neuronal damage [7].

4. Genetic factors

    - While most cases of AD are sporadic, a small percentage is associated with specific genetic mutations. Mutations in genes such as APP, PSEN1, and PSEN2 are linked to familial forms of AD.

    - These genes are involved in the production and processing of Aβ [3, 5].

5. Mitochondrial dysfunction

    - Impaired mitochondrial function has been observed in AD. Mitochondria play a crucial role in energy production and maintenance of cellular health.

    - Dysfunction in mitochondria may contribute to increased oxidative stress and damage to neurons [3, 5].

6. Synaptic dysfunction and neuronal loss

    - Synaptic dysfunction occurs early in the course of AD, leading to impaired communication between neurons.

    - Progressive neuronal loss, particularly in regions critical for memory and cognitive function, is a characteristic feature of AD [3, 5].

7. Vascular factors

    - Vascular risk factors, such as hypertension and atherosclerosis, have been associated with an increased risk of developing AD.

    - Vascular dysfunction may contribute to decreased blood flow and nutrient supply to the brain, impacting neuronal health [3, 5].

8. Environmental and lifestyle factors

    - Several environmental factors, such as education, diet, physical activity, and social engagement, may influence the risk of developing AD.

    - Chronic stress, traumatic brain injury, and exposure to certain toxins have also been studied in relation to AD risk.

The interaction and interplay of these factors likely contribute to the complex pathogenesis of AD. Research is ongoing to better understand these mechanisms, and potential therapeutic strategies are being explored to target various aspects of the disease process. Early diagnosis and intervention remain important areas of focus for improving outcomes and developing effective treatments for AD [3, 5].

3. Pathogenesis of Parkinson's disease (PD)

PD is a neurodegenerative disorder characterized by the progressive degeneration of dopamine-producing neurons in the brain. The exact cause of PD is not fully understood, and it likely involves a combination of genetic and environmental factors. Here are key aspects of the pathogenesis of PD [5].

1. Dopaminergic neuron degeneration

    - PD primarily affects a region of the brain called the substantia nigra, where dopaminergic neurons are located. These neurons are responsible for producing dopamine, a neurotransmitter crucial for motor control and coordination.

- Progressive degeneration of these dopaminergic neurons leads to a reduction in dopamine levels, resulting in the motor symptoms characteristic of PD [3, 5].

2. Alpha-synuclein accumulation

   - The abnormal accumulation of a protein called alpha-synuclein in the form of Lewy bodies is a pathological hallmark of PD.

   - These aggregated proteins are believed to interfere with normal cellular function and contribute to the degeneration of dopaminergic neurons [3, 5].

3. Mitochondrial dysfunction

   - Mitochondria, the cellular organelles responsible for energy production, play a role in the pathogenesis of PD.

   - Dysfunction in mitochondrial activity, including oxidative stress and impaired energy metabolism, may contribute to neuronal damage and cell death [3, 5].

4. Genetic factors

   - While most cases of PD are sporadic, a small percentage is associated with specific genetic mutations. Mutations in genes such as SNCA (encoding alpha-synuclein), LRRK2, PARK2, and PINK1 have been linked to familial forms of PD.

   - Genetic factors can influence the susceptibility to PD and may contribute to its pathogenesis [3, 5].

5. Oxidative stress

   - Increased oxidative stress, resulting from an imbalance between the production of reactive oxygen species (ROS) and the ability of cells to neutralize them, is implicated in PD.

   - Oxidative stress can damage cellular structures, including proteins, lipids, and DNA, leading to neuronal dysfunction and death [3, 5].

6. Inflammation

   - Neuroinflammation, involving the activation of microglia and other immune cells in the brain, is associated with PD.

   - Inflammatory processes may contribute to the degeneration of dopaminergic neurons and the progression of the disease [3, 5].

7. Environmental factors

    - Exposure to certain environmental toxins has been implicated in the development of PD. For example, pesticides, herbicides, and industrial chemicals may contribute to an increased risk.

    - Traumatic brain injury and viral infections have also been suggested as potential environmental triggers [3, 5].

8. Autophagy dysfunction

    - Autophagy, a cellular process responsible for removing damaged or dysfunctional cellular components, is impaired in PD.

    - Dysregulation of autophagy may contribute to the accumulation of alpha-synuclein and other cellular abnormalities.

Understanding the multifaceted nature of PD pathogenesis is essential for the development of targeted therapies. Research efforts continue to investigate these mechanisms and identify potential interventions to slow or halt the progression of the disease. Early diagnosis, symptomatic management, and ongoing research are critical components of PD care [7, 8].

4. Pathogenesis of Huntington's disease (HD)

Huntington's disease (HD) is a hereditary neurodegenerative disorder caused by a mutation in the HTT gene, leading to the production of an abnormal form of the huntingtin protein. The pathogenesis of HD involves a range of cellular and molecular mechanisms that result in progressive damage to specific areas of the brain. Here are key aspects of the pathogenesis of HD [5]:

1. Genetic mutation

    - HD is caused by an expanded CAG repeat sequence in the HTT gene. The CAG repeat leads to an abnormally long polyglutamine stretch in the huntingtin protein.

    - Individuals with a higher number of CAG repeats tend to exhibit an earlier onset and more severe symptoms [3, 5].

2. Mutant huntingtin protein aggregation

    - The mutant huntingtin protein has a tendency to misfold and aggregate, forming insoluble clumps within neurons. These aggregates are known as inclusion bodies.

    - The accumulation of these aggregates is believed to interfere with normal cellular function and contribute to neuronal dysfunction and death [9].

3. Neuronal degeneration

    - The regions of the brain most affected by HD include the striatum (especially the caudate nucleus and putamen), cerebral cortex, and other subcortical structures.

    - Progressive degeneration of neurons in these brain regions, particularly GABAergic medium spiny neurons in the striatum, is a characteristic feature of the disease [7].

4. Excitotoxicity

    - Dysregulation of neurotransmitters, particularly excessive release of glutamate, may lead to excitotoxicity. Excessive glutamate can overstimulate neurons, causing damage and cell death.

    - The imbalance in neurotransmitter signaling contributes to the neurodegenerative process [7].

5. Mitochondrial dysfunction

    - HD is associated with mitochondrial dysfunction, including impaired energy production and increased oxidative stress.

    - Dysfunctional mitochondria may contribute to neuronal damage, especially in regions with high energy demands [3, 5].

6. Impaired axonal transport

    - The mutant huntingtin protein disrupts the normal intracellular transport of various cellular components, including vesicles and organelles, along neuronal axons.

    - Impaired axonal transport contributes to the dysfunction of neuronal processes and the accumulation of toxic substances [7].

7. Transcriptional dysregulation

    - Mutant huntingtin affects gene transcription, leading to alterations in the expression of various genes involved in neuronal function and survival.

    - Transcriptional dysregulation contributes to the overall disruption of cellular processes in HD [9].

8. Autophagy impairment

    - Autophagy, a cellular process responsible for clearing damaged or dysfunctional cellular components, is impaired in HD.

- Dysfunction in autophagy contributes to the accumulation of mutant huntingtin protein and other cellular abnormalities.

Understanding the intricate details of HD pathogenesis is crucial for developing targeted therapies. While there is currently no cure for HD, ongoing research aims to identify potential interventions that could modify the course of the disease or alleviate symptoms. Genetic testing and counseling are important components of managing the risk of HD within families [7].

5. Pathogenesis of amyotrophic lateral sclerosis (ALS)

Amyotrophic Lateral Sclerosis (ALS), also known as Lou Gehrig's disease, is a progressive neurodegenerative disorder that primarily affects motor neurons in the brain and spinal cord. The pathogenesis of ALS is complex and involves a combination of genetic and environmental factors. Here are key aspects of the pathogenesis of ALS [10]:

1. Motor neuron degeneration

    - ALS is characterized by the selective degeneration of both upper motor neurons (located in the brain) and lower motor neurons (located in the spinal cord and brainstem).

    - The loss of these motor neurons disrupts the communication between the brain and muscles, leading to muscle weakness, atrophy, and eventually paralysis [7].

2. Genetic factors

    - Approximately 5–10% of ALS cases are considered familial, meaning they have a clear genetic component. Mutations in several genes have been associated with familial ALS, including:

    - C9orf72: The most common genetic cause of familial ALS.

    - SOD1 (superoxide dismutase 1): Mutations in this gene are associated with a significant proportion of familial ALS cases.

    - TARDBP (TDP-43): Abnormalities in the TDP-43 protein are found in both familial and sporadic ALS cases [3, 5].

3. Protein aggregation

    - Misfolded and aggregated proteins, including TDP-43 and FUS, are found in the cytoplasm of affected motor neurons in many ALS cases.

    - These protein aggregates may disrupt normal cellular function and contribute to neurodegeneration.

4. Excitotoxicity

    - Dysregulation of glutamate, a neurotransmitter, can lead to excitotoxicity, where excessive glutamate signaling causes damage to motor neurons.

    - Glutamate-mediated excitotoxicity is thought to play a role in the selective vulnerability of motor neurons in ALS [9, 10].

5. Mitochondrial dysfunction

    - Impaired mitochondrial function and energy metabolism have been implicated in ALS.

    - Mitochondrial dysfunction may contribute to oxidative stress, a process that damages cells through the production of reactive oxygen species [3, 5].

6. Oxidative stress

    - Elevated levels of oxidative stress, resulting from an imbalance between the production of reactive oxygen species and the body's ability to neutralize them, are observed in ALS.

    - Oxidative stress contributes to cellular damage and may be involved in the death of motor neurons [3, 5].

7. Glia involvement

    - Glial cells, including astrocytes and microglia, play a role in ALS pathology. Dysfunction in these support cells can contribute to neuroinflammation and the progression of the disease.

    - The activation of astrocytes and microglia may contribute to the release of inflammatory molecules and the removal of damaged neurons [3, 7].

8. RNA processing abnormalities

    - Disruptions in RNA processing and transport have been implicated in ALS pathogenesis.

    - Mutations in genes like C9orf72 can lead to abnormal RNA processing, affecting the function of motor neurons [3, 7].

9. Neuroinflammation

    - Activation of the immune system within the central nervous system contributes to neuroinflammation in ALS.

    - Inflammatory processes involving microglia and astrocytes may exacerbate neuronal damage and accelerate disease progression [7].

Understanding the underlying mechanisms of ALS is crucial for developing effective therapies. While there is currently no cure for ALS, research is ongoing to identify potential targets for intervention and improve the management of the disease. Multidisciplinary care, supportive therapies, and assistive devices are currently used to enhance the quality of life for individuals living with ALS [8, 11, 12].

Although rare neurodegenerative diseases are particularly challenging for both research and drug development, encouraging progress has been made in the development of drugs for many of these diseases.

6. Amyotrophic lateral sclerosis (ALS)

So far, only four drugs have been used, Riluzole (an antiglutamatergic drug), dextromethorphan hydrobromide and quinidine sulfate (DHQ) (a non-competitive NMDA receptor antagonist), edaravone (an antioxidant drug), and sodium phenylbutyrate and Taurursodiol (PB/TUDCA) is a cellular stress signaling blocker approved by the FDA for ALS [13].

6.1 Current treatment options

6.1.1 Riluzole

Riluzole is the only treatment available for people with ALS. The goal is to reduce excitotoxicity, specifically glutamate. Riluzole was approved by the FDA in 1995 and then by the EMA in 1996. Riluzole is an effective drug and side effects such as fatigue, nausea, stomach problems, and elevation of intestinal and liver enzymes have been detected [14].

6.1.2 Edaravone

Following the approval of Riluzole, no new drugs entered the market for several years until edaravone was approved in Japan and South Korea in 2015. FDA approval in 2017 was followed by the Chinese NMPA and Switzerland, followed by entry in 2019, Indonesia in 2020, and finally Malaysia and Thailand in 2021. Edaravone has been used for many years in Japan for stroke prevention, reducing oxidative depression and neuroinflammation by eliminating free radicals. Common side effects of edaravone treatment are bruising, gait disturbance, headache, and skin irritation [15].

To date, the dose of edavalone is 60 mg/day. Once the first dose was given for a period of 14 days, it was given for 10 days each subsequent month. However, this treatment is less suitable than oral medication. A total of 105 mg/day oral suspension will be approved by the FDA in 2022. Meanwhile, Ferrer (TRICALS) is conducting a Phase III trial evaluating the safety and effectiveness of FNP122, another oral form of edaravone [15].

6.1.3 Sodium phenylbutyrate and taurursodiol

Recently, sodium phenylbutyrate and Taurursodiol (also known as PB-TURSO or PB-TUDCA) have been introduced in a combination. The drug is currently approved by the FDA and Canada, both of which have previously been approved for medical use. Both have been identified as inhibitors of neuronal apoptosis, and their synergistic effects are thought to reduce cell death and oxidative stress by reducing endoplasmic reticulum (ER) stress and mitochondrial dysfunction [15].

The most common side effects in the Phase II trial were diarrhea, abdominal pain, nausea, and upper respiratory tract infection. Gastrointestinal tract-related adverse events occur more frequently in the first 3 weeks of treatment [13].

Sodium phenylbutyrate/ Taurursodiol is formulated as an oral suspension and powder to be mixed with hot water. The dose is 3 g of sodium phenylbutyrate and 1 g of Taurursodiol; start taking it once a day for 3 weeks, then twice a day [15].

6.1.4 Anakinra and Fingolimod

Arterial inflammation is now recognized as a possible pathology in ALS. Therefore, inhibitors of neuroinflammatory pathways may be helpful [16].

Anakinra is an IL-1 receptor inhibitor whose protective effects have been studied in experimental and clinical studies. Anakinra has been shown to extend life expectancy in SOD1-G93A mice [17].

Additionally, Fingolimod (Gilenya) acts as an anti-inflammatory drug by inhibiting lymphocyte influx from lymphoid tissue and reducing circulating lymphocytes associated with sphingosine-1-phosphate receptor (S1PR) inhibition. Experimental studies in SOD1-G93A mice showed that fingolimod improved survival. In addition to its effects in multiple sclerosis (MS), fingolimod is a safe and tolerable drug in ALS patients. Side effects include bradycardia at the initial dose, mild decrease in FEV1, macular edema, and progressive multifocal leukoencephalopathy [18].

6.1.5 Masitinib

Masitinib is a selective tyrosine kinase inhibitor that exerts neuroprotective effects by modulating the immune system and microglia activity [19].

Masitinib is a selective tyrosine kinase inhibitor and is unique compared to other ALS drugs in targeting the immune system in the central and peripheral nervous system, including microglia, macrophages, and mast cells. It is used orally and has antitumor, neuroprotective and anti-inflammatory activities. It regulates mast cell survival, migration, and degranulation by inhibiting important growth and differentiation pathways (and indirectly regulating various proinflammatory and vasoactive mediators that cells can release) [20].

Masitinib has a favorable safety profile with no significant toxicity at a daily dose of 7.5 mg/kg. Side effects of masitinib are similar to other tyrosine kinase (TK) inhibitors. Long-term use of masitinib may cause gastrointestinal (nausea, vomiting), hematological (anemia, lymphopenia, neutropenia, thrombocytopenia), dermatological (eyebrow and facial edema, rash) and other disorders (fever, jaundice, dehydration, symptoms, deterioration of body health, hypokalemia and thrombosis). Liver function should be carefully controlled in these patients [13].

7. Alzheimer's disease (AD)

The goal of therapy in AD is to symptomatically treat cognitive impairment and preserve patient's function for as long as possible. Other goals include managing psychiatric and behavioral sequelae. Current treatments for AD do not seem to prolong life, cure AD, or halt or reverse the pathophysiologic processes of the disease [21].

7.1 FDA-approved therapies

Many medications can cause psychosis in people with dementia, but some medications are more common. Benzodiazepines and other sedative-hypnotics, anticholinergics, and antipsychotics have been associated with cognitive impairment. Additionally, H2 receptor antagonists, corticosteroids, and opioids such as pethidine have been associated with delirium or altered consciousness. Because medication use is associated with a return of cognitive symptoms, medication review and management are important [22].

The US Food and Drug Administration (FDA) has approved six drugs for treatment: tacrine, donepezil, rivastigmine, galantamine, memantine, and lecanemab. Although aducanumab was quickly approved by the FDA on June 7, 2021, its long-term safety and tolerability require further monitoring and approval. The above FDA-approved treatments are intended to improve symptoms only. Therefore, treatment-modifying strategies are needed to slow, modify, and control the progression of AD [23].

There is interest in developing various drugs that address many aspects of AD pathology, including prevention of Aβ accumulation, tau phosphorylation, oxidative stress, and mitochondrial autophagy dysfunction. Many of these drugs are currently in clinical trials [24].

7.2 Drugs under investigation

7.2.1 β-Secretase inhibitor

Beta-secretase inhibitors often reduce beta-amyloid production. However, clinical trials of β-site APP-cleaving enzyme 1 (BACE1, also known as β-secretase 1) have been unsuccessful. Verubecestat, Lanabecestat, and Atabecestat are some of the acyl-guanidine class molecules that have entered late clinical trials. However, they failed to reach the market due to toxicity or lack of appropriate treatment [25].

7.2.2 γ-Secretase inhibitors

Semagacestat is a non-selective small molecule γ-secretase inhibitor whose mechanism of action is identical to that of a β-secretase inhibitor and is designed to reduce Aβ amyloid deposition. In a later phase III trial, the trial was stopped due to greater weight loss in patients taking semaacestat compared to the placebo group and side effects such as skin cancer and infection. Similarly, a phase II study of avagacestat in patients with mild-to-moderate AD was discontinued due to AEs such as cerebral microbleeds, diabetes, and cancer [26].

7.2.3 Anti-tau drugs

The role of Tau is not fully understood, but studies have shown that it plays an important role in the assembly and stability of cytoskeletal microtubules. Abnormal hyperphosphorylation of Tau (p-tau) reduces its binding affinity to microtubules, and abnormal phosphorylation of Tau causes aggregation and formation of NFTs. Anti-tau therapy mainly involves three aspects: preventing excessive phosphorylation and accumulation of tau, stabilizing microtubules, and ensuring the removal of tau [23].

7.2.4 GSK-3β inhibitor

GSK-3β inhibitors prevent hyperphosphorylation of tau protein. Studies have shown that GSK-3β can reduce abnormal Tau phosphorylation and amyloid production *in vitro* and *in vivo*, making it a promising treatment-modifying therapy for AD. Lithium was first used in psychiatry, discovered by Australian psychiatrist John Cade in 1949 and was widely used in the treatment of manic episodes [27].

In recent years, lithium has been shown to be an inhibitor of GSK3, which is involved in glucose metabolism, cell signaling and proliferation, and control of glial cell function. Lithium prevents amyloid formation and tau hyperphosphorylation. Long-term use of lithium therapy is associated with serious adverse events (SAEs), and it requires constant monitoring of lithium concentration in the blood. There is a medical need for safer and better lithium [23].

7.2.5 Tau aggregation inhibitor

Tau protein accumulation is associated with neuron loss. Tau aggregation inhibitors such as methylene blue chloride (methblue) and hydromethanesulfonate (LMTM) can reduce Tau accumulation. Methylene blue chloride (methylene blue) is also a drug with a long history of use, mainly in the treatment of malaria, hyperferremia and carbon monoxide poisoning, and as a histological stain.

In a 24-week phase II study, methylene blue chloride failed to show clinical benefit in AD [28].

7.2.6 "Multi-target" agents on AD

7.2.6.1 γ-Carbolines

Dimebon is a gamma-carboline derivative compound combined with methylene blue. Dimebon is a multi-purpose drug. Its activities include protecting neurons from death, reducing protein synthesis, and increasing autophagy [23].

However, owing to a lack of statistically significant efficacy, the use of dimebon for AD was not confirmed through a phase II clinical trial [29].

7.2.6.2 Phenothiazine

Phenothiazine-based theranostic compounds inhibit Aβ aggregation in a double transgenic mouse model of AD and can serve as near-infrared fluorescence (NIRF) imaging probes of amyloid plaques in AD [30].

Unfortunately, there are currently no reports of phenothiazine studies for the treatment of AD in the PubMed database.

7.2.6.3 Carbazoles

P7C3 is a neuroprotective aminopropylcarbazole found during postnatal hippocampal neurogenesis studies. P7C3, named P7C3 because it is the third compound (C3) in the seventh pool (P7), protects young hippocampal neurons and prevents neuron death. It has also been shown to inhibit cognitive function in terminally aged mice. Unfortunately, there are no reports of clinical studies of P7C3 in the treatment of AD in the PubMed database [23].

7.2.6.4 5-HT

Idalopirdine is a novel selective 5-HT6 receptor antagonist that binds to ChEI, improving central acetylcholine levels and neuronal activity and improving cognition in animal models. A phase II proof of concept (PoC) study combining successful treatment of AD with idalopirdine plus donepezil showed significant improvement in cognitive functions in AD, such as ADAS-implant and MMSE scores [31].

On the other hand, Phase III development of idalopidine ("OLEX", idalopidine alone and "MEMOLEX", idalopidine plus memantine) for the treatment of AD did not demonstrate significant benefit. AVN-101 is a potent 5-HT7 receptor antagonist. AVN-101 shows good oral bioavailability, increases blood-brain barrier permeability and has low toxicity and reasonable efficacy in animal models of central nervous system disease [23].

7.2.6.5 Tyrosine kinase inhibitor

Masitinib is an oral tyrosine kinase inhibitor that exerts neurodegenerative effects in neurodegenerative diseases such as multiple sclerosis by inhibiting mast cell and microglia/macrophage activity [32].

Recently, a phase III clinical trial of masitinib in AD was completed and showed that masitinib improved ADAS-cog and ADCS-ADL scores [33].

8. Huntington's disease (HD)

8.1 Current therapeutic options for Huntington's disease

The most commonly used HD medications are designed to reduce chorea. One of the main features of HD is degeneration of the basal ganglia, especially the striatum, which is associated with the development of chorea [34].

Patients with chorea whose daily activities are not affected should be recognized and educated. If chorea requires medical treatment, drug options may be considered. Dopamine receptor blockers such as haloperidol, risperidone, and olanzapine have been used in the past and have additional benefits in treating depression and behavioral disorders. However, the disadvantage of atypical and atypical drugs is that they increase the risk of sudden death and the use of drugs for PD [35].

Since its approval, tetrabenazine has been frequently used to treat chorea, but its use is generally limited due to the risk of side effects. In a clinical trial, deutetrabenazine, approved by the FDA in April 2017, showed a statistically significant improvement in chorea in 90 HD patients compared to placebo [36].

The most common side effect in the deutetrabenazine group was drowsiness. Events such as depression and akathisia were similar between the drug and placebo groups. Amantadine has also been reported to have an effect on chorea. Anticholinergic drugs, such as benztropine, do not help treat chorea because they are actually prodopinergic drugs [34].

Depression is the most common symptom associated with HD, and most experts agree that it can be treated with serotonin reuptake inhibitors. Patients with obsessive-compulsive disorder, anxiety, and depression may also respond to this medication. Valproic acid and carbamazepine can help reduce anxiety and depression [37].

Both typical and atypical antipsychotics may be useful in treating mental illness, mood swings, and anxiety, but doses should be kept to a minimum to minimize the risk of extrapyramidal side effects [38].

Riluzole is a CNS glutamate neurotransmission inhibitor that exhibits neuroprotective effects in clinical models of HD and HD transgenic mice [39].

Ifenprodil, a specific antagonist of NR2B (NMDAR isoform), reduces excitotoxic cell death in medium spiny neurons in HD transgenic and wild-type mice after exposure to NMDA [40].

Minocycline, a second-generation tetracycline that inhibits the caspase pathway, has shown some benefit in mouse models of HD. Meclizine exerts neuroprotective effects and inhibits apoptosis in mouse models [41].

9. Parkinson's disease (PD)

PD is a neurodegenerative disease caused by the death of a type of neuron that plays a fundamental role in the production of dopamine in the brain. There is no cure for PD, but therapies including drugs, surgery and rehabilitation can reduce symptoms. The medicine that increases the amount of dopamine in the brain, is the most common medication for PD [42].

9.1 Management of motor symptoms

Current treatment is mainly based on restoring dopamine levels, with levodopa considered the main option. However, levodopa administration has limitations due to the occurrence of side effects, of which dyskinesia is a significant problem [43].

Additionally, as the disease progresses, patients become less responsive to dopaminergic medications and require increasingly frequent doses of dopaminergic medications [44].

Therefore, current levodopa formulations contain decarboxylase inhibitors, either carbidopa or benserazide. Decarboxylase inhibitors work by preventing the peripheral metabolism of dopamine and increasing the bioavailability of the drug [45].

However, to avoid problems caused by using too much of one drug, it is recommended to give levodopa simultaneously with other drugs [46].

These medications include rasagiline, safinamide, selegiline, and monoamine oxidase B (MAOB) inhibitors, which have been shown to increase dopamine levels [47].

Catechol-O-methyltransferase (COMT) inhibitors such as entacapone and tolcapone have also been used. These tools improve dopamine levels and increase physical activity because they promote the absorption of levodopa in the intestine, where most of this enzyme is located [43].

Another class of drugs are dopamine agonists, such as ropinirole and pramipexole, which have been described as safe and effective as monotherapy and in combination with levodopa. In this group, rotigotine is available as a transdermal patch that provides continuous dosing, while apomorphine is available as an injection or subcutaneous infusion to rescue potency change in patients with systemic disease [43].

9.1.1 Invasive treatment options for motor symptoms

Advanced treatments are available for patients with motor disorders or dyskinesias that cause dysfunction and do not improve even with appropriate drug therapy. Deep brain stimulation (DBS), levodopa-carbidopa enteral suspension, and continuous subcutaneous infusion of apomorphine are the best-known alternatives [43].

DBS reduces downtime and improves patients' quality of life more than any other treatment. National Institute for Health and Care Excellence (NICE) guidance recommends use in the final stages of the disease [48].

Although concurrent dopaminergic therapy is necessary, sometimes the dose can be reduced by 60% after starting treatment [49].

Currently, DBS has proven to be one of the most promising and safe methods of treating PD. Although proven to be safe, surgery is not without risks; the most important being seizures associated with DBS implantation [50].

However, this technology has changed a lot in the last 20 years, the number of side effects has decreased and more targeted treatment of the needed areas has been enabled, supported by clinical pathology. Therefore, DBS appears to be an improved treatment modality for various neuropathologies, including PD [51].

Moreover, Levodopa-Carbidopa Enteral Suspension is another surgical method that can provide safety by placing a permanent tube through percutaneous endoscopic gastrostomy (PEG) connected to a portable external device. This treatment prevents changes in levodopa levels, thus shortening drug withdrawal times and reducing the risk of dyskinesia. However, adverse outcomes and costs led 34% of patients to discontinue the study after 4 years [52].

Finally, continuous subcutaneous infusion of apomorphine allows continuous administration and has the advantage of not requiring surgery. Additionally, this type of treatment does not require the use of high doses of levodopa every day, and some cases in which levodopa administration is not necessary are described. However, a study found that after the first year, half of patients abandoned treatment due to ineffectiveness and poor quality [49].

9.2 Management of nonmotor symptoms

Cognitive impairment, depression, sleep disorders, and functional impairments are non-motor problems in PD. The most common medications used to treat psychosis are acetylcholinesterase inhibitors such as donepezil, galantamine, and rivastigmine [43].

For depression, people with PD are often treated with serotonin/norepinephrine reuptake inhibitors (SNRIs), such as duloxetine, desvenlafaxine, milnacipran, and venlafaxine. Other treatments include benzodiazepines (e.g., alprazolam, clonazepam, diazepam, and lorazepam), selective serotonin reuptake inhibitors (SSRIs) (e.g., fluoxetine and sertraline), tricyclic compounds such as amitriptyline (e.g. amitriptyline, imipramine, and other antitriptyline), imipramine and nortriptyline), buspirone, propranolol, quetiapine and trazodone) [53].

For sleep disorders, amitriptyline, clonazepam, doxepin, eszopipine, melatonin, mirtazapine, and trazadone are frequently used in affected patients. But it is important to consider behavioral therapy as a good option to improve sleep hygiene, reduce stress pressure, and improve depression [54].

Patients with orthostatic hypotension can be treated with fludrocortisone, pyridostigmine, and droxidopa. There are four main groups of medications for reducing urinary incontinence: anticholinergics such as darifenacin, oxybutynin, solifenacin, and tolterodine; Beta-3-agonists, mainly mirabegron; Alfuzosin, silodosin, tamsulosin and more importantly, Alpha-1A Blockers; and SNRIs such as duloxetine. In people with PD, on the other hand, salivation usually occurs due to slow swallowing and can be treated with atropine drops, botulinum toxins A and B, glycopyrrolate, or scopolamine patches [55].

Finally, digestive problems such as constipation are often treated primarily with non-pharmacological measures such as dietary changes (such as consuming high-fiber foods and plenty of fluids). However, in cases where this does not work, medications such as lubiprostone and polyethylene glycol can be given. For other conditions such as nausea and vomiting, the most common treatment options are ondansetron and trimethobenzamide [56].

9.3 Treatments under investigation

Recent research into the genetic basis of PD has led to a better understanding of the pathophysiology of the disease, leading to new therapeutic targets and possible treatments. The difficulty in diagnosing PD is an important problem in terms of its treatment. PD is diagnosed when symptoms occur. As mentioned earlier, not everyone with PD may show symptoms, at least in the early stages of the disease [43].

Additionally, PD can cause symptoms similar to dementia. In this sense, the specific dementia caused by PD should not be confused with the development of AD. It has even been said that the combination of Lewy pathology and Alzheimer's pathology (beta-amyloid plaques and neurofibrillary tangles) is the strongest correlate of PD dementia [57].

The pathophysiological relationship between these two diseases has led to numerous clinical studies examining the combination of the two diseases (PD and AD) [43].

On the other hand, another limitation of PD treatment is the difficulty of drugs reaching dopaminergic neurons in the nigrostriatal region. The blood-brain barrier filters molecules into the brain, allowing molecules that are smaller or have specific pathways to enter [58].

This phenomenon limits the pharmacological options available for the treatment of neurological diseases. Much research now focuses on increasing the permeability of this barrier to allow entry of molecules that cannot enter the central nervous system. In this sense, the use of forced ultrasound to open the blood-brain barrier to deliver the virus to alpha-synuclein and improve the child's neurotrophin has been shown to reduce PD-related pathology in the trial model, but the results of this study are limited [43].

One of the biggest problems hindering the control of these diseases is the lack of more complete animals that include important factors such as aging and peripheral diseases, which can also reduce the value of preclinical results [59].

As a result, clinical trials testing potential drugs to alter the progression of PD have yielded mixed results. These results can be attributed to many factors, including the diversity of pathophysiology and clinical manifestations of PD, the difficulty of identifying PD in the early stages, and the lack of targets and outcomes to evaluate drug use [60].

Moreover, we can now only evaluate the effects of the disease by observing the symptoms that are the result of neuronal degeneration (motor and non-motor) and the indirect signs of degeneration (e.g., visual function). Similarly, patients in clinical trials often receive dopaminergic drugs with significant symptoms, making it difficult to see the disease-modifying effects of other treatments. These limitations make it difficult for studies to demonstrate disease modification [61].

Author details

Ali Gamal Al-kaf[1,2]* and Ali Abdullah Al-yahawi[3,4]

1 Faculty of Pharmacy, Medicinal Chemistry Department, Sana'a University, Yemen

2 Faculty of Medical Sciences, Department of Pharmacy, National University, Yemen

3 Pharmacy department at Saba University, Yemen

4 Clinical pharmacy faculty-21 September University for Medical and Applied Sciences, Yeman

*Address all correspondence to: alialkaf21@gmail.com; alialkaf@national-univ.net

References

[1] Pillai JA, Cummings JL. Neurodegenerative Diseases: Unifying Principles. USA: Oxford University Press; 2016

[2] Orphanet. Available from: www.orpha.net

[3] De Jonghe P et al. Genetics of neurodegenerative diseases. Cold Spring Harbor Perspectives in Biology. 2012:719-736

[4] Chia K, Klingseisen A, Sieger D, Priller J. Zebrafish as a model organism for neurodegenerative disease. Frontiers in Molecular Neuroscience. 2022;**15**:940484

[5] Nunomura K et al. Molecular mechanisms and genetics of oxidative stress in Alzheimer's disease. Archives of Biochemistry and Biophysics. 2009;**72**:981-1017

[6] Mocanu MM, Nissen A, Eckermann K, et al. The potential for beta-structure in the repeat domain of tau protein determines aggregation, synaptic decay, neuronal loss, and coassembly with endogenous Tau in inducible mouse models of tauopathy. The Journal of Neuroscience. 2008;**28**:737-748

[7] Klionsky DJ et al. Autophagy: Cellular and molecular mechanisms. Physiological Reviews. 2021;**221**:3-12

[8] Menzies K et al. Autophagy in neurodegenerative diseases: From mechanism to therapeutic approach. Molecular Neurodegeneration. 2015;**38**:381-389

[9] Sarkar R et al. Autophagy in neurodegenerative diseases: A hunter for aggregates. Cell Cycle. 2007;**21**:3369

[10] Abrahao A, Abath Neto O, Kok F, Zanoteli E, Santos B, Pinto WB, et al. One family, one gene and three phenotypes: A novel VCP (valosin-containing protein) mutation associated with myopathy with rimmed vacuoles, amyotrophic lateral sclerosis and frontotemporal dementia. Journal of the Neurological Sciences. 2016;**368**:352-358. DOI: 10.1016/j.jns.2016.07.048

[11] Palikaras K, Tavernarakis N. Mitophagy in neurodegeneration and aging. Frontiers in Genetics. 2012;**3**:297. View at: Publisher Site | Google Scholar

[12] Ciuffa R, Lamark T, Tarafder AK, Guesdon A, Rybina S, Hagen WJH, et al. The selective autophagy receptor P62 forms a flexible filamentous helical scaffold. Cell Reports. 2015;**11**:748-758. DOI: 10.1016/j.celrep.2015.03.062

[13] Ketabforoush AHME, Chegini R, Barati S, Tahmasebi F, Moghisseh B, Joghataei MT, et al. Masitinib: The promising actor in the next season of the amyotrophic lateral sclerosis treatment series. Biomedicine & Pharmacotherapy. 2023;**160**:114378. DOI: 10.1016/j.biopha.2023.114378. Epub 2023 Feb 10

[14] Saitoh Y, Takahashi Y. Riluzole for the treatment of amyotrophic lateral sclerosis. Neurodegenerative Disease Management. 2020;**10**(6):343-355. DOI: 10.2217/nmt-2020-0033. Epub 2020 Aug 27

[15] Tzeplaeff L, Wilfling S, Requardt MV, Herdick M. Current state and future directions in the therapy of ALS. Cells. 2023;**12**(11):1523. DOI: 10.3390/cells12111523

[16] Liu J, Wang F. Role of neuroinflammation in amyotrophic lateral sclerosis: Cellular mechanisms and

therapeutic implications. Frontiers in Immunology. **2017**;**8**:1005

[17] Meissner F, Molawi K, Zychlinsky A. Mutant superoxide dismutase 1-induced IL- 1β accelerates ALS pathogenesis. Proceedings of the National Academy of Sciences. 2010;**107**(29):13046-13050

[18] Berry JD, Paganoni S, Atassi N, Macklin EA, Goyal N, Rivner M, et al. Phase IIa trial of fingolimod for amyotrophic lateral sclerosis demonstrates acceptable acute safety and tolerability. Muscle & Nerve. 2017;**56**(6):1077-1084

[19] Mora JS, Genge A, Chio A, Estol CJ, Chaverri D, Hern'andez M, et al. Masitinib as an add-on therapy to riluzole in patients with amyotrophic lateral sclerosis: A randomized clinical trial. Amyotrophic Lateral Sclerosis and Frontotemporal Degeneration. 2020;**21**(1-2):5-14

[20] Adenis A, Blay J-Y, Bui-Nguyen B, Bouch'e O, Bertucci F, Isambert N, et al. Masitinib in advanced gastrointestinal stromal tumor (GIST) after failure of imatinib: A randomized controlled open-label trial. Annals of Oncology. 2014;**25**(9):1762-1769

[21] Fillenbaum GG, Peterson B, Morris JC. Estimating the validity of the clinical dementia rating scale: The CERAD experience. Consortium to establish a registry for Alzheimer's disease. Aging (Milano). 1996;**8**(6):379-385

[22] 2019 American Geriatrics Society Beers Criteria® Update Expert Panel. American Geriatrics Society 2019 updated AGS beers criteria® for potentially inappropriate medication use in older adults. Journal of the American Geriatrics Society. 2019;**4**:674-694

[23] Peng Y, Jin H, Xue Y-h, Chen Q, Yao S-y, M-q D, et al. Current and future therapeutic strategies for Alzheimer's disease: An overview of drug development bottlenecks. Frontiers in Aging Neuroscience. 2023;**15**:1206572

[24] Athar T, Al Balushi K, Khan SA. Recent advances on drug development and emerging therapeutic agents for Alzheimer's disease. Molecular Biology Reports. 2021;**48**:5629-5645

[25] Patel S, Bansoad AV, Singh R, Khatik GL. BACE1: A key regulator in Alzheimer's disease progression and current development of its inhibitors. Current Neuropharmacology. 2022;**20**:1174-1193

[26] Willis BA, Zhang W, Ayan-Oshodi M, Lowe SL, Annes WF, Sirois PJ, et al. Semagacestat pharmacokinetics are not significantly affected by formulation, food, or time of dosing in healthy participants. Journal of Clinical Pharmacology. 2012;**52**:904-913

[27] Lovestone S, Boada M, Dubois B, Hull M, Rinne JO, Huppertz HJ, et al. A phase II trial of tideglusib in Alzheimer's disease. Journal of Alzheimer's Disease. 2015;**45**:75-88

[28] Tucker D, Lu Y, Zhang Q. From mitochondrial function to neuroprotection-an emerging role for methylene blue. Molecular Neurobiology. 2018;**55**:5137-5153

[29] Doody RS, Gavrilova SI, Sano M, Thomas RG, Aisen PS, Bachurin SO, et al. Effect of dimebon on cognition, activities of daily living, behaviour, and global function in patients with mild-to-moderate Alzheimer's disease: A randomised, double-blind, placebo-controlled study. Lancet. 2008;**372**:207-215

[30] Dao P, Ye F, Liu Y, Du ZY, Zhang K, Dong CZ, et al. Development

of phenothiazine-based theranostic compounds that act both as inhibitors of b-amyloid aggregation and as imaging probes for amyloid plaques in Alzheimer's disease. ACS Chemical Neuroscience. 2017;**8**:798-806

[31] Wilkinson D, Windfeld K, Colding-Jørgensen E. Safety and efficacy of idalopirdine, a 5-HT6 receptor antagonist, in patients with moderate Alzheimer's disease (LADDER): A randomised, double-blind, placebo-controlled phase 2 trial. Lancet Neurology. 2014;**13**:1092-1099

[32] Vermersch P, Brieva-Ruiz L, Fox RJ, Paul F, Ramio-Torrenta L, Schwab M, et al. Efficacy and safety ofMasitinib in progressive forms of multiple sclerosis: A randomized, phase 3, clinical trial. Neurology Neuroimmunology & Neuroinflammation. 2022;**9**:e1148

[33] Dubois B, López-Arrieta J, Lipschitz S, Doskas T, Spiru L, Moroz S, et al. Masitinib for mild-to-moderate Alzheimer's disease: Results from a randomized, placebo-controlled, phase 3, clinical trial. Alzheimer's Research & Therapy. 2023;**15**:39

[34] Ferguson MW, Kennedy CJ, Palpagama TH, Waldvogel HJ, Faull RLM, Kwakowsky A. Current and possible future therapeutic options for Huntington's disease. Journal of Central Nervous System Disease. 2022;**14**:11795735221092517

[35] Ray WA, Chung CP, Murray KT, et al. Atypical antipsychotic drugs and the risk of sudden cardiac death. The New England Journal of Medicine. 2009;**360**(3):225-235

[36] Frank S, Testa CM, Stamler D, et al. Effect of deutetrabenazine on chorea among patients with Huntington disease: A randomized clinical trial. Journal of the American Medical Association. 2016;**316**(1):40-50

[37] Reilmann R. The pridopidine paradox in Huntington's disease. Movement Disorders. 2013;**28**:1321e4

[38] Gelderblom H, Fischer W, McLean T, et al. ACTION-HD: A randomized, doubleblind, placebo-controlled prospective crossover trial investigating the efficacy and safety of bupropion in Huntington's disease. Neurotherapeutics. 2013;**10**(1):180-181

[39] Rosas HD, Koroshetz WJ, Jenkins BG, Chen YI, Hayden DL, Beal MF, et al. Riluzole therapy in Huntington's disease (HD). Movement disorders. Official Journal of the Movement Disorder Society. 1999;**14**(2):326-330

[40] Tang TS, Chen X, Liu J, et al. Dopaminergic signaling and striatal neurodegeneration in Huntington's disease. The Journal of Neuroscience. 2007;**27**:7899-7910

[41] Varma H, Voisine C, DeMarco CT, et al. Selective inhibitors of death in mutant huntingtin cells. Nature Chemical Biology. 2007;**3**:99-100

[42] DeMaagd G, Philip A. Parkinson's disease and its management: Part 1: Disease entity, risk factors, pathophysiology, clinical presentation, and diagnosis. Pharmacy and Therapeutics. 2015;**40**(8):504-532

[43] Pardo-Moreno T, García-Morales V, Suleiman-Martos S, Rivas-Domínguez A, Mohamed-MohamedH,Ramos-RodríguezJJ, et al. Current treatments and new, tentative therapies for Parkinson's disease. Pharmaceutics. 2023;**15**:770

[44] Chou KL, Stacy M, Simuni T, Miyasaki J, Oertel WH, Sethi K, et al. The Spectrum of "off" in Parkinson's disease:

What have we learned over 40 years? Parkinsonism & Related Disorders. 2018;**51**:9-16

[45] Müller T. Catechol-O-Methyltransferase inhibitors in Parkinson's disease. Drugs. 2015;**75**:157-174

[46] Dhanawat M, Mehta DK, Gupta S, Das R. Understanding the pathogenesis involved in Parkinson's disease and potential therapeutic treatment strategies. Central Nervous System Agents in Medicinal Chemistry. 2020;**20**:88-102

[47] Oertel W, Schulz JB. Current and experimental treatments of Parkinson disease: A guide for neuroscientists. Journal of Neurochemistry. 2016;**139**(Suppl. 1):325-337

[48] Nijhuis FAP, Esselink R, de Bie RMA, Groenewoud H, Bloem BR, Post B, et al. Translating evidence to advanced Parkinson's disease patients: A systematic review and meta-analysis. Movement Disorders. 2021;**36**:1293-1307

[49] Dijk JM, Espay AJ, Katzenschlager R, de Bie RMA. The choice between advanced therapies for Parkinson's disease patients: Why, what, and when? Journal of Parkinson's Disease. 2020;**10**:S65-S73

[50] Atchley TJ, Elsayed GA, Sowers B, Walker HC, Chagoya G, Davis MC, et al. Incidence and risk factors for seizures associated with deep brain stimulation surgery. Journal of Neurosurgery. 2020;**1-5**:279-283

[51] Fox SH, Katzenschlager R, Lim S-Y, Barton B, de Bie RMA, Seppi K, et al. Movement Disorder Society evidence-based medicine committee. International Parkinson and Movement Disorder Society evidence-based medicine review: Update on treatments for the motor symptoms of Parkinson's disease. Movement Disorders. 2018;**33**:1248-1266

[52] Afentou N, Jarl J, Gerdtham U-G, Saha S. Economic evaluation of interventions in Parkinson's disease: A systematic literature review. Movement Disorders Clinical Practice. 2019;**6**:282-290

[53] Pontone GM, Mills KA. Optimal treatment of depression and anxiety in Parkinson's disease. The American Journal of Geriatric Psychiatry. 2021;**29**:530-540

[54] Egan SJ, Laidlaw K, Starkstein S. Cognitive behaviour therapy for depression and anxiety in Parkinson's disease. Journal of Parkinson's Disease. 2015;**5**:443-451

[55] Schapira AHV, Chaudhuri KR, Jenner P. Non-motor features of Parkinson disease. Nature Reviews. Neuroscience. 2017;**18**:435-450

[56] Park A, Stacy M. Non-motor symptoms in Parkinson's disease. Journal of Neurology. 2009;**256**(Suppl. 3):293-298

[57] Hosp JA, Dressing A, Blazhenets G, Bormann T, Rau A, Schwabenland M, et al. Cognitive impairment and altered cerebral glucose metabolism in the subacute stage of COVID-19. Brain: A Journal of Neurology. 2021;**144**:1263-1276

[58] Zhao Y, Gan L, Ren L, Lin Y, Ma C, Lin X. Factors influencing the blood-brain barrier permeability. Brain Research. 2022;**1788**:147937

[59] Folke J, Ferreira N, Brudek T, Borghammer P, Van Den Berge N. Passive immunization in alpha-Synuclein preclinical animal models. Biomolecules. 2022;**12**:168

[60] Paolini Paoletti F, Gaetani L, Parnetti L. The challenge of disease-modifying therapies in Parkinson's disease: Role of CSF biomarkers. Biomolecules. 2020;**10**:335

[61] Athauda D, Foltynie T. Challenges in detecting disease modification in Parkinson's disease clinical trials. Parkinsonism & Related Disorders. 2016;**32**:1-11